Different Bodies

Different Bodies

Essays on Disability in Film and Television

Edited by MARJA EVELYN MOGK

McFarland & Company, Inc., Publishers
Jefferson, North Carolina, and London

LIBRARY OF CONGRESS CATALOGUING-IN-PUBLICATION DATA

Different bodies : essays on disability in film
and television / edited by Marja Evelyn Mogk.
p.   cm.
Includes bibliographical references and index.

ISBN 978-0-7864-6535-4
softcover : acid free paper ∞

1. People with disabilities in motion pictures.
2. People with disabilities on television.
I. Mogk, Marja editor of compilation.
PN1995.9.H34D54 2013   791.43'6527—dc23   2013022270

BRITISH LIBRARY CATALOGUING DATA ARE AVAILABLE

On the cover: Tekki Lomnicki plays herself in a romantic dream
sequence featuring Paris in Jeffrey Jon Smith's *The Miracle* (2007).

Manufactured in the United States of America

*McFarland & Company, Inc., Publishers
Box 611, Jefferson, North Carolina 28640
www.mcfarlandpub.com*

For all those who are
new to disability studies

Table of Contents

Acknowledgments

Eunjung Kim and Michelle Jarman's essay ("Modernity's Rescue Mission") first appeared in the *Canadian Journal of Film Studies/Revue Canadienne d'Études Cinématographique* 17.1 (2008) and is reprinted here with permission.

My special thanks to Cynthia Miller for her support of the Different Bodies area, which I inaugurated and chaired at the Film & History conferences of 2008 and 2010, and for encouraging me to proceed with a new collection of essays on the topic. This project has brought me a number of new friends and colleagues, among them Nicole Markotić, whose good cheer and sound, generous advice on the process of editing a book made a difference. I am also grateful for my sabbatical leave in 2010–11 from California Lutheran University, which allowed me to conceive of this project and work through its initial stages, and for the support of the wonderful members of my department and colleagues at the university. Last but not least, all my love and gratitude to my family.

Introduction

An Invitation to Disability

A few years ago I pitched the idea of a special edition on disability to a film journal. The editor-in-chief was not persuaded. He didn't think there would be anything to write about outside of identifying a few disabled characters here and there, and how would that constitute a viable collection of substantive essays? Disability is a critical non-starter. So instead I pitched the idea for a book, and it was accepted. The journal editor's response is not unique to him — it participates in a larger social phenomenon of disability misperception that is central to the complex functions of disability in film, culture and language. The fact is that there are many more disabled characters than most viewers realize in film and television, and they have more culturally critical roles than we recognize. Beyond disabled characters themselves, disability contributes to characterizations of the nondisabled, it shapes storylines on a range of topics, facilitates genre and metaphor, reflects deeply held social beliefs and values, and constructs difference across a range of matrices. Yet like the journal editor, we tend not to see it.

The question of why we don't see disability is a longstanding one in disability studies. In the earliest landmark essay on disability and film, "Screening Stereotypes: Images of Disabled People in Television and Motion Pictures," written in 1985, Paul K. Longmore asks: "Why are there so many disabled characters and why do we overlook them so much of the time? Why do television and film so frequently screen disabled characters for us to see, and why do we usually screen them out of our consciousness even as we absorb those images?" (132).

A quarter century later, there is still comparatively little criticism on disability in film even when protagonists with disability appear, as they frequently do in Academy-lauded productions. As Tobin Siebers observes, playing a disabled character has become a familiar path for nondisabled actors to an Oscar nomination. *The English Patient* (1996), *Sling Blade* (1996), *Shine* (1996), *A Beautiful Mind* (2001), *I Am Sam* (2001), *Iris* (2001), *Frida* (2002), *Ray* (2004), *The Aviator* (2004), *Million Dollar Baby* (2004), *Away from Her* (2007) and *The King's Speech* (2010) come to mind. Even those attending to disability can be unaware of its prevalence in popular culture. "After a decade of working in disability studies, I still find myself surprised by the presence of disability in narratives I had never considered to be 'about' disability," Michael Bérubé reflected in 2005, "in animated films from *Dumbo* to *Finding Nemo*; in literary texts from *Huckleberry Finn* to Joan Didion's *Play It As It Lays*; and, more curiously, even in the world of science fiction and superheroes" (568).

So why don't we see disability? First, as Longmore points out, we are culturally trained to individualize it, to perceive it as the isolated condition of a particular person. Moreover, our perception of disability as personal is story-driven. We think of disability solely as a feature of biography. We think about blindness, for example, in terms of someone who was born blind, became blind, overcame blindness or was thwarted by it. "Disability immediately becomes part of a [...] time-sequenced narrative," observes Lennard J. Davis. "By narrativizing an impairment, one tends to sentimentalize it and link it to the bourgeois sensibility of individualism and the drama of an individual story [...] so deafness, a physical fact, becomes deafness a story, with a hero or a victim" (Davis 3–4). As a result, we do not perceive experiences of disability as connected to each other or generated by the social environment. Therefore we do not perceive them as stories of a society, as we do stories of gender, race, ethnicity or sexual orientation. Consequently, we do not perceive disability as offering its own valuable perspectives on that society beyond individual life lessons (Mitchell and Snyder, *The Body* 2).

There is a second related reason why we do not see disability: because we use it as a narrative device. As many disability critics have observed, disability turns out to be among the most powerful vehicles of expression and narrative structure that we have. Our stories frequently use impairment or disability as a kind of shorthand to spice characters and convey internal qualities or plot functions vividly and efficiently through an alchemy of representational equivalents. We recognize the monstrous villain by the movements of his palsied body (Grendel in *Beowulf* 2007) or his halting gait and facial scars (the Joker in *The Dark Knight* 2008), which make his alienation and moral corruption visible. We assume we recognize the victim because he has a gentle persona coupled with a limp, which renders him vulnerable among hardnosed criminals (Verbal Kint in *The Usual Suspects* 1995). We recognize the hero because of his paraplegia: this acquired impairment telegraphs his outsider status in a testosterone-fueled military and lends explanatory verisimilitude to his acceptance of an indigenous people with different bodies in a narrative that is not ostensibly about disability, but about genocide in the name of resource acquisition and the bankruptcy of Western values in relationship to the natural environment (*Avatar* 2009). We do not see disability; we see the personal and social qualities that disability makes visible. That is why disability is one of the most persuasive tools of cinematic language in the Western tradition.

Disability works as storytelling shorthand because we think in metaphors (see Lakoff and Johnson) and metaphors of the body are familiar, evocative, moving, humorous, and terrifying for us. Without realizing it, we often rely on metaphors of impairment to articulate everyday experiences and frustrations. We say we were *blind*sided, she was *deaf* to his pleas, I was *left without a leg* to stand on, they're *freaks*, or he's *dumber than a doornail*. Disability functions for us as a wellspring able to make vivid any number of qualities or abstract concepts. David T. Mitchell and Sharon L. Snyder call this dependency on disability the *materiality of metaphor* for the way in which disability is able to literalize the ideas we want to communicate. They call our reliance on disability as a medium of characterization and as a metaphorical device *narrative prosthesis*— disability as enabler of rhetoric and representation itself. The more we use disability metaphorically, the more we lean on its potency to tell stories, the less we are aware that we do so, and the less we are inclined to consider disability as a lived, social or political experience beyond applying the meanings to it that have become familiar to us from using it to tell our own stories (*Narrative* 47–8).

There is a third even more powerful reason why we do not see disability: because we use bodily difference to define ourselves and others. A number of scholars have noted that disability has long been the medium through which populations have been categorized as inferior. To the degree that identities of gender, class, race, ethnicity, nationality or nation of origin, sexual orientation and so forth are constructed as less than, these constructions are achieved predominantly through disability. To claim that a person is inherently less capable is inevitably to use the language of the body — to use concepts and imagery of impairment and disability. This pattern is ubiquitous in the United States, as Douglas C. Baynton discusses in his essay "Disability and the Justification of Inequality in American History." It was foundational to slavery and appears in civil rights and immigration discourses, in the association of femininity with hysteria and in feminist tracts, in the pathologization of homosexuality and so forth.

Given the pervasiveness of disability's use as a medium of social control and stratification, Mitchell and Snyder posit that "rather than add disability to the theoretical matrices of other marginalized peoples," it is essential to perceive that "disability has become the keystone in the edifice of bodily based inferiority rationales built up since the eighteenth century" (*Narrative* 2, 12). As Siebers puts it, disability functions as "a symbolic mode different from other representations of minority difference. It is as if disability operates symbolically as an *othering other*. It represents a *diacritical marker of difference* that secures inferior, marginal or minority status, while not having its presence as a marker acknowledged in the process" (6, emphasis added).

Disability's cultural function as the "master trope of human disqualification" (Mitchell and Snyder, *Narrative* 3) is so established and naturalized that it has gone largely unnoticed and unquestioned. As a result, disability has had a problematic and unacknowledged relationship with other movements of equality. "As feminist, race, and sexuality studies sought to unmoor their identities from debilitating physical and cognitive associations, they inevitably positioned disability as the 'real' limitation from which they must escape" (2). Mitchell and Snyder call this *the representational double-bind of disability*: "While disabled populations are firmly entrenched on the outer margins of social power and cultural value, the disabled body also serves as the raw material out of which other socially disempowered communities make themselves visible" through dissociation (*The Body* 6–7). As Lennard J. Davis points out, it has not occurred to most of us that even as we protest recognized forms of social exclusion such as racism, sexism and classism, "the very foundations on which [our] information systems are built, [our] very practices of reading and writing, thinking, and moving are themselves laden with assumptions about hearing, deafness, blindness, normalcy, paraplegia, and ability and disability in general" (4–5).

On the topic of disability itself, there is often silence in academia. Curricula, for example, continue to address disability predominantly or exclusively in applied fields as a category of medicine, rehabilitation services or educational specialization. While North American diversity course requirements typically define diversity to include race and ethnicity, gender, and increasingly sexual orientation, disability is omitted (see Linton). As Davis point out, this is striking given the focus on the social construction of the body in the humanities and social sciences over the last quarter century. "Alternative bodies people this discourse: gay, lesbian, hermaphrodite, criminal, medical, and so on. But lurking behind these images of transgression and deviance is a much more transgressive and deviant figure: the disabled body" (Davis 5).

Still largely unacknowledged, disability remains at the heart of how we tell stories in Hollywood and Bollywood and in our homes, how we construct difference, and how we understand ourselves.

Considering disability in film and television requires some familiarity with basic concepts in disability studies, just as considering gender or race would require some familiarity with basic concepts in those disciplines of inquiry. This section is intended to provide a brief gloss of a few key ones. For a more comprehensive introduction, see Appendix II: Selected Readings in Disability Studies.

Impairment vs. Disability

Many people use the words impairment and disability interchangeably, but distinguishing between them is a prerequisite for understanding much of Anglo-American disability studies. Schematically, think of impairment as a physiological feature _of a body_, such as vision loss or paralysis. Think of disability on the other hand as a dynamic resulting from one or more features _of an environment_— social, cultural, political, historical, material or physical — that act as barriers or create exclusion, such as inaccessible stairs, poor lighting or prejudice. Thus disability is not a characteristic of an individual, but of a _social reality_. Take the hypothetical example of a six-year-old boy with dyslexia. He has an impairment, but whether he has a disability depends upon where he lives. If he attends first grade in Michigan under an educational imperative to learn to read, he may experience disability and be considered learning disabled. But if he lives in a traditional Amazonian culture under an imperative to acquire nonliterary skills, such as hunting, he would not experience disability nor be considered disabled. The point is that bodies and environments are both diverse and when they converge they generate a range of dynamics we call ability and disability.

I do not mean to oversimplify the distinction between impairment and disability. Its strictest articulation arises from its original definition in the 1970s by the British Union of Physically Impaired Against Segregation (see Oliver). It is analogous to the distinction made by second-wave feminism between sex and gender — between physiology and sociology — a distinction that enabled an entirely different way of thinking about "male" and "female," "men" and "women." So, too, the distinction between impairment and disability enabled and still enables an entirely different way of thinking about physiological difference. That said, there are varying views within disability studies about the viability or even desirability of maintaining a strict distinction between these two terms. Many have argued that they are not so easily separable. Impairment is not wholly individual. Our physiology is intrinsic to each of us, but it is also environmentally impacted from conception. Much impairment is generated by environmental factors: prenatal exposures, nutrition, chemical toxins, industrial collateral damage, natural disasters, poverty and warfare. Disability is not wholly social. It may depend upon culture for its existence, but it is constructed and experienced in the context of particular bodies with particular impairments. As Tom Shakespeare puts it, "There can be no impairment without society, nor disability without impairment [...] impairment is always already social, while disability is almost always intertwined with impairment effects" (34–35). Nonetheless, the distinction between impairment and disability continues to be fundamental to much of British disability studies and present in various ways within North American disability studies.

The Medical Model of Disability

The medical model or personal tragedy theory of disability is the most culturally dominant and therefore the most familiar. The name invokes a clinical or institutional relationship to disability in which the focus is on the physiological cause, cure and care of impairment, all of which locate the "problem" of disability in a person and the solution in treatment and rehabilitation. The medical model either does not effectively distinguish between impairment and disability or situates both predominantly within a personal framework. Disability becomes "an individual defect lodged in the person, a defect that must be cured or eliminated if the person is to achieve full capacity as a human being" (Siebers 3). Disability is thus always construed as a pathology.

Contemporary media is so saturated with this model that it has become naturalized and seems like common-sense, but it is deeply cultural. It provides the story arc for our most popular narrative about disability: the overcoming narrative in which a disabled protagonist struggles with impairment, usually alone or with the help of nondisabled characters, ultimately surmounting his or her *personal* limitations — both psychological and physical — to triumph over great odds and realize something about life that is inspiring to nondisabled viewing audiences. As a model for storytelling it is captivating. As a model for understanding the lived experience of disability it is inadequate at best and — of course — itself a source of disability insofar as it constructs and reinforces culturally disabling concepts of different bodies and what it means to live with one.

The Social Model of Disability

The social model of disability arose in the United Kingdom and constitutes a seismic shift in the understanding of disability from a form of stigmatized personal embodiment to a form of social injustice. The social model holds that disability is culturally perceived and shaped, much like gender, race, class and sexuality. You may have female sex organs, light skin, or no arms, all of which are distinguishable physical characteristics, but what each of those possibilities *means*— the ways others will perceive you, the opportunities and roles you will be permitted or denied, the significance attached to your body — is entirely cultural. From a social model perspective, therefore, the "cure" for disability is not the medical or rehabilitative treatment of individuals or the elimination of those with impairment, but the inauguration of significant social change in attitudes, institutions and human designed environments, which have been built for the nondisabled (Siebers 3). In other words, the "cure" is not the prescribing of prosthetics or a medical miracle; it's political change.

Social approaches to disability, most prominently the social model and social oppression theory (see Shakespeare 9–28), enabled the disability rights movements of the United Kingdom and the United States, which arose in the 1960s in tandem with the civil rights and women's rights movements, and evolved on either side of the Atlantic with different emphases. The discourse in British disability rights tends to be grounded in the country's experience with entrenched class stratification, framing disability as group social oppression and focusing on systems of access and material conditions. The U.S. discourse tends to be grounded in the country's experience with race discrimination, framing disability as a minority identity and focusing on individual civil rights (Shakespeare and Watson 4). In the United States, the disability rights movement led to the enactment of the Americans with Disabilities Act (ADA) in 1990, which was modeled after the Civil Rights Act of 1964 and ostensibly offers analogous protections, including equal employment opportunities and greater access to public facilities and services.

Disability studies scholars have since debated the strengths and limitations of the social model, especially insofar as it insists on a strict distinction between impairment and disability. In *Cultural Locations of Disability*, Snyder and Mitchell discuss another option: the cultural model, which has emerged in the United States. It holds that the construction of disability is not strictly a process of exclusion, oppression or the enforcement of difference. It is not even strictly social at all. Rather it is "a site of phenomenological value." In other words, social experiences — including obstacles — and physiological experiences — including impairment — coexist and are co-constructed in the lived experiences of disabled people so that "the definition of disability must incorporate both the outer and inner reaches of culture and experience as a combination of profoundly social and biological forces" (7). In this way, "the cultural model has an understanding that impairment is both human variation encountering environmental obstacles *and* socially mediated difference that lends group identity and phenomenological perspective" (10). Disability becomes not simply a site of social oppression, but a synthesized source of embodied insight and a "productive locus for identification" (10). The cultural model "imbricates the physicality of disability with the social and imagines the two always working in concert" (Chivers and Markotić 10).

Disability Studies

Disability studies in the humanities and social sciences arose subsequent to the disability rights movement, as did critical race studies after the civil rights movement and gender studies in the wake of second-wave feminism. In addition to developing its own critical and theoretical frameworks, it has drawn widely from race, gender and queer studies, recognizing that many of the insights of these fields — including the pernicious effects of stigma, the social dynamics of passing, the reification of biological essentialism, the reliance on binaries, the politics of segregation and so forth — occur with disability as well (Snyder and Mitchell 12). Disability studies, like the disability rights movement, has remained committed to the larger goal of interrogating the "widespread belief," as Siebers puts it, "that having an able body and mind determines whether one is a quality human being" (3–4).

In terms of media, as Mitchell and Snyder lay out in "Representations and Its Discontents: The Uneasy Home of Disability in Literature and Film" (*Narrative Prosthesis* 15–45), early disability studies in film took an image-analysis approach as reflected in Longmore's essay and the work of Martin F. Norden. They examined the proliferation of negative or stereotyped disabled characters who typically appear as isolated, psychologically enmeshed figures in medical model plotlines. Stock characters like the disabled waif or victim, the disabled villain or avenger, and the disabled "supercrip" — the ordinary person who achieves extraordinary feats of personal redemption and acceptable social reintegration by overcoming his or her own tragic disability — are all there.

The related social realist approach evaluates whether representations accurately reflect the specifics of lived experiences of disability or reinforce misperceptions with either negative or positive image, occluding social contexts. Both approaches interrogate the ways in which stylized, distorted representations of disability become naturalized, functioning to achieve a range of narrative effects. The work of both the image-analysis and social-realist approaches openly combines cultural inquiry with social change advocacy. At its heart is the larger quest of identifying sites at which disability becomes suppressed, manipulated, conflated or constructed in ways that are inimical to the full inclusion of people with disability or the recognition of the rich complexity of their experiences, or that furthers the mythologies of ableism and normalcy.

The New Historicist approach explores disability's representation in relation to specific contexts, complicating assessments of "positive" and "negative" or "realistic" or "unrealistic" by examining the complex ways in which any given representation has functioned in the cultures and eras in which it has been consumed. It traces patterns of social ideology, revealing a multitude of ways in which disability has been excluded or integrated, used to explain phenomena or teach principles, deployed as a tool for critiquing the dehumanizing qualities of social institutions or as articulation in various ways of nondisabled social experience. As Mitchell and Snyder observe, "Historical revisionist efforts produced interpretations that situated disability as both a perpetual social obsession in the West and as the object of complex cultural beliefs" (27).

Subsequent approaches have drawn from a range of critical and theoretical frameworks, including disability studies, genre studies, literary and film theory, queer theory, postcolonial theory and auto/biographical studies.

Disability: Positive or Negative?

Disability is a charged word with a range of valences. As a minority identity, it is not negatively inflected — at least it should not be. "The use of disability to disparage a person has no place in progressive, democratic society," Siebers reminds us, "although it happens at present all the time" (4). Within disability studies the term disability may appear positively, negatively or neutrally charged, often within the same critical discussion or even the same sentence, depending upon the context or referent. We talk about disabling culture (negative) and disability perspectives (neutral or positive). We recognize that disability as an excluded social position is the result of pernicious dynamics, while disability as a perspective offers valuable contributions to cultural understanding. Disability and impairment as lived experiences have complex evaluative associations, as does most of life. Negotiating these different valences and perceiving their intersections while remaining focused on the core value of disability studies — to "speak about, for, and with disabled people" towards a more inclusive and aware society — is a feature of the field (5).

The Invention of Normal

The term normal is so ubiquitous in our lives that we take its parameters for granted. But it is only about 160 years old. As Lennard J. Davis explains in *Enforcing Normalcy: Disability, Deafness and the Body*, "normal" as we know it — along with *the norm, normalcy, normative, average* and *abnormal*—entered the English language and our way of understanding ourselves and others between 1840 and 1860 courtesy of the new science of statistics. Before that point, "normal" was simply a technical carpentry term that meant perpendicular. Instead of the concepts of "normal" and "abnormal," there existed the ideal and the grotesque. The ideal was exactly that — the imaginative realization of perfected aesthetic beauty, reserved for deities such as Aphrodite and sculptures such as Michelangelo's David, if it could be realized in the human form at all. People were not expected to attain the ideal, especially not in this age before orthodontics, plastic surgery and digital enhancements, although the wealthy aspired to it in idealized portraiture. The grotesque saturated culture. It was a feature of humanity that was widely shared. All humans participated to some degree in the grotesque with their mortal flesh, bodily functions, and structural flaws alongside gargoyles with their bulging eyes and clawed feet. In its carnivalesque forms, the grotesque had life-affirming celebratory qualities that playfully and pointedly inverted social hierarchies (25).

The norm swept the ideal and the grotesque away, instituting a new imperative where there had been none quite like it before. "The concept of a norm, unlike that of an ideal, implies that the majority of the population must or should somehow be part of the norm," Davis points out. "In a society where the concept of the norm is operative, then people with disabilities will be thought of as deviants," which is "in contrast to societies with the concept of an ideal in which all people have non-ideal status" (29). This new imperative was not an accidental byproduct. The norm was created as a foundational term and concept of statistics, which was developed as a science of social improvement engineering, specifically eugenics. Eugenics was not a fringe ideology in Anglo-American culture during the nineteenth and most of the twentieth centuries. Supporters included Alexander Graham Bell, Margaret Sanger, and W.E.B. Du Bois. By the late 1930s half the states in the Union had compulsory sterilization laws. California's program became a model for the Third Reich.

We have largely retained our eugenics heritage in our internalization of "normal" as an evaluative standard that we see as self-evident and biological. We have also retained it in our discomfort with disability as "abnormal." As Davis notes, "Repulsion is the learned response on an individual level that is carried out on a societal level in actions such as incarceration, institutionalization, segregation, discrimination, marginalization, and so on. Thus the 'normal,' 'natural' response to a person with disabilities is in reality a socially conditioned, politically generated response" (13).

Within disability studies, normalcy studies has developed to interrogate "normal" and its camouflage as a neutral, empirical term. Scholars such as Davis and Rosemarie Garland-Thomson have shown that normal is a culturally specific term constructed in a binary relationship to its supposed opposite in a process that remains imbricated in a eugenicist ethos and is endemic in contemporary culture. As Michael Warner observes in *The Trouble with Normal: Sex, Politics, and the Ethics of Queer Life*, "Nearly everyone wants to be normal. And who can blame them, if the alternative is being abnormal, or deviant, or not being one of the rest of us?" (53). Normal has long been the most prominent example of a concept that relies on disability for its definitional existence and that has been wielded to label, control or exclude other populations. In *Crip Theory*, Robert McRuer proposes a theory of *compulsory able-bodiedness* in which he argues that "the system of compulsory able-bodiedness, which in a sense produces disability, is thoroughly interwoven with the system of compulsory heterosexuality that produces queerness: that, in fact, compulsory heterosexuality is contingent on compulsory able-bodiedness and vice-versa" (McRuer 2).

We were perhaps primed for normal by an older concept that is also implicated in the development of disability: equality. As Jacques Stiker surveys in *A History of Disability*, Western disability arose within Western democratic traditions that strongly associate equality with similarity, creating a precursor imperative to normal. Consider the words *handicap*, *disability* and *rehabilitation*, all of which link equality to similarity either by eliminating differences (handicapping), identifying dissimilarity that precludes equality, or indicating the mechanism of the restoration of similarity for the purposes of equality. We perceive equality as an entirely liberatory term, but Stiker recognizes its potential dangers in cultural practice when it comes to similarity. The story of political equality in the United States is not just a story of hard-won rights, but of the hard cultural work of connecting the concepts of equality and diversity. Disability stands at the epicenter of that story and we are still writing it.

The Instability of Disability

Disability as a category is uniquely "unstable": its existence varies among cultures, its boundaries are contested and its membership fluid, even within disability studies. Western definitions of disability are closely derived from Western medicine, industrial wage labor practices, and the high value placed on individual autonomy. We consider epilepsy a disability, but not infertility. Why? Because the former potentially interferes with employment and functional independence, while the latter does not. These criterion may seem self-evident, but they are not universal. Within traditional Hmong communities, as Anne Fadiman documents in *The Spirit Catches You and You Fall Down: A Hmong Child, Her American Doctors, and the Collision of Two Cultures*, epilepsy is not perceived as disability in the Western sense (although it may entail impairment), but as evincing a privileged relationship to the sacred. Eliminating it would involve the destruction of that relationship. Among the Punan Bah of Central Borneo where personhood is closely tied to intergenerational relatedness, infertility condemns one to a liminal state of child-adult, never becoming fully mature, a stigmatized, marginalized and dependent status similar to Western disability (Nicolaisen 50), which has also been characterized as liminal (Murphy, Scheer, Murphy and Mack).

In fact, the category of disability itself does not exist in many cultures as we understand it and the word is not easily translatable. Types of impairment are recognized — one can be blind or deaf or lame — but there is no equivalent to disability as a single, stigmatized category (Ingstad and Whyte 7). Instead there exists a variety of conceptual frameworks for understanding differences in physiology, whether from impairment or not (see Ingstad and Whyte). These include concepts of personhood or maturity, as among the Punan Bah, which appear to have much more in common with the pre-normal concepts of the ideal and the grotesque than with our now-dominant normal. Even within Western cultures disability has differing connotations, qualities and boundaries. For example, the distinction between disability and impairment is difficult to translate into Nordic languages "because there are not separate words which can capture the sense of individual bodily experience and social-contextual experience" (Shakespeare 25).

Not everyone who is supposedly disabled would define themselves thus. From the perspective of the Deaf community — in which Deaf is an identity conferred by cultural and linguistic fluency in American Sign Language (ASL) along with deafness — the Deaf are a linguistic minority. If we all spoke ASL and our environments were bilingually designed there would be still be sensory difference, but where would the disability be? There is historical precedence in the nineteenth century for this model of Deafness in the bilingual community of Martha's Vineyard where hereditary deafness and hearing were two equally accepted forms of embodiment. But the historical disavowal by the hearing of ASL as a language equal linguistically and neurologically to spoken languages, which we now know that it is, has disallowed the linguistic minority model.

Where disability starts and stops is another element of its instability in which the hand of history, cultural tradition, and even politics is obvious. The definition of blindness in the United States for government statistics, program eligibility, and membership as a blind person in national blind organizations is political. It was set by Congress in the 1930s — an origin reflected in the term "legally blind" — based on cut-off scores in either of two measurements, acuity or field (20/200 acuity or less or 20 degree field or less). But as we now know, acuity by itself is poorly correlated to functional vision. Additionally, these parameters exclude other aspects of vision loss, such as scotoma pattern (pattern of blind spots) or contrast sensitivity loss, which today have significant impacts for North Americans with visual impairment because of changes in the leading cause of vision loss and in demographics.

Then there is the question: does everyone get to be disabled? Many in disability studies point out that disability is not actually a minority category because it encompasses a majority of the population over time. But this claim rests on including impacts from disease processes and impairment in later life in the category of disability. Not everyone would agree to do so. The counter-argument is that illness is not disability because it is a typically temporary state with its own very different trajectory that leads to a resolution either in recovery or death, giving it a distinctive place *inside* the culture, as the many memoirs of illness in bookstores demonstrate. Conversely, disability is not incompatible with health and is a permanent state of being held *outside* the cultural mainstream. Impairment acquired at older ages from whatever cause is arguably not disability because it is socially normative, however undesirable or life-changing for the individual. Older adults who become impaired aren't *abnormal,* which means that they aren't disabled. They're simply even *older.* As Mitchell and Snyder write:

> While categories such as illness and aging also come replete with associations of physical debility and social suspicions of diminished productivity, disability bears the onus of permanent biological conditions such as race and gender from which the individual cannot extricate him- or herself [...] The ill or aged participate in a natural cycle of biological processes and breakdowns, but people with disabilities possess a biology that does not conform to even the most radical operations of normalization [4].

While recognizing the importance of grasping this point, this volume takes an inclusive view of disability in light of evolving concepts of both disability and aging. Moreover, recognizing patterns of stigma across forms of physical difference involving impairment would seem key to deconstructing their potency. From this perspective, disability's greatest instability is rooted in the vicissitudes of our lives. Disability is perhaps our only temporally contingent minority category: anyone can join at any time. The possibility of impairment — or additional impairment — is presumably daily and lifelong for all of us, although we often choose not to recognize it. As Tobin Siebers observes in *Disability Theory,* "I know as a white man that I will not wake up in the morning as a black woman, but I could wake up a quadriplegic [...] Able-bodiedness is a temporary identity at best, while being human guarantees that all other identities will eventually come into contact with some form of disability identity" (5). If nothing else, this reality should make us all interested in understanding how we perceive disability — really, how we create it.

There is a gulf between film studies and disability studies. Few film scholars appear familiar with disability studies. Some disability studies scholars have a depth of experience in film theory, technical terminology or practice but more are needed. Anthony Enns and Christopher R. Smit make this observation in the introduction to their 2001 publication, *Screening Disability: Essays on Cinema and Disability,* and it still holds largely true. It explains the relative paucity of scholarship on disability in film and television. *Different Bodies* invites film scholars, students and viewers to narrow the gulf by exploring the essays herein, and becoming familiar with disability studies and prior scholarship on disability in film and television through the recommended readings provided in Appendix II.

This collection offers nineteen essays on contemporary film and television by authors from the United States, Canada, the United Kingdom, Australia and India. Recognizing the global nature of cinematic media and of disability, the scope of the collection is international, including films from those countries as well as from France, China, South Korea and Thailand. Almost all the works addressed are readily available and can be screened in combination with reading selections for class discussion or independent study. The essays are offered as starting points for debate and inquiry into the issues they raise. Part I: Disability on the Screen opens with nine essays that consider a range of dynamics and drivers in relation to disability in film, including genre, community, commodification, modernity, and globalization. Four essays on contemporary television series follow that consider disability in relation to narrative function, curing, satire, and competitive reality shows. Part II: Disability in Production and Reception offers six essays that consider autobiographical film and television representations of disability produced in partnership with disabled people, disability biopics, and disabled viewer responses. Abstracts follow below.

Part I: Disability on the Screen

Timothy E. Wilson's essay, "Deaf Sexy: Genre and Disability in *Read My Lips*" (*Sur mes lèvres*, 2001), draws on disability theory and genre studies to parse the ways in which the film's portrayal of deafness as disability is determined by the requirements of its two genres, melodrama and the thriller, and conversely the ways in which this portrayal facilitates the transition between them and lends them verisimilitude. In doing so, Wilson observes the film's participation in what Tobin Siebers has called disability drag, its representations of deafness (as impairment) and Deafness (as identity and linguistic minority), as well as its highly structured intersections of disability, sexuality, and pathology. Associating deafness first with asexual social inferiority and insecurity and later with eroticized hyper-skilled social transgression, *Read My Lips* relies on deafness for its dramatic unity and affective thrill, ultimately offering a protagonist who isn't so much deaf as she is deaf-sexy.

In "Punk Will Tear Us Apart: Performance, Liminality and Filmic Depictions of Disabled Punk Musicians," David Church observes that disability has been one of the most fundamental yet least explored tropes of the punk genre and subculture. Distinguishing between the liminality of disability — the ways in which disability is figured as an unintegrated, non-normative state held at the borders of dominant culture and awareness — and the liminoid performances of the freak show and punk concert that construct abnormality as entertainment and socio-political alternative, Church notes the ways in which musicians and fans align themselves with both. Yet this dynamic has problematic implications for artists with disabilities, as Church explores in three films: the biopic *Control* (2007), the mockumentary *Brothers of the Head* (2005) and the comedy-drama *Bad Boy Bubby* (1993). In each case, genre-driven audience expectations of disability's liminality shape the narrative consequences for disabled musicians, ultimately limiting both their artistic lives and punk's actual political efficacy.

Heather Warren-Crow's essay, "Acquired Community: Leigh Bowery and *Hail the New Puritan*'s Mise-en-Scène of AIDS," explores the ways in which avant-garde pioneer Bowery's influential costume designs — particularly his iconic polka dots — responded to the AIDS crisis and the repressive public reaction it generated by exploring anxieties while performing an aesthetic of community that countered institutional and cultural efforts to curtail queer networks. Turning to *Hail the New Puritans*, an iconoclastic hybrid of screen dance, fiction and documentary that focuses on Bowery's friend and colleague, Scottish choreographer and dance celebrity Michael Clark, and for which Bowery designed the costumes, Warren-Crow considers the ways in which the film represents bodily contamination in the context of community. Ultimately Bowery and his peers modeled a form of belonging that countered Margaret Thatcher's regime of heteronormativity and privatization in 1980s Britain.

In "Razzle-Dazzle Heartbreak: Disability Promotion and Glorious Abjection in Guy Maddin's *The Saddest Music in the World*," Nicole Markotić argues that Maddin offers a new positioning for disability in contemporary media. Situating the film in relation to David Mitchell and Sharon Snyder's notion of narrative prosthesis in which disability is understood to function as a narrative device that enables potent plotlines that generate affective experience, often at the expense of representations of disability itself, Markotić points out that Maddin's film troubles this paradigm. By both raising and sidestepping depictions of disabled characters as naturalized figures of pathos, instead depicting them as both happy and fraught, displaying their disabilities on their own terms, and participating in the commodification and packaging of their own bodies alongside other products in a film that invokes and mocks disability tropes, Maddin moves one step beyond the traditional usage of disability.

Sally Chivers' essay, "Seeing the Apricot: A Disability Perspective on Alzheimer's in Lee Chang-dong's *Poetry*," takes up another counter to disability as narrative prosthesis in considering the depiction of early stage Alzheimer's in this award-winning South Korean drama. Demographic changes in industrialized countries have generated an increasing interest in forms of dementia as reflected in a number of films released within the last decade. Chivers argues that *Poetry* offers an alternative depiction to the typical "movie Alzheimer's" in which the condition functions as the narrative forge for nondisabled caregivers' difficult choices and self-development. Drawing on the aesthetics of the pastoral, *Poetry* sidesteps the monolithic portrayal of Alzheimer's as dependency, instead exploring the condition's effect on language and perception, suggesting a new view of memory. However, as Chivers points out, the film's innovative perspective is achieved in part through negatively charged depictions of other forms of disability, complicating its representation.

Sarah Dauncey's essay, "Breaking the Silence? Deafness, Education and Identity in Two Post-Cultural Revolution Chinese Films," considers Sun Zhou's *Breaking the Silence* (2000) and Ning Jingwu's *Silent River* (2000), both dramas critically acclaimed within China. Dauncey argues that assessing these films from a disability studies perspective—which was developed in the West and remains steeped in Western constructions of disability and identity—without an understanding of their specific Chinese contexts risks misunderstanding their cultural complexity and significance. Situating these films within the evolution of disability in Chinese films since the early twentieth century, Dauncey negotiates between Western expectations and the depiction of disability within China. As issues of deaf identity in China intersect those of disability in general, these films provide a case study not only for considering the implications of Chinese educational choices for deaf children in an era of social mobility, but for considering shifting notions of disability itself.

In "Modernity's Rescue Mission: Postcolonial Transactions of Disability and Sexuality," Eunjung Kim and Michelle Jarman draw from disability studies critiques of the evolution and enforcement of the concept of normalcy through systems of charity, rehabilitation and institutionalization that have been central not only to the construction of disability but also of modernity. Focusing on the Japanese film *Princess Mononoke* (Mononoke Hime, 1997) and the Australian film *The Good Woman of Bangkok* (1991), Kim and Jarman argue that

Western or modern efforts to rescue people with disabilities in non–Western or "pre-modern" locations play a critical role in enshrining hierarchies of development within and between nations. Both films feature female protagonists who resist and in doing so reveal the violence inherent in modernity's benevolent efforts of inter- and intra-cultural rescue. Through their stories the films reflect the ways in which disability has been deployed to sentimentalize marginalized people as a condition for Western intervention and for maintaining hierarchical relationships between nations and cultures.

Russell Meeuf's essay, "*Chocolate*'s Ass-Kicking Autistic Savant: Disability, Globalization and the Action Cinema," examines an alternative case in the filmic intersection of disability and modernity, arguing that Thai director Prachya Pinkaew's creation of a twelve-year-old heroine with autism disrupts the normative representations of the body in the action genre, invoking disability anxieties that are conventionally repressed beneath the muscled able-bodied adult male hero. In doing so, the film invites an uncomfortable awareness of the realities of impairment and inequality within globalization. While ambivalent about disability and steeped in pathos highlighted by its hybrid action-melodrama structure, *Chocolate* nonetheless troubles modernity as the source only of solutions. However, the film reins in its generic disruptions and critique of capitalism with its final shots, which return its heroine to the protective care of her Japanese father against a horizon of wind turbines, symbols of an imagined clean, pan-geographic globalization.

Joyojeet Pal offers the first comprehensive topography of disability in Indian film in his essay "Physical Disability and Indian Cinema," providing a companion work to Martin F. Norden's groundbreaking survey of disability in Western film, *Cinema of Isolation*. Examining more than 200 films from 1936 to the present, Pal observes that Indian cinema participates in the full panoply of disability stereotypes familiar to Western culture. However, many of its representations have culturally specific roots in Indian social practices and sacred texts, including the *Mahabharata*, the *Ramayana* and the Upanishads. Pal isolates and discusses four prominent patterns of disability representation — disability as punitive, disability as dependence, disability as disequilibrium, and disability as maladjustment — tracing the appearance of each to traditional figures, storylines and teachings within Indian literature and scripture. Turning to twenty-first century film, Pal considers films that depart from these patterns in the context of social change and what the future may promise for the depiction of disability in India.

In "Extra-Textual Reveals: Disability, (Sort of) Queer Sexuality and a Military Coup in *Battlestar Galactica*," Alyson Patsavas points out that the few films that feature disabled queer characters tend to use disability to further articulate queer sexual difference or to reinforce able-bodied heterosexuality. Similarly, *Battlestar Galactica* and its separate but allied web series, *Battlestar Galactica: Face of the Enemy*, use communications officer Lt. Felix Gaeta's disability and sexuality, represented as queer only in the latter, to achieve a particular narrative function: explaining Gaeta's leadership role and motivations in a key military coup. However, by reading these two narratives together — effectively "cripping" the series by interrogating its deployment of disability to construct Gaeta as both an embodiment of larger social tensions and to personalize his motive, and "queering" the webisodes by interrogating its use of queer sexuality — Patsavas argues that they present a tangentially queer, disabled character whose function exceeds the stock characterization of each narrative.

Johnson Cheu's essay, "Healer? Assassin? Ben Hawkins, 'Cure,' 'Disability' and Missions in HBO's *Carnivàle*" considers another character central to a series whose relationship to disability troubles its standard narrative use and representation: Hawkins who heals by drawing life energy from another living source. The figure of the healer in Western medical discourse is grounded in a duality between the body as sick or impaired versus the body as cured or repaired such that healing becomes by definition a gain. Illness and disability follow as negatives with their opposites as positives, a paradigm that has significant implications for how disabled and nondisabled people may view one another. While not discounting medicine nor invalidating the lived experience of desiring a cure, Cheu argues that with Hawkins the series disrupts this dominant duality, raising an alternative view of the power of healers and of curing in relation to disability along with the startling question: if curing involves a loss, what exactly do we lose? Ultimately, *Carnivàle's* paradigm reminds us that the body and its treatment is socially understood, as is the quality, meaning and value of our own lives.

In "'Are they laughing at us or with us?' Disability in Fox's Animated Series *Family Guy*," Simon McKeown and Paul A. Darke argue that unlike most television fare, *Family Guy*— despite being rife with stereotypes and raw humor — doesn't recycle stereotypical representations of disability or offer typically exploitative viewer relationships to it. Instead, the series participates in the long tradition of progressive cartoon satire not dissimilar from Britain's *Punch* magazine, which lambasted the predilections of nineteenth century Londoners. Observing that *Family Guy* features a remarkable array of characters with disability and has garnered a fan following among disabled viewers, McKeown and Darke focus particularly on the now infamous episode "Extra Large Medium," which includes Down syndrome in its storyline, to explore the ways in which series creator Seth MacFarlane undermines nondisabled certainties, challenges his audience to develop a different relationship to disability, and even includes some disability-centric jokes along the way.

Heath A. Diehl's essay, "Choreographing Disability: Stigma, Handicapability and *Dancing with the Stars*," serves as an opposing case study to the previous essay. Diehl points out that while *Dancing* promises the opportunity for self-representation and the opportunity for achievement on a level stage so to speak, it reinscribes dominant narratives of disability as a function of its own generic needs. As with all reality series, *Dancing* relies upon a combination of stock characterizations and the titillation of risk to generate the story arcs that power each season. These are achieved through editing, clip packages that offer carefully crafted contestant backstories and rehearsal sessions, and judges' comments. Diehl examines the ways in which Marlee Matlin's appearance on the show in season six reflects this dynamic, despite Matlin's longstanding media presence in counter-stereotypical roles, including a skit on *Family Guy Presents Seth & Alex's Almost Live Comedy Show*.

Part II: Disability in Production and Reception

In "Don't Film Us, We'll Film You: Agency and Self-Representation in the *Joined for Life* Television Documentaries," Ellen Samuels considers the two televised documentaries that conjoined twins Abigail and Brittany Hensel made as adolescents about their lives, *Joined for Life* (2001) and *Joined for Life: Abby and Brittany Turn Sixteen* (2006). The sisters have stated that their intention was to create a non-exploitative media presence that provided their own perspective as a context for their public interactions. Given the complexities of twenty-first century media production and distribution, Samuels considers a range of questions in relation to these films, including the images they convey in relation to historical representations of conjoined twins, the ways in which agency functions in and through these film, and the ways in which they create, reinforce or challenge perceptions of extraordinary bodies, particularly the Hensels'.

Veronica Wain's essay, "The Making of *18q-*: Parental Advocacy, Disability and the Ethics of Documentary Filmmaking," reflects on her own experience as the mother of daughter Allycia, who was born with a rare deletion on the 18th chromosome known as 18q-, and as the filmmaker of the first full-length documentary to explore the experience of children born with this genetic difference and their families, *18q-: A Different Kind of Normal*, which features Wain and her family. Wain recognizes that autobiography is a prominent yet contentious form of disability advocacy that becomes additionally complex in the context of parental control. Considering various practice models, Wain evaluates her own filmmaking process and the decisions she faced in crafting her daughter's and her family's appearance on screen, ultimately focusing on the ethical responsibility of the advocate filmmaker to maintain the child-subject's relationships with others and to create or strengthen communities dedicated to social change.

In "Overcoming the Need to 'Overcome': Challenging Disability Narratives in *The Miracle*," Terri Thrower discusses Chicago performance artist Tekki Lomnicki's 2007 autobiographically inspired film, which was based on her successful stage play *Thanksgiving* and culminates in the depiction of a pilgrimage with her devout mother to Lourdes, France, ostensibly for a miracle that would provide Lomnicki with a "normal" embodiment. Parsing six different ways in which the film overturns the culturally dominant and expected narrative of overcoming that the film's title invokes, Thrower argues that Lomnicki, who plays herself, and director Jeffrey Jon Smith offer a model of disability autobiographical storytelling that has powerful potential for representing and constructing first-person narratives that counter the hegemonic expectation of individual overcoming in disability dramas.

Martin F. Norden's essay, "*Born on the Fourth of July*: Production and Assessment of a Turbulent Text," traces the rocky development of the film from its inception as Vietnam veteran Ron Kovic's memoir in 1969 to its release as a blockbuster Tom Cruise vehicle with a classic three-act Hollywood script structure in 1989. This transformation came at the cost of distortions of the historical record and a repackaging of the representation of disability. Norden situates *Born* in relation to other post–World War II films about disabled war veterans and "Civilian Superstar" films — highly adapted biopics of prominent Americans who experienced disability — contending that as a result of its production process, *Born* falls most clearly in the latter category. It offers a traditional "overcoming" narrative generated by its script structure, which reinforces medical-model understandings of disability and popular American mythologies of individualism.

In "Deafness as *Peripeteia*: 'Beethoven' and *Immortal Beloved*," Dawne C. McCance points out that Bernard Rose's 1994 biopic of Beethoven is prototypical of the ways in which the composer's deafness has been cast as a dramatic turning point: either as precipitating the tragic fall of a great man or the rise of a hero who — in an epic form of the overcoming narrative — transcends disability itself to liberate music and the human spirit. But these versions of "Beethoven" require considerable falsifications of historical record and elisions of medical knowledge. McCance considers *Immortal Beloved* in relation to this troubled history of "Beethoven" production, parsing not only the ways in which the film deviates from fact, but the ways in which it ultimately is not so much a Beethoven biopic as a disability drama. It offers a highly fictionalized story that collapses aesthetics and biography into myth by manipulating the representation of deafness.

Katie Ellis' essay, "'This isn't something I can fake': The Discourse of Disability Surrounding *Glee!*," takes up the polarized viewer responses to the season one episode

"Wheels" of Fox Broadcasting's popular comedy-drama. The series has received numerous Teen Choice, Golden Globe and Emmy Awards and has been praised for its sensitive representation of disability and interrogation of disability issues, especially accessibility and social inclusion. While mainstream media commentators for *E! Online* and the *Los Angeles Times* laud the episode, a cluster of prominent bloggers with disability perceive it as highly problematic for a number of reasons that reveal the extent to which disability remains framed and contained by culturally dominant representations within popular media. The disparity of these responses reinforces the importance of attending to social media in order to access and recognize the diversity of viewer perspectives in relation to disability representation.

Works Cited

Baynton, Douglas C. "Disability and the Justification of Inequality in American History." *The New Disability History: American Perspectives*. Eds. Paul K. Longmore and Lauri Umansky. New York: New York University Press, 2001. 33–57. Print.

Bérubé, Michael. "Disability and Narrative." *PMLA* 120.2 (2005): 568–76. Print.

Chivers, Sally, and Nicole Markotić, eds. *The Problem Body: Projecting Disability on Film*. Columbus: Ohio State University Press, 2010. Print.

Davis, Lennard J. *Enforcing Normalcy: Disability, Deafness and the Body*. New York: Verso, 1995. Print.

Enns, Anthony, and Christopher R. Smit, eds. *Screening Disability: Essays on Cinema and Disability,* Lanham, MD: University Press of America, 2001. Print.

Fadiman, Anne. *The Spirit Catches You and You Fall Down: A Hmong Child, Her American Doctors, and the Collision of Two Cultures*. New York: Farrar, Straus and Giroux. 1998. Print.

Ingstad, Benedicte, and Susan Reynolds Whyte, eds. *Disability and Culture*. Berkeley: University of California Press, 1995. Print.

Lakoff, George, and Mark Johnson. *Metaphors We Live By*. Chicago: University of Chicago Press, 2003. Print.

Linton, Simi. *Claiming Disability: Knowledge and Identity*. New York: New York University Press, 1998. Print.

Longmore, Paul K. "Screening Stereotypes: Images of Disabled People in Television and Motion Picture." *Why I Burned My Book and Other Essays on Disability*. Philadelphia: Temple University Press, 2003. 131–148. Print.

McRuer, Robert. *Crip Theory: Cultural Signs of Queerness and Disability*. New York: New York University Press, 2006. Print.

Mitchell, David T., and Sharon L. Snyder. *The Body and Physical Difference: Discourses of Disability*. Ann Arbor: University Michigan Press, 1997. Print.

_____, and _____. *Narrative Prosthesis: Disability and the Dependencies of Discourse*. Ann Arbor: University of Michigan Press, 2000. Print.

Murphy, Robert F., Jessica Scheer, Yolanda Murphy, and Richard Mack. "Physical Disability and Social Liminality: A Study in the Rituals of Adversity." *Social Science and Medicine* 26.2 (1988): 235–242. Print.

Nicolaisen, Ida. "Persons and Nonpersons: Disability and Personhood among the Punan Bah of Central Borneo." *Disability and Culture*. Eds. Benedicte Ingstad and Susan Reynolds Whyte. Berkeley: University of California Press, 1995. 38–55. Print.

Oliver, Michael. *Understanding Disability: From Theory to Practice,* 2d ed. New York: Palgrave Macmillan, 2009. Print.

Shakespeare, Tom. *Disability Rights and Wrongs*. New York: Routledge, 2006. Print.

_____, and Nicholas Watson. "The Social Model of Disability: An Outdated Ideology?" *Research in Social Science and Disability* 2 (2002): 9–28. Print.

Siebers, Tobin. *Disability Theory*. Ann Arbor: University of Michigan Press, 2008. Print.

Snyder, Sharon L., and David T. Mitchell. *Cultural Locations of Disability*. Chicago: University of Chicago Press, 2006. Print.

Stiker, Henri-Jacques. *A History of Disability*. Ann Arbor: University of Michigan Press, 2000. Print.

Warner, Michael. *The Trouble with Normal: Sex, Politics, and the Ethics of Queer Life*. Cambridge: Harvard University Press, 1999. Print.

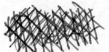

Deaf Sexy

Genre and Disability in *Read My Lips*

TIMOTHY E. WILSON

"Sometimes loneliness can be deafening," reads the first of a series of captions in the Magnolia Pictures preview for the U.S. release of *Read My Lips* (*Sur mes lèvres*, 2001), directed by Jacques Audiard. "Until a stranger opens your eyes," the captions continue: "She taught him good manners...he taught her bad ones." These cryptic snippets establish that "she" is deaf and "he" is an ex-con; "she" is lonely and innocent but he will "open her eyes," she obeys the rules and he breaks them, creating a terminological framework that yokes deafness to sexual inexperience, solitude, vulnerability, tutelage, and ultimately criminality — a seductive melding of disability, delinquency and danger. A cliché tagline then flashes onto the screen, one word at a time: "Don't Believe Everything You Hear." Next come a pair of quotes from prominent critics: "A brilliant Hitchcockian thriller," observes Stephen Holden, of *The New York Times*; "A deliciously sinister thriller," confirms Leslie Camhi, of *The Village Voice*. Two things are thus made abundantly clear: first, *Read My Lips* is about a deaf woman and a criminal,[1] and second, whether full-on Hitchcockian or merely sinister, it promises to thrill. The purpose of this essay is to investigate the intersection of the two genres that successively structure *Read My Lips*, melodrama and thriller, the ways in which they determine the film's portrayal of deafness as disability, and conversely the ways in which this portrayal conducts the film's tempo and facilitates its transition from the first genre to the second. Thus, although *Read My Lips* ostensibly contends with the complexities of representing deafness, imperatives of genre ultimately hold sway.

The film's plot traces the tense relationship between Carla (Emmanuelle Devos) and an ex-con, Paul Angeli (Vincent Cassel). Carla, neither attractive nor homely, works in a secretarial capacity for a property development company. She is deaf but navigates the hearing world with relative ease thanks to a pair of clunky hearing aids that she takes pains to keep buried under her hair. She hires Paul as her office assistant. When his debts catch up with him, the film changes direction and Carla is drawn into Paul's world of club music and crime. The film's second half revolves around a heist plot that ends with a double-cross and a getaway, the curtain falling firmly in thriller territory. Audiard had blueprinted a conventional thriller: "I wanted to make a genre film, and it was very constructed. The plot was complex, edgy, crammed to the brim."[2] Later, the film's talented stars, Devos and Cassel, intervened in the creative process, eventually compelling Audiard to rethink *Read My Lips* as "purely and simply a love story" (Rigoulet and Pomares). The result is a film balancing melodramatic romance with hardboiled robbery, a hybrid Vincent Malausa would later describe as "un tango malade."

The choice of a deaf protagonist is unique to Audiard's work as a feature film director, but it was not the first time he filmed deafness. In 1996, he directed a music video for the French rock band Noir Désir based on the group's track "Comme elle vient." The clip stars a diverse cast of women fluent in French Sign Language (Langue des signes française, or LSF) who dance, sign, and fingerspell their way through the song's esoteric lyrics. LSF also appears in *Read My Lips*, but it is coded in a very different and much more negative fashion. While Carla waits for her friend Annie (Olivia Bonamy) in a café, a young man approaches her, soliciting money in exchange for keychain lights and cards for learning the alphabet in LSF. He somehow[3] realizes that Carla can understand him and becomes more animated as he tries to get her to sign back to him. Uncomfortable, she pretends to ignore him. When she does eventually gesture back, her body language appears calculated to end the encounter as quickly as possible. He departs, but leaves a keychain light with Carla (he takes the card back, which she obviously doesn't need). With the young man's departure, this trinket takes on a new meaning: it is now an emblem of Carla's alienation from Deaf culture.

Indeed, the key to understanding what is at stake in this scene is bound up with the orthographic differentiation between deaf and Deaf, wherein deaf refers to a physiological difference and Deaf refers to a socio-cultural identity. As Lennard J. Davis explains, the Deaf are "people who are deaf (that is, without a significant degree of hearing) and also culturally Deaf," meaning that they "[belong] to a community of deaf people who share a similar language (American Sign Language, British Sign Language, etc.), a common community, a similar education in a Deaf setting, and a common cultural and social history (172). It is therefore significant that Carla is fluent in LSF, which suggests that Carla's participation in the hearing world and concurrent rejection of the Deaf community is not due to a lack of access to the latter; rather, it is self-imposed. Carla has apparently experienced Deaf culture—here represented as a culture of unemployment—and has elected to distance herself from it. When she is presented with the trinket, she accepts it with a nod, briefly recognizing the Deaf community in the person of the young man, who makes no request for a donation from her. In doing so, she temporarily acknowledges her position as an "insider" in this context, yet this tiny show of comradeship is just as quickly denied. As the young deaf man leaves the café, Carla fiddles with the keychain light he gave her and preemptively mutters, "It doesn't work." Actually, it does work (as Carla soon realizes), but her going assumption is that a product from a member of the Deaf community will malfunction. In her only encounter with Deaf culture in the film, Carla presupposes failure.

After Annie's arrival, the young deaf man passes by again and waves goodbye to Carla. She mumbles a barely coherent "Bye," avoiding eye contact as much as possible. This prompts Annie to ask, "Do you know him?" Carla's reply to this is so immediate and acidic—"No, why? Because he's deaf?"—that Annie is startled (subtitles).[4] This scene effectively excludes any alternative representation of the Deaf community by stressing the apparent quality of Carla's long-standing experience with Deaf culture: hesitation, awkward acknowledgement, and renunciation. She is deaf, not Deaf.

Ultimately, the film constructs her deafness in only two contexts, both hearing—the office and the nightclub — which are unmistakably linked to the melodrama and the thriller respectively. Reviewers have not addressed the relationship between disability and genre in *Read My Lips*,[5] although Annie Coppermann (*Les Échos*) noticed that the film "uses the heroine's disability like an extraordinary motor, charged at times with a strange sensuality," ultimately praising it as "un vrai bon film."[6] To say that genre "constructs" disability in *Read My Lips* is to engage with the social model of disability.[7] In *Digital Disability*, Gerard Goggin and Christopher Newell summarize this model, which "entails a distinction between 'impairment' and 'disability'" that divorces impairment, or "the irreducible, material, biological condition that inheres in an individual's body," from disability, a construction produced by society (21). This concept is important to understanding *Read My Lips*, for the film never seriously represents Carla as deaf. She does adjust her earpieces a few times, but these throwaway moments simply function to reinforce the stigma of deafness that the film posits as inherent to Carla's character as a deaf person: impairment and disability are one and the same in the film.

Tom Shakespeare has argued that disabled people are routinely objectified by cultural representations, which positions them as "passive" and "akin to animals, objects rather than subjects." Drawing on Mike Oliver, who theorized disability as "a relationship between people with impairment and a disabling society," Shakespeare points to the failure of cultural representations to give voice to experiences of impairment. *Read My Lips* participates in this historical trend, which Shakespeare dates to the seventeenth century (287), by avoiding engagement with impairment through the casting of a hearing actress and through its depiction of a deaf woman who is, for all intents and purposes, hearing. The film's concentration on Carla's hearing aids as the sole indicator of her deafness and the determining mediator of her disability subtracts her hearing interlocutors from the equation, making her simply a hearing person who needs hearing aids — and yet is also imbued with vulnerability and a naturalized stigma that deserves sympathy.[8] Indeed, as Shakespeare would no doubt point out, in this case the problem is written into the term itself, "hearing aid": "Disabled people [...] are viewed as passive and incapable people, objects of pity and of *aid*" (288, *my emphasis*).

But what the sciences and social sciences measure, fiction improvises, and because feature filmmaking has traditionally been prohibitively expensive, bankable dominant ideologies tend to distort the physical and social phenomena represented in film fictions. It is thus not surprising that when Susan Gregory and Gillian Hartley examined the discrepancies between lived social constructions of deafness and fictions of deafness, they identified a general lack of correlation:

> It appears [...] that film and fiction, rather than reflecting popular views of the lives and culture of deaf people, appropriate deafness to their own ends and use it as a device within essentially hearing contexts. They almost invariably create a simplistic view of deaf people, who are generally portrayed as either totally good or totally bad, as stupid or as having amazing powers of lipreading [293].

This dynamic is apparent in *Read My Lips*, which begins with ethical certainty in the figure of Carla, whose chaste longsuffering is facilitated and emphasized by her deafness, but slips into ethical ambiguity as the film changes genres. In the melodrama, Carla is a fundamentally blameless victim whereas Paul is a fundamentally tainted ex-con; in the thriller, as their roles within that genre dictate, both characters are mixtures. Gregory and Hartley also found that deafness is often exoticized, as when deaf characters are made stranger and more exciting through their "amazing powers of lipreading." Carla very obviously exemplifies this pattern. Her "amazing powers" are not only the fulcrum for the film's generic shift but also the crux of the diegetically prominent heist plot.

Throughout the first half of *Read My Lips*, Carla's deafness modulates the film's melodrama. She is seen mainly in her workspace, where her male coworkers habitually ignore her, belittle her, and slander her behind her back. Her clothes are noticeably bland and overly modest. She has no friends at work. When she faints in the office at one point, crying out softly and collapsing to the ground, no one notices, not even the man on the phone within feet of her, who appeared placed there to underscore Carla's invisibility. On three occasions coworkers casually leave a cup of coffee on Carla's desk as if her workspace were a designated receptacle for waste. One of these cups spills, damaging papers and soaking into Carla's chair, to her distress and embarrassment. A senior colleague steals credit for a project she has been working on for months; when she objects, he responds with thick condescension before brusquely dismissing her to answer his phone.

Carla's sexual sheepishness and social isolation are further accentuated when we meet her friend Annie, who presents a striking contrast. Our first encounter with Annie is carefully choreographed. Carla has just brushed off the young deaf man mentioned earlier — the distributor of sign language alphabet cards and keychain lights — when Annie enters. She is slimmer than Carla, wears a leather jacket over a fitted pink sweater, sports a tan and a vibrant smile, and moves quickly, pushing a stroller. Annie appears sexier and more socially confident than Carla. She is also a mother, but the limiting stereotypes of motherhood are deemphasized as the carriage of the stroller is kept below the camera frame. As Annie sits down and strips off her jacket, the lens hugs her body, lingering on the bare skin of her shoulder. She speaks quickly and uses slang, dashing off an excuse for being late — something about the woman who blow-dried her hair — before racing through some babysitting notes for Carla, stopping on a dime with a breezy "Okay?" to make sure that Carla has registered her instructions. Their conversation focuses on Annie's marriage, which has gotten rocky: "I feel dead. We haven't fucked in six months." Carla, who is inexperienced in these matters, struggles to find an adequate response to such frank sex talk, eventually settling for the safety of a maxim tantamount to incomprehension: "Married life is tough." Annie's casual fashion chic, easy sociability, status as a mother, romantic potential, and nightlife (she says she might go out salsa dancing later) all serve to intensify our impression that Carla's life is limited and uninteresting.

The film provides no concrete explanations for Carla's exaggerated modesty, social isolation, routine victimization at work, or the awkward asymmetry of her relationship with Annie. The viewer is given just two connected grains of information about Carla's childhood from which to make causal inferences about the formation of her personality: she was profoundly deaf when she was younger and has since chosen to live among the hearing. It is thus only too easy to suppose that Carla has internalized deafness as socially stigmatized disability; she is modest, awkward, solitary, and ultimately victimized because her life experience has been that of a deaf person among the hearing. Indeed, it could be said that Carla embodies the social model's critique of the construction of disability. She has accepted her deafness as disability, defect, and deficit, and learned to internalize the hurtful ideas about deafness the hearing world has always fed her. The film quietly imputes every detail of Carla's personality to the fact of her deafness. It is her core characteristic. She is pure pathology, a bundle of tics and traits. Her personality is shaped and motivated by a set of fictionalized psychological ramifications presumably attributable to a lifetime of persecution and social isolation.

Most prominently, Carla's desexualization by deafness and comorbid loneliness are reinforced by her idealization of romantic love, which is associated with her lipreading and thereby dutifully tied back to her hearing impairment within the diegesis. She reads lips alone and without Paul's prodding only twice in the film: once before she meets Paul and again during a period later in the narrative when they are separated without any indication that they will be drawn back together. Her designated love interest absent, Carla inhabits a kind of romantic escapist vacuum in both scenes, eavesdropping on nearby hearing intimacies by choosing both times to read the lips of a woman in private dialogue with a man. We see only the mouths of the speakers on the second occasion, but on the first the incidence of idealization is transparent. Carla intently watches the lips and hands of a young couple at a nearby table in the office cafeteria. The lovers smile as they speak to each other. As the clatter of the cafeteria dissolves, Alexandre Desplat's haunting score creeps in to fill the silence. The man reaches out to touch the woman's cheek and she kisses the palm of his hand. This couple represents a model of romance that is reinforced in the pages of the magazine Carla flips through as the scene begins, full of polished photos of beautiful people.

In his essay "Disability as Masquerade," Tobin Siebers observes that "the best cases of disability drag are found in those films in which an able-bodied actor plays disabled," a dynamic that *Read My Lips* exemplifies with its casting of Emmanuelle Devos, a hearing actress, as Carla (16). Siebers argues that "the modern cinema often puts the stigma of disability on display, except that films exhibit the stigma not to insiders by insiders, as is the usual case with drag, but to a general public that does not realize it is attending a drag performance." Of course, on the surface, Emmanuelle Devos's performance as Carla in *Read My Lips* is anything but bombastic. But for Siebers, this is beside the point, for in his view, "Dustin Hoffman's performance in *Rain Man* is as much a drag performance as his work in *Tootsie*." The difference is decided by the audience: "They know the first performance is a fake but accept the second one as Oscar worthy" for its realism (17). Predictably, Devos's Carla won best actress at the 2002 César Awards.[9]

Disability drag wins awards, Siebers says, because "it prompts audiences to embrace disability," yet at the same time, it contorts and transforms the realities of disability, for casting nondisabled actors — as in the case of *Read My Lips*—"not only keeps disability out of public view but transforms its reality and its fundamental characteristics." Bluntly put, disability drag "renders disability invisible because able-bodied people substitute for people with disabilities, similar to white performers who put on blackface at minstrel shows or to straight actors who play 'fag' to bad comic effect" (18). Devos' scrupulously patterned gestures and glances give Carla a recognizable set of habits and mannerisms that line up plausibly with hearing expectations, making them seem inherent, natural — believable — regardless of their highly constructed, stereotypically skewed, and generically utilitarian quality. The actress dons the character's disability like a comfortable second skin, and her success is measurable: if "the audience perceives the disabled body as a sign of the acting abilities of the performer," then she has mastered her role. The audience knows that she "will return to an able-bodied state as soon as the film ends," and that is the point. As the pathologized deaf protagonist of a melodrama, the fictional Carla "acts as a lure for the fantasies and fears of able-bodied audiences and reassures them that the threat of disability is not real, that everything was only pretend" (Siebers 18). Before this happens, however, the film will modulate from the restrained theatrics of a melodrama to the accelerated energy of a thriller, and Devos's Carla will move with it.

The shift in genre is announced by the introduction of a heist plot. Earlier, Paul stole a file from Keller at Carla's request. Now he asks her to return the favor and she agrees, on the condition that he come back to work in the office as her assistant. Days of answering phones and making copies are followed, in Paul's case, by nights spent working as a bartender in a seedy nightclub to pay off an old debt and, in Carla's, by colder, lonelier nights posted on the roof of the building facing the nightclub. The nightclub's owner, Marchand (Olivier Gourmet), holds Paul's debt. He is also planning a big score with the dangerous Carambo brothers (David Saracino and Christophe Vandevelde). Carla's job is to eavesdrop on their discussions by reading their lips through the windows of Marchand's studio above the club. She does this from two stories up, across the street, using binoculars.

As a thriller character, Carla is a casebook example of a fictional deaf person with "amazing powers of lipreading." Even a skilled lipreader can only be expected to grasp about 30 percent of spoken language without contextual cues, but Carla is called upon to read lips with more accuracy than this not only without contextual clues, but at an absurd distance, an absurd angle, and through multiple layers of glass (Lenel 22). Yet this is not all. Later, Carla's "amazing powers" are diversified. Marchand and the Carambos' operation a success, they temporarily store the cash in Marchand's studio above the nightclub. Paul goes to look for it but can't find it, so Carla takes the makeshift key he made from a wax impression of the original, and sneaks upstairs. Marchand walks in while she is still there, so she hides in the bedroom closet and turns up the volume on her hearing aids, significantly enhancing her hearing. She listens closely as Marchand moves around the studio, nervously checking on the money. When he leaves, she uses aural cues to reconstruct the path he took and find her way to the payload. A comparison of this new, criminally active Carla with the meek office drone of the film's opening scenes immediately exposes a palpable difference. Once passive, submissive, and preyed upon, Carla now stalks the very people who prey on society at large.

When Carla turns to Paul to take revenge on Keller, the film mobilizes a trope common to many film representations of disability — that of the "disabled avenger" — which the film's thriller segment then extends and elaborates. In *Narrative Prosthesis: Disability and the Dependencies of Discourse* (2000), Snyder and Mitchell interpret the disabled avenger as a representational heirloom of the long-refuted nineteenth-century science of physiognomy, by which physical appearance is "a mirror to the intangible workings of psychology" (97). According to Snyder and Mitchell, twentieth-century film narratives reactivate received (though disproved) knowledge of physiognomic principles whenever they "rely upon an audience's making connections between external 'flaws' and character motivations in a way that insists upon corporeal differences as laden with psychological and social implications" (96). Films use "distortions of the physical surface [to] provide a window on the soul of motivation, desire, and physic 'health'" (97). The disabled avenger targets those responsible for their disfigurement. In Carla's case, the disfigurement is social and cultural: hearing normativity has stigmatized her, ridiculed her, and denied her assimilation. Logically, she revenges herself by transgressing the social and legal structures that organize and legitimize the culture that refused her full membership.

Meanwhile, the film has radically revised the cluster of meanings associated with Carla's deafness, which are arguably rewritten through a kind of incidental apprenticeship in crime. Martin Rubin observes in his book *Thrillers* that "the thriller's practice of removing the everyday world from its familiar context is often underscored by the introduction of elements that are literally foreign and unfamiliar — that is, exotic" (21). The introduction of a thriller plot to *Read My Lips* recodes Carla's deafness as precisely this exotic element.

Paul's heist scheme hinges on her impossible lipreading skills and on her ability to prosthetically amplify her hearing. Apparently, Carla's efforts to integrate herself into the hearing world coincidentally equipped her for a life of crime. Thanks to her struggles with stigmatization, she now possesses a specialized set of skills that make her indispensable to Paul's risky scheme.

Moreover, the unique status she enjoys in her newfound niche boosts her confidence and makes her more aggressive.[10] Upon discovering that Paul has purchased a one-way ticket out of the country, she quickly deduces his design to ditch her and make off with the stolen cash. Later, she coolly wields this knowledge against him. By this point, she has definitively discarded the socially mandated construction of deafness that she embodied earlier in the film (deafness as disability) and replaced it with a socially transgressive appetite for action, an improbable talent for lipreading, and uncommonly sensitive hearing made possible by prosthetics. These unusual attributes make Carla peculiar and enticing. She is a criminal like no other, an alluring rarity. The fact of Carla's deafness now serves to guarantee the unexpected, to fulfill the trailer's dictum "Don't Believe Everything You Hear." Her hearing impairment is the "foreign and unfamiliar" element of *Read My Lips*, the element of the exotic that promises to thrill.

Carla's transformation in service of the film's generic modulation is enacted in her relationship to love: romance is replaced with eroticism. On a surface level, this is accomplished by the absence of any further traces of romantic love. In fact, an ambiguous domesticity-gone-wrong subplot follows Paul's parole officer Masson (Olivier Perrier), an ostensibly well-adjusted husband, who nonetheless murders his own wife despite claiming to love her. But we also see Carla slowly shed the strict inhibitions that governed her sexuality when she was a character of melodrama. This process is carried through incrementally, giving Audiard a chance to show off his eye for detail. It occurs primarily across a series of three scenes, all of which show Carla alone in her bedroom, dressing and/or undressing in front of an old mirror.[11] In the first scene, Carla ceremonially straps on a pair of red high-heeled shoes then strips completely naked. In the second, she undresses first then dons a shirt stained with Paul's dried blood. In the third scene, she sports a pair of low-top sneakers in the style of those she has seen on younger girls at the nightclub. The first scene is dreamlike and insulated: the red high-heels appear only in this scene. The second breaks this seclusion, as Paul's bloodied shirt cuts across the boundary separating Carla's public life from her private sexual fantasies. The third scene reverses, reiterates, and thereby completes the traversal, for when Carla puts on her new trainers she is actually dressing up to go out to Marchand's club. These three scenes reframe Carla's erotic identity to fit the demands of a thriller. Secretly sexy at first, she becomes openly so. Even Annie notices the difference. Violence, another trademark of the thriller, is also part of Carla's metamorphosis: her handling of Paul's bloodied shirt is powerfully fetishized and Carla's youthful footwear attracts the wrong type of admirers at Marchand's club, forcing Paul to fight off a would-be rapist.

Thus, although *Read My Lips* begins as a melodrama with Emmanuelle Devos's "disability drag" performance at its center, when the film later veers away from melodrama and becomes a thriller, Carla's deafness is imbued with a fresh set of meanings that respond directly to the change in genre. Devos's "disability drag" performance acts as a masquerade that assembles exaggerated postulations about the psychological ramifications that disability may potentially have, cultivating associations between Carla's deafness and lip reading, her social isolation and disempowerment, and her idealization of romantic love. However, when the film remakes itself as a thriller, Carla's ability to read lips becomes the defining characteristic of her new personality as a debutante criminal. Concurrently, she abandons idealized romance and gives freer expression to her erotic sensibility, enabling *Read My Lips*' thriller genre linking of deafness, crime, and eroticism. As a deaf character in a melodrama, Carla desires but is denied romantic love. The kind of love that becomes accessible to her — erotic love — requires that she reinterpret her marginality by passing from melodrama to thriller, trading in ostracization for transgression.

Yet these conclusions are incomplete, for *Read My Lips* does not present Carla's deafness as impairment but rather through a paired set of fictions about disability that work in tandem, the second reinforcing the realism of the first. The mechanism is clever: because Carla's thriller persona is obviously unrealistic, the pathology of deafness that the film develops in its melodrama mode is unlikely to be recognized for what it is — stylized "disability drag." Carla's superhuman lip-reading skills in the second half of the film render her awkward persona and social marginalization in the first half entirely plausible. The film's narrative structure thus reifies the realism of Devos's "disability drag" performance, which comes to serve as the mundane "normal" from which the thriller heroine emerges. This narrative ploy, by which the thriller's excesses naturalize the melodrama's logic of pathologization is reminiscent of Paul Darke's distinction between the "good cripple" and the "bad cripple" in fictions about disability. For Darke, "the 'good cripple' for culture comes across on film as the cripple who does his/her utmost to overcome his/her abnormality of body, in contrast to the 'bad cripple' who is happy to be a cripple" (Chivers and Markotić 106).

On one level, *Read My Lips* appears to realize this dichotomy, with the Carla of the melodrama figuring as the "good cripple" and the Carla of the thriller as the "bad cripple." However, in the case of *Read My Lips* the pressures of generic coding complicate a direct application of Darke's paradigm. Carla never stops trying to overcome her deafness. Instead, she finds herself relocated generically such that her melodramatic "abnormality" is rewritten as thriller "normality." Intriguingly, the mystery surrounding Carla's motivations is sidelined in the film by the enigmatic subplot involving Paul's parole officer, Masson, whom Carla and Paul see being arrested as they make their final getaway. This subplot, structured like a murder mystery and largely ignored by reviewers, consists of a handful of short segments that show Masson at home alone or asking others whether they've seen his missing wife. The clues are few and far between: in the first scene, Masson comes up from the basement of his house in an undershirt, sweaty, washes his hands and takes a swig from a bottle of wine. Later, the police visit his home at his request and ask about the basement, though they don't seem particularly suspicious. Finally, when Masson is arrested, Carla reads his lips from inside a car as Paul drives them by the police vehicle containing Masson: "I loved her," he says.

Thus, while Carla becomes increasingly trite as a character as the film solidifies a comprehensible psychological profile for her, the mystery surrounding Masson's inner life intensifies. Seen beside the shroud of irrationality that envelops Masson as the film concludes, Carla's trajectory fits that of a "good cripple" story with a happy ending. She finds acceptance in the criminal margins of hearing society whereas Masson falls from his privileged position as a symbol of authority and becomes a dangerous aberrance that must be locked away. The film offers prosthetically "corrected" deafness as a socially nontoxic, legitimate criminal identity by contrasting it with tragic and inexplicable homicidal behavior that threatens the safety of the family home and the sanctity of romance itself.

Synchronously, the film's naturalization of Emmanuelle Devos's disability drag provides the thriller's reworking of Carla's deafness with a rationalization that is simple and powerful:

Carla's profound deafness, confirmed and embodied by Devos' drag performance, lends her fantastic lip reading skills the modicum of realism required to suspend disbelief until the credits roll. Meanwhile, deafness as a context for the construction of Carla's interactions with the hearing is systematically ignored or denied and the question of impairment is left unaddressed. Instead, *Read My Lips* offers up a pair of fictions about deafness, representing it first as internalized, pathologized disability then as externalized, super-skilled criminality. In the melodrama, Carla's fictional deafness deepens the film's dramatic texture by adding overtones of pathology. In the thriller, it adds an element of the exotic, a hint of the "foreign and unfamiliar" that is elaborated and intensified by adding overt sexualization. Like a rare spice, deafness is kneaded into *Read My Lips* for intrigue and excitement. Ultimately, Carla Behm isn't so much deaf as she is deaf sexy.

Notes

1. The symbiosis of disability and delinquency developed in *Read My Lips* is echoed, not coincidentally, by the choice of cover art for Sharon L. Snyder and David T. Mitchell's book *Cultural Locations of Disability* (2006): Vincent Van Gogh's "Prisoners' Walk," which invokes the prison to symbolize the relegation of disability to high-surveillance cultural locations.

2. All translations are mine unless otherwise noted.

3. Carla's hearing aids are covered entirely by her hair, so it is unclear how the man could have known that Carla understands sign language. Arguably, the film posits Carla's deafness as inherently visible, noticeable even when carefully hidden.

4. Carla's feeling of embarrassment at being publicly addressed in LSF is appropriate to the legal standing of LSF in France at the time. It was not until 2005 that deaf children were actually granted the right to choose a bilingual education (French and LSF) over a French-only education (Loi n°2005–102 du 11 février 2005 — art. 19 JORF 12 février 2005). In contrast, by 2005 similar rights had been active in the United States for 30 years, beginning in 1975 with the Education for All Handicapped Children Act, which has since undergone several revisions, including a change of name in 1990 to the Individuals with Disabilities Education Act. As a case-law review of this law in action for children with hearing impairment shows, progress has come in fits and starts, but in France progress has just begun (Kreisman and John).

5. Although reviewers across the board failed to critique the determinative role genre plays in *Read My Lips*'s depiction of deafness, the *Cahiers du cinéma* critic Vincent Malausa did employ a rather strikingly opportunistic vocabulary. He suggests that Carla's "deficient perception" fills *Read My Lips* with "an autistic sensuality" disrupted only by the "brutal straightness" of Paul's movements. Besides the obvious sexual metaphor, Malausa's use of non-specific autism as a metonym for the sexual tension between Carla and Paul powerfully demonstrates how the film's own metonymic ploys cultivate a pathologizing gaze.

6. The French is retained in this instance to highlight the author's inclusion of the word "vrai," which is used here somewhat atypically as an adverb meaning "truly" but also has the adjectival usage "true." Of course, to say that the film is "truly" good is not necessarily to claim that it is "true"; however, the atypical turn of phrase employed here does lend itself to precisely that layering of meanings.

7. As Sharon L. Snyder and David T. Mitchell note in the introduction to *Cultural Locations of Disability*, "the social model [of disability] developed largely in the United Kingdom, beginning with the history of the Union of the Physically Impaired Against Segregation" (6). In a 1997 essay entitled "Defending the Social Model," Tom Shakespeare and Nicholas Watson pointedly recall these politically charged origins, writing that "it is important to note that this ideological position [that of the social model] should be properly located in British disability politics: the movement [*sic*] in other countries, while adopting a social or minority group approach, have not built their campaign and self-definition around the social model" (293).

8. In *Read My Lips*, "the split in the term impairment" proposed by Snyder and Mitchell is not enacted. Aside from a few fleeting reminders that Carla's hearing aids are not a perfect solution — she adjusts them in public a couple of times — the film, like the social model of disability, "casts off" impairment. Or, more often, recasts impairment as convenience. In one instance, Carla takes her hearing aids out to muffle the sound of Annie's baby, who begins to cry while she tries to comfort it. (Her failure to do so is also not insignificant.) She also removes her prosthetics when she enters the nightclub for the first time. Most telling for the film's overall characterization of deafness as oh-so-convenient is the scene in which Carla climbs into the passenger seat of her car and complains to Paul that he is playing the stereo too loud, to which he retorts, "You just have to take out your hearing aids." In a way, then, *Read My Lips* both justifies and

critiques the social model. Carla embodies disability as social construction, but in this screen incarnation the social model's tactical evasion of impairment becomes distinctly problematic.

9. In the introduction to *The Problem Body: Projecting Disability on Film* (2010), Sally Chivers and Nicole Markotić cite Siebers' "Disability as Masquerade" essay in a discussion of a *Kids in the Hall* skit called "The Academy Awards," in which four actors, three of whom played characters with disabilities and one of whom played Hamlet, receive nominations for Best Actor at the Oscars (5). The result is a three-way tie ("Everybody but the Hamlet guy!"). Chivers and Markotić use the development of this skit to redirect critical attention away from what is represented onscreen and instead toward the "spectatorship, meaning, and normative gaze that settle upon what we call 'the problem body' on film," a reorientation that has particular poignancy in the case of *Read My Lips* (7).

10. Carla's aggressiveness is more assured in the second half of the film, but not absent from the first half. Indeed, she is assigned a sort of allegorical animality by the opening frames, which show her licking water out of her hands, something Paul will do later, when the pair's morning routine synchronizes during the build-up to the thriller payoff. Also, when Carla sits down to eat lunch with Paul on his first day at the office, she politely asks, "Can I ask you a question?" and receives a similarly toned-down "Yeah, sure" from Paul. The question that follows, however — "Why were you in prison?" — is accompanied by such an exaggerated burst of aggression (she speaks louder, fast, adds a gruff "Hein?" after the question, and maintains direct eye contact) that Carla herself immediately recoils from her own barb by lowering her voice, casting her eyes downward, and trails off at the end of "No, no, that was dumb, I never should have..." However, psychological manipulation and physical violence remain sharply separated, and Carla only ever responds to bodily aggression with alarm and acute discomfort.

11. These voyeuristic episodes actualize the powerful and oft-cited overlap of disability studies and feminist theory within film criticism. In their introduction to *The Problem Body*, Chivers and Markotić draw on Laura Mulvey (and Michel Foucault) to argue that "spectatorship ... allows audience members to take on the unique and contradictory position of what we call the 'panopticon viewer'" (3). In *Cultural Locations of Disability*, Snyder and Mitchell make a similar observation: "To a significant degree, film produces interest in its objects through the promise of providing bodily differences as an exotic spectacle" (157). While Carla's body is not outwardly "excessive" (Snyder and Mitchell's term), the mirror scenes in *Read My Lips* offer up intimate knowledge of Carla's psychological particularities by performing the side effects of her supposed internalization of hearing impairment as social stigmatization. Carla's body and mind thus both become objects of a kind of clinical voyeurism that "hinges on securing audience interest through the address of that which is constructed as 'outside' a common visual field" (158).

Works Cited

Audiard, Jacques. Interview by Laurent Rigoulet and Claire Pomares. *Télérama.fr*. Telerama. 28 Feb. 2010. Web. 11 Feb. 2011.

Camhi, Leslie. "All About Their Mothers." Rev. of *Read My Lips* [*Sur mes lèvres*]. *Village Voice* 12 Mar. 2002: 124. Web. 1 May 2011.

Chivers, Sally, and Nicole Markotić, eds. *The Problem Body: Projecting Disability on Film*. Columbus: Ohio State University Press, 2010. Print.

Coppermann, Annie. "Une histoire trouble." Rev. of *Read My Lips* [*Sur mes lèvres*]. *Les Échos* 17 Oct. 2001: 53. Web. 1 May 2011.

Ebert, Roger. "Souls Connect in Tale of Rare Depth." Rev. of *Read My Lips* [*Sur mes lèvres*]. *Chicago Sun-Times* 19 July 2002: Weekend Plus; 33. Web. 1 May 2011.

Frodon, Jean Michel. "Tous les sens en éveil; *Sur mes lèvres*. Jacques, admirablement épaulé par ses acteurs, signe un film troublant." Rev. of *Read My Lips* [*Sur mes lèvres*]. *Le Monde* 17 Oct. 2001. Web. 1 May 2011.

Goggin, Gerard, and Christopher Newell, eds. *Digital Disability: The Social Construction of Disability in New Media*. Lanham, MD: Rowman & Littlefield, 2003. Print.

Gregory, Susan, and Gillian Hartley, eds. *Constructing Deafness*. London: Continuum; Milton Keynes: Open University Press, 2002. Print.

Hoberman, J. "Suspended Animation." Rev. of *Read My Lips* [*Sur mes lèvres*]. *Village Voice* 9 July 2002: 99. Web. 1 May 2011.

Kreisman, Brian M., and Andrew B. John. "A Case Law Review of the Individuals with Disabilities Education Act for Children with Hearing Loss or Auditory Processing Disorders." *Journal of the American Academy of Audiology* 21.7 (2010): 426–440. Web. 26 June 2011.

Loi n°2005–102 du 11 février 2005 pour l'égalité des droits et des chances, la participation et la citoyenneté des personnes handicapées. Article L112–2–2. *Legifrance.gouv.fr*. Web. 26 June 2011.

Lenel, N. "Les communications alternatives." *Les surdités de l'enfant.* Eds. M. Mondain and V. Brun. *Rencontres en rééducation* 25. Issy-les-Moulineaux: Elsevier Masson, 2009. 20–26. Print.

Malausa, Vincent. Rev. of *Read My Lips* [*Sur mes lèvres*]. *Cahiers du cinéma* no. 561 (Oct. 2001): 91. Print.

Mitchell, David T., and Sharon L. Snyder. *Narrative Prosthesis.* Ann Arbor: University of Michigan Press, 2000. Print.

Read My Lips [*Sur mes lèvres*]. Dir. Jacques Audiard. Perf. Emmanuelle Devos and Vincent Cassel. 2001. Columbia TriStar Home Entertainment, 2003. Film.

Rubin, Martin. *Thrillers.* Cambridge: Cambridge University Press, 1999. Print.

Sarris, Andrew. "Lip-Reading Her Way Through An Ingenious French Thriller." Rev. of *Read My Lips* [*Sur mes lèvres*]. *New York Observer* 15 July 2002: Arts & Entertainment, 21. Web. 1 May 2011.

Scott, A.O. "If Work Doesn't Pay, There's Always Crime." Rev. of *Read My Lips* [*Sur mes lèvres*]. *The New York Times* Late Edition (Final) 5 July 2002: E1. Web. 1 May 2011.

Shakespeare, Tom. "Cultural Representation of Disabled People: Dustbins for Disavowal?" *Disability & Society* 9.3 (1994): 283–299. Web. 30 June 2011.

_____, and Nicholas Watson. "Defending the Social Model." *Disability & Society* 12.2 (1997): 293–300. Web. 30 June 2011.

Siebers, Tobin. "Disability as Masquerade." *Literature and Medicine* vol. 23 no. 1 (Spring 2004): 1–22. Web. 11 Feb. 2011.

Snyder, Sharon L., and David T. Mitchell. *Cultural Locations of Disability.* Chicago: University of Chicago Press, 2006. Print.

Tranchant, Marie-Noëlle. "Association de mal-aimés." Rev. of *Read My Lips* [*Sur mes lèvres*]. *Le Figaro* 17 Oct. 2001. Web. 1 May 2011.

Punk Will Tear Us Apart

Performance, Liminality and Filmic Depictions of Disabled Punk Musicians

DAVID CHURCH

In the decades since the generic development of punk rock in the mid-to-late 1970s, numerous films have depicted performers, fans, and assorted denizens of this musical sub-culture and its various offshoots. Despite punk's steady mainstreaming over those same decades — achieved precisely through popular media like film — a rebellious sense of social deviance has remained a central subcultural ideology, rooted in punk's loud and disorderly musicality. Amid the constellation of identity factors that intersect with performances of subcultural belonging, disability has been one of the most foundational — and yet, one of the least explored — representational tropes of the punk milieu. In particular, punk musical performance has drawn upon the history of freakery and the traditional freak show's semiotic inseparability from potentially disabling forms of corporeal difference. In drawing upon this symbolic reservoir for subcultural distinction, musicians and fans alike implicitly align themselves with disability's social liminality, especially during the live concert's blurring of boundaries between performers and audience members. Yet, this mode of performance has problematic implications for punk musicians with actual disabilities, depending on how audience reception frames the concert experience. In this essay, I will explore the audience/performer dynamics in three films that take punk musicians with very different disabilities as their lead subjects: *Control* (Anton Corbijn, 2007), *Brothers of the Head* (Keith Fulton and Louis Pepe, 2005), and *Bad Boy Bubby* (Rolf de Heer, 1993). In contrasting these texts, this essay seeks spaces where disability's stigmas paradoxically open up grotesque interconnections between bodies in the spirit of music.

Disability, Freakery, and Liminality

Victor Turner describes a culture's rites of passage as a tripartite process involving an initial *separation* from one's prior social status, a liminal state of *transition*, and an eventual *incorporation* into one's changed social status (56). During the transitional stage, liminal figures are placed outside society and seem to blur a variety of social categories: "They are

28

... associated with life and death, male and female, food and excrement, simultaneously, since they are at once dying from or dead to their former status and life, and being born and growing into new ones" (58–59). Given Turner's emphasis on the liminal figure's "uniformity, structural invisibility, and anonymity" (59), liminality has proven a fruitful concept for discussing the state of people with disabilities. Robert F. Murphy et al. compare disability to a permanent "in-between state, for the person is neither sick nor well, neither fully alive nor quite dead," resulting in social isolation, exclusion, and presumed asexuality or sexual deviance (238, 240). Indeed, the disabled body is rendered invisible yet regarded as a potentially contaminating threat (often by violating taboos about requisite control over one's own body); in common social situations, for example, "we are treated to the paradox of nobody 'seeing' the one person in the room of whom they are most acutely, and uncomfortably, aware" (239). Yet, unlike the temporary liminality of the initiate in traditional societies, Jeffrey Willett and Mary Jo Deegan describe the person with disabilities as unable to ever be (re)incorporated back into our hypermodern society, except "with death, and the accompanying funeral rites" that resolve disability's supposed potential to pollute normative bodies (142, 145). However, they also argue that "because of the permanent liminality of disability, the arbitrariness and hostility of the disabling society can be revealed and shattered," thus embodying the potential for social change (147). Consequently, I will focus on the political potential of freaks — extraordinarily non-normative people who do not remain invisible, but who deliberately insist upon public visibility.

Although the public exhibition of non-normative bodies has been used as an entertainment spectacle for centuries, Rosemarie Garland-Thomson, Rachel Adams, and Michael M. Chemers note that our contemporary conceptions of the traditional freak show descend from nineteenth-century traveling sideshows and museums. Common exhibits included both "born freaks" (performers with congenital disabilities) and "self-made freaks" (able-bodied performers voluntarily positioning their bodies as "abnormal"). The boundaries between these categories routinely blurred as Freak Show exhibits framed performers through elaborate costuming and mise-en-scène. Nevertheless, apparently "authentic" teratological displays remained privileged in the cultural imagination by virtue of their rarity, especially after the genetically "abnormal" or disabled body was removed from public visibility with the decline of the freak show in the twentieth century and the medicalization of physical difference (Garland-Thomson 78). While this has meant that "freakishness" remains a lingering, stigmatizing connotation carried by many visible disabilities even today, we should be careful to distinguish between a person with disabilities and the figure of the "freak," as the latter involves "the intentional performance of constructed abnormality as entertainment" (Chemers 24). Freakery is therefore less a permanent embodied state than a deeply capitalistic process of investing oneself with (and being invested by) a plethora of cultural discourses about the body.

Spectators of the traditional freak show sought the promised pleasures of wonder, horror, and pity at the sight of so-called human oddities. As Garland-Thomson argues, "Invested with the liminality that Victor Turner suggests threatens both to transform and to disrupt the social order, extraordinary bodies carry a range of attributed cultural meanings projected onto them by astonished onlookers" (70). Serving as both an intentional performance by a distinctive individual irreducible to pure corporeal difference, and as a template for the projection of spectators' normative attitudes, the freak becomes a figure at the intersection of selfhood and otherness. In this respect, Garland-Thomson argues that the freak's liminality — like Mikhail Bakhtin's discussion of the grotesque carnivalesque body — makes him/her a greater figure of potentiality than the disabled body described by Murphy et al. as primarily marked by adversity and lost/unattainable social status (Garland-Thomson 113).

The traditional freak show's appeal transmogrified into new cultural forms as twentieth-century attitudes privileged the spectacle of freakish bodies safely contained within a medical or institutional context. How, then, can the freak's status as a publicly visible individual who performatively revels in his/her physical difference be reconciled with arguments about people with disabilities as socially invisible, anonymous, and lacking social status? Complicating Garland-Thomson's discussion of the freak as "liminal," I would argue that Turner's differentiation between "liminal" and "liminoid" phenomena clarifies this distinction. Liminal in this context refers to a congenital or acquired embodiment of difference or transformation kept at the margins of social culture, often out of sight. Liminoid is an assumed embodiment of visible difference or transformation performed in the limelight. In traditional societies, it is obligatory for the entire community to observe and respect the liminal space/time set apart from everyday life during transitional rites of passage — from puberty to adulthood is the classic example. In today's post-industrial societies, however, we have largely lost these ritual liminal spaces. Instead, we have participation in symbolic inversions like carnivalesque play or performative genres, which are voluntary entertainments indulged in by smaller segments of the population (74). This generation of the liminoid as its own sphere largely rose as industrialization separated work and leisure as distinct segments of social existence (67–69). Because participation in liminoid leisure genres like music, art, and cinema remains optional, "great public stress is laid on the individual innovator, the unique person who dares and opts to create" (74–75).

Therefore, if people with disabilities continue to occupy a liminal status that renders them largely invisible and anonymous through the socially shared and obligatory ableism that Robert McRuer terms "compulsory able-bodiedness" (8), the figure of the freak remains highly individuated as a distinctive and unique performer. The historical freak show was a liminoid genre, spawning freakery's more recent diffusion into a plethora of other liminoid cultural genres. As Garland-Thomson argues, freak shows can offer "a counternarrative of peculiarity as eminence, the kind of distinction described by Bakhtin's and Foucault's notions of the particularized pre–Enlightenment body." They manifest a "tension between an older mode that read particularity as a mark of empowering distinction and a newer mode that flattened differences to achieve equality" (17). Broadly speaking, then, the freak show has generically served as a sort of historical "rite of passage," its evolution staging a series of changes between early-modern and hypermodern notions of embodiment. If disability is routinely stigmatized and contained as Otherly in modern societies, then aesthetic genres can all the more safely use it as a key trope in exploring the body's (oft-repressed) potential for openness and becoming. Yet, because actual disability remains stigmatized, recognizing it for itself rather than electively taking it on as a rich form of representation available for self-expression can limit its aesthetic usefulness for the non-disabled. If disability's ambiguously liminal status comes to the forefront, it may drain its playful function within liminoid genres. As Turner puts it, recognizing actual disability risks "the acme of insecurity, the breakthrough of chaos into cosmos, of disorder into order" (77).

Punk Performance as Liminoid Phenomenon

For Turner, the realm of leisure is an in-between time/space composed of electively chosen activities set apart from the obligations of both work and familial/civic responsibility

(71). The rock concert is a prime example, as rock is a musical genre that has ideologically retained its emphasis on attendance of the "authentic" live performance as a requisite ritual for any self-respecting fan (Thornton 70). Turner cites rock music as a leisure genre that playfully assembles cultural raw material "in random, grotesque, improbable, surprising, shocking, usually experimental combinations" (71). Emerging in the United States and Britain during the mid–1970s, the subgenre of punk rock exemplifies these qualities in its raw, loud, and simplistic chord progressions, its lyrical emphasis on shock value and grotesquerie, and its overall reaction against refined musical talent. Meanwhile, musical subcultures often form through a perceived sense of "underground" distinction from the "mainstream," with fans commonly attempting to build "subcultural capital," or a sense of hipness that "confers status on its owner in the eyes of the relevant beholder" (Thornton 11).

The strictness of these intra-subcultural norms is particularly ironic, given the prescribed unruliness and spontaneity of the punk rock concert itself, in which performances of subcultural belonging wildly intermingle with onstage performances, and one can become temporarily swept up in a chaotic atmosphere with little time to contemplate careful subcultural distinctions. Punk shows encourage actively disruptive and even violent audience participation (pogoing, moshing, stage diving) that erodes the boundaries between band and audience, especially if the performers' deliberately amateurish musical acumen makes the privileged onstage role seem accessible to everyday fans. Both onstage and off, bodies crash into one another, sometimes extending beyond their limits in grotesque ways (spitting, vomiting, bleeding). Early punk bands such as the Sex Pistols even recalled the Bakhtinian carnival's "Lords of Misrule," lyrically and performatively motivated by "an impulse to disgust and appall by reducing the sublimations of serious artists and musicians to a celebration" of lower bodily processes like drinking, sex, and death (Brottman 14–15). This sense of disorder is amplified by the sheer cacophony within the small clubs where punk concerts often occur.

Amid punk's inversion of social taboos, the genre's rough, open, and unfinished musical style evokes qualities similarly associated with disabled bodies. Punk rock could thus seem especially conducive to disability-related issues, but its subcultural ideology of supposed rebellion and nonconformity more specifically associates it with freakery's spectacularly non-normative bodies, given the continuing stigmatized link between physical difference and social deviance. These attitudes largely descended from members of the 1960s counterculture (including rock musicians), who honorifically self-identified as "freaks" by detaching that term from its associations with born freakery and rearticulating it with self-imposed marginalization and ostracism as an anti-establishment challenge over the limits of social possibility demarcated by the taboo (Fiedler 300–05, 313–15). Even if punk rejected much of the hippie-era counterculture, it retained the image of rock star as self-made freak, paradoxically flaunting his/her "rebellious" social deviance onstage to build subcultural credibility and thus avoid the erasure from public visibility that such deviance usually incurs. As many medical institutions shuttered in the late twentieth century (particularly in the English-speaking countries that were concurrently experiencing punk's birth), people with disabilities increasingly moved into public spaces but were still often treated as socially invisible; consequently, punk expresses defiance by moving these bodies back to center stage, insisting upon their prominence. Early punk and post-punk performers often drew upon signifiers of bodily excess and disorder, modeling their carnivalesque stage presence after sideshow freaks and disabled characters in film and literature (McKay 355–56; Church, "Welcome").

Yet, most punk musicians were able-bodied, not people whom audiences understood as actually disabled. This means that the freak's liminoid capacity to ambivalently blur the boundaries between self and other, normative and non-normative, is potentially limited by fans' reception of freakery as ostensibly "resistant" to mainstream tastes, and therefore a source of subcultural capital. If freakery (and, by extension, disability) continues to be read as irreconcilable with wider society, then fans' reactions can place constraints upon the political impact of leisure rituals featuring punk performers who have actual disabilities — extending even to films that depict them. While film viewing may not impact the body as forcefully as live music, nor be as tightly linked to the authenticity of lived performance, our bodies still react to onscreen imagery in visceral ways that blur the boundaries between spectator and spectacle (much as the freak show does), especially when enveloped and stimulated by music during concert scenes. By looking at these live concert interactions in three films portraying disabled performers, we can see how audience perceptions of disability inform the narrative consequences for punk musicians with disabilities.

Control

A biographical picture based on the life of Ian Curtis, singer of the English post-punk band Joy Division, *Control* details Curtis's (Sam Riley) burgeoning musical career, his disintegrating marriage after an affair with a Belgian journalist, and his struggles with grand mal epilepsy. Having formed after attending a Sex Pistols concert, we first see his band (then called "Warsaw") performing at a Manchester punk club in 1977. The band nervously plays a simple, undistinguished punk song while the subdued crowd listens. Curtis stands awkwardly with both hands fixed to the microphone stand, barely moving as he sings. Later, during the band's first performance as Joy Division, Curtis begins loosening up onstage, starting to move his lanky arms, while the crowd responds with greater enthusiasm; the band's distinctive sound also emerges by this second concert scene, with brooding bass lines taking the place of lead guitar. Earning a new manager, record deal, and TV appearance following this scene, *Control* thus frames the band's potential success as perhaps more dependent on the singer's onstage performance than any other factor. Indeed, the band's subsequent TV performance is of much longer duration than the relatively brief concert footage previously shown, and Curtis's stage persona is far more frenetic (arms flailing in circles as he dances and stalks the microphone), suggesting that the imagined televisual audience compensates for the absence of a crowd within the TV studio. The film's focus on his stage presence, arguably inspired by punk's generic emphasis on performing a sort of self-made freakery (especially to stand out in a late–1970s musical milieu filled with derivative punk groups), becomes an indicator of the band's capacity to affect audiences.

Curtis's epilepsy first manifests itself as a seizure during the drive back to Manchester after the band's poorly attended London premiere, narratively suggesting a consequence of the sub-par concert. This implies that even if the band's emergent visibility is tied to their increasingly distinctive performances, the singer's emergent epilepsy also foreshadows the threat of failure for the young group. Recommending plenty of sleep and no alcohol, Curtis's doctor prescribes a range of anti-seizure medications, but is not forthcoming about possible side effects until Curtis directly asks. While the doctor seems unconcerned about side effects, Curtis is visibly worried, later staring at the row of medicine bottles above his bathroom sink; evidence suggests that the medication exacerbated his depressive states, contributing to his later suicide (Church, "Welcome"). His diagnosis is particularly ironic, given Curtis's day job as an employment exchange officer for people with disabilities, including a young woman with epilepsy. After she dies during a seizure, Curtis writes the epilepsy-themed song "She's Lost Control," which is performed in the next concert scene. By this point in the band's short career, Curtis's frenzied dancing "had become a distressing parody of his off-stage seizures ... an accurate impression of the involuntary movements he would make. Only the seething and shaking of his head was omitted" (Curtis 74). Yet, audiences did not know about his condition until several years after his death, as his epilepsy was never made public; audiences (mis)perceived his increasingly bleak and introspective lyrics through the more recognizable artistic trope of tortured Romantic outsider, rather than as a reflection of his private disability experience (Waltz and James 371–73).

The film's key concert scene occurs as Curtis's marriage is falling apart but the band's popularity is surging. Performing before a lively and appreciative crowd, a seizure surfaces as Curtis dances between verses, and he collapses into the drum set before being whisked away by several roadies. Evoking the strobe effects that can trigger seizures, the camera rapidly cuts back and forth between a frontal shot of Curtis dancing onstage and a shot looking out at the crowd from behind him, suggesting that his powerful connection with the audience was a factor in exceeding his seizure threshold. Recovering backstage, a mortified Curtis asks if anyone saw the seizure, and is told that everyone did—though the rest of the band seems relatively unconcerned, as his onstage seizures had apparently become an unsurprising occurrence. Curtis seems caught in a paradoxical position between lyrically and physically performing his disability experience in coded ways—by covertly mimicking his seizures as a means of "enfreaking" himself onstage—yet also trying to keep his condition secret, out of fears of stigmatization (Church, "Welcome"). Although cinematically depicted as important to the band's success, the pressure to perform a "freakish" role becomes an investment in subcultural capital, a marker of supposed authenticity recognized by patrons of the live concert.

However, the fact that epilepsy is a largely invisible disability, not marked by the obvious signifiers of bodily difference associated with the traditional freak show, limits the degree to which Curtis's audience understands and empathizes with his liminal position as an actual disabled person beneath the liminoid freak role embodied onstage. For example, Curtis is expected to perform mere days after a failed suicide attempt, but is too distraught to perform the first song and is replaced by the singer of a supporting band. The rowdy crowd immediately turns against the replacement singer, and Curtis briefly appears to wild applause before vanishing again, leading to a violent riot as the audience begins throwing bottles and attacking Joy Division's remaining band members. Sitting amid the rubble of the trashed venue after the show, a self-loathing Curtis blames himself for the violence, confessing that he thinks everyone hates him. The film's titular theme of control extends from Curtis's potential to lose control over his own body onstage to losing control over the audience itself. In the unruly atmosphere of the punk concert, the bodies of performers and fans chaotically intermingle, but because disability has been kept secret from the crowd, they have no empathy for corporeal struggles that are simply seen as all part of the show. The unacknowledged status of Curtis's violent seizures leads from personal threat to collective threat as violence spills across the footlights in both directions, with freakery displacing the potential for wider disability awareness.

While the epilepsy subplot takes center stage in the live performance scenes, Curtis's love affair and marriage troubles form the crux of the offstage scenes, replaying the common rock mythology about musicians' relationships being destroyed by a romance with a fan. When Curtis eventually hangs himself in May 1980, it seems more closely linked to this love triangle than epilepsy, though a last-minute seizure is depicted as if a deciding factor.

While "binding disability and creativity tightly together permits the 'triumph over adversity' narrative" so common to disability-themed biopics, *Control* uses disability as a tragic trope, adopting it as "a mark of authenticity in an industry that finds such evidence in increasingly thin supply" (Waltz and James 374, 375). Curtis's own rite of passage from able-bodied to disabled status may have failed by ending in death, but still fits Willett and Deegan's assertion that death symbolically "solves" disability's liminality (142). His disability may garner more sympathy when posthumously highlighted by the film, since we know more about it than the diegetic audience, but the privileged knowledge offered by film's biographical lens nevertheless reasserts distance between the disabled performer and our own role as participant-viewers of the filmed concert scenes. We may be viscerally and emotionally moved by such scenes, but the film's retrospective lens ultimately positions us as coroners clinically analyzing Curtis's life and work for signs of illness.

Brothers of the Head

Although *Control*'s basis in real events constrains how viewers may respond to its concert scenes, the unstable relationship it depicts between performer and fans serves as a prime point of comparison with the heavily stylized mockumentary, *Brothers of the Head*, which is composed of contemporary interviews and ersatz documentary footage. Set largely in 1975 England, it centers on Tom and Barry Howe (Luke and Harry Treadaway), fictional twins conjoined at the chest, who have been effectively sold to Zak Bedderwick (Howard Attfield), a sleazy music impresario (reminiscent of Sex Pistols manager Malcolm McLaren) trying to assemble a hit punk band. Asserting that he "didn't exploit anyone who didn't want to be exploited," Bedderwick sends the Howes to a secluded manor where the band (dubbed "The Bang Bang") rehearses for long hours as Tom learns guitar and Barry sings. Meanwhile, a documentarian has been hired by Bedderwick to film the proceedings, suggesting that much of the footage we see is inspired by the same capitalistic imperative to frame the twins as abnormal spectacle. Indeed, Bedderwick even indicates his approval of the band's progress by sending them sheet music to "Every Little Moment," a song originally performed in vaudeville shows by real-life conjoined twins Daisy and Violet Hilton.

Unlike Ian Curtis's covert disability representations, the Howes' visible disability lets them perform freakery in highly exoticized ways. As recollected by interviewees, the Bang Bang met a harsh crowd at their first concert (shown mostly in still photos), with patrons initially mocking the frontmen of the unknown band as gay because of how the brothers hold onto each other. In response to this scorn, Barry begins furiously screaming the lyrics like never before, then taunting the crowd by starting to lift his shift to show the band of skin conjoining the brothers. The crowd starts calling for them to show it altogether, and the brothers oblige. This atmosphere raises the question of whether the performance is a defiant act of bodily eminence or simply a throwback to the traditional freak show. We are told, for example, that Barry seemed to be "fighting for his life" while performing, seeking a sense of power and desirability. The next concert footage depicts a much more enthusiastic and even sympathetic crowd of young people, particularly young women (unlike the predominately male audiences in *Control*). After the show, several fans breathlessly address the camera, with several young men remarking that the Howes prove that it "doesn't matter what you look like," since their example makes it seem as if one "can do anything." Of course, these comments assume that such a disability would otherwise disqualify the Howes from doing just "anything," so the twins' visual appearance does indeed matter considerably in the inspirational role they seem to play for subcultural members identifying with the twins' apparent nonconformity.

Female fans are most prominent in the concert scenes, with women coming up to touch the skin conjoining the brothers, and perhaps being rewarded with a kiss. Unlike the supposedly desexualizing liminality of disability itself, the liminoid status of the uniquely distinguished freak plays into the potential for eroticization. As Leslie Fiedler notes, "All Freaks are perceived to one degree or another as erotic," with nondisabled viewers' desire for them "itself felt as freaky" for wanting to transgress corporeal boundaries (137). Songs like "Two-Way Romeo" link eroticism and danger, while others address the issue of blurred bodies and identities with great angst. Meanwhile, in their offstage lives, ethnographer Laura Ashworth (Tania Emery and Diana Kent) has arrived to write an article about "exploitation of the physically impaired," but instead falls in love with Tom. As in *Control*, a female outsider threatens to fragment established relationships — with Laura's presence leading to talk of the twins surgically separating. When the band subsequently starts falling apart and Laura is kicked out of their lives, more men than women are shown at the concerts, recalling the threat of violence from their first gig; indeed, in a reversal of the concert riot in *Control*, Barry throws bottles at the crowd, leading to a violent melee that leaves the twins injured. Unlike Curtis's self-loathing, the Howes have no refuge in masquerading as able-bodied, thus forcing them to project their performative violence back toward the unruly crowd itself.

The final concert scene comes as Bedderwick arranges a showcase to exhibit The Bang Bang to record executives. The Howes contemptuously dedicate a punk rendition of "Every Little Moment" to the impresario, but the executives seem less than pleased, their presence calling into question just how subculturally resistant to dominant capitalist imperatives the prefabricated band's "underground" status really is. As the concert proceeds, the film's editing becomes more violent to match the building intensity of the onstage performance. As a song climaxes with Barry repeatedly screaming the lyrics "Are you you, or are you me?," the twins descend into the crowd, enveloped in a sea of writhing arms and bodies, as if their growing desire to tear apart from one another has been offered to the audience. This moment exemplifies the punk concert's liminoid potential to chaotically blur the boundaries between performers and other participants, but also its potential dangers. Amid the crowd, Barry is struck by Tom's guitar and badly injured; the twins leave the band, are taken back home by their sister, and later found dead from the head trauma.

A film about the grotesque blurring of bodies depicts the embrace of this logic as inevitably fatal — but only for those already marked as irretrievably different. Like the film's own viewers, able-bodied concert attendees may identify as "freaks" in this liminoid ritual that viscerally moves the body beyond distanced contemplation — yet they retain the privilege of reasserting their normative status when the lights come back up. Like *Control*, the film narratively resolves its most fascinating contradictions through a turn toward tragedy. While framed as if documenting a real band, the fact that the Howes are entirely fictional creations helps this film avoid some of the clinical dynamic set up by films based on reality. Yet, the film's impressionistic visual style also exaggerates the apparent abnormalcy of their offstage bodies through fragmentary glimpses of their torsos and various bizarre images that evoke an atmosphere of strangeness throughout. Like Bedderwick, the filmmakers exoticize freakery for commercial gain, or at least for the subcultural capital surrounding the consumption of "hip" and outré art films. As with *Control*, *Brothers of the Head* seems unable to imagine disabled punk musicians whose enfreaked role does not lead to self-destruction — but here, disability's spectacular visibility prevents the band's audience from reading it as anything but freakish, thus losing sight of the humanity beneath the onstage role the Howes have been enjoined to play.

Bad Boy Bubby

Bad Boy Bubby is a comedy/drama about an eponymous thirty-something Australian man (Nicholas Hope) who has been locked in a decrepit apartment for his entire life, suffering sexual and psychological abuse at his mother's hands. Threatening that God will punish him for disobedience and explaining that the outside world is full of toxic gas, Bubby's mother's neglect has left him psychologically impaired, able only to repeat back the phrases that he hears. When Bubby's father, a conman who has been posing as a priest, finds them and attempts to reconcile after many years, Bubby suffocates his parents to death with plastic wrap and cautiously ventures into the world. Just after escaping, he sees a Salvation Army band singing on the street corner, and becomes immediately fascinated by this first encounter with music. After a series of altercations with local townspeople, he is adopted as an "apprentice roadie" by an unsuccessful rock band, but is soon arrested for the murders.

Upon his release from prison, Bubby encounters a church organist who explains that humans are simply assemblages of subatomic particles, and that our duty is to insult God and think him out of existence in order to take full responsibility of our lives while creating our own order and harmony through achievements like music. Bubby takes this philosophy to heart by becoming more responsible, and wearing a clerical collar inspired by his father. After assuming this "grown-up" role, he stumbles across the same rock band in a bar and reunites with them onstage mid-song as a few patrons confusedly applaud. His lyrics during the bridge between verses are a seemingly random collage of angry cat noises and insults or admonitions he has previously heard. Like the Howe brothers, he seems energized by the audience members and the sudden ability to hurl abuses back at them, even if less cognizant of the words' full meaning. Like a blank slate for the frequently obscene phrases he has heard, his lyrics and inarticulate sounds recontextualize language in disruptive and unruly ways, exposing the uglier side of interpersonal discourse while forming assemblages from the chaos of potential linguistic sounds and fragments heard over a lifetime. Bubby is depicted as innocently unaware of social conventions, achieving punk's shock effect by naively reflecting society's prejudices back toward the audience while onstage. Even the few hecklers seem satisfied by the song's end, and Bubby is later invited to join the band's nightly gigs at the bar.

Because of his sensitivity to fellow social outsiders and his lack of learned ableist prejudices (Ellis 98–99), Bubby is invited to live at a hospital for people with cerebral palsy, where he tenderly assists with their daily lives, translates for a disabled woman, and begins a romantic relationship with nurse Angel (Carmel Johnson). His next concert features his vocal reproduction of the patients' nonverbal articulations; while Angel seems shocked by this freakish public performance of disability, it also "demonstrates his total acceptance of [the patients] by mimicking the disabled in his punk routine in exactly the same way he mimics everyone else he has met" (Ellis 99). As if musically resonating with the disorderly expressions caused by Bubby's psychological disability, the band itself moves from blues toward more of a punk sound once Bubby joins and his popularity grows. Outlandish but autobiographical props become part of his stage act — from beating a plush cat with a wooden spoon to wearing a gas mask to holding a blow-up sex doll with cartoonishly large breasts — all signifiers of grotesquely exaggerated features, bodies, and actions.

By the film's final concert scene, the other band members wear full-head masks made of plastic wrap, giving them a monstrous appearance, while fans imitate Bubby by wearing clerical collars and gas masks and chanting along in call-and-response style. Although it is unclear to what extent the adoring audiences understand or empathize with Bubby's disability, the film has come full circle, with able-bodied viewers now mirroring his profane language and unusual stage persona, much as he had earlier mimicked able-bodied people. His wildly celebratory concerts may suggest the non-normative body's grotesque openness, but they do not necessarily lead to the self-destruction depicted in the other films; they remain a carnivalesque form of controlled chaos, not situations where severe physical violence remains a threat to all parties. His performances have become more standardized over time, leading to a sense of mutual acceptance between performers and concert participants who collectively enfreak themselves as a means of playfully subverting the ableist social decorum that the liminal body visibly disrupts (Iocco and Hickey-Moody 132).

Confirming this achieved unity, the final concert scene smoothly transitions to Angel giving birth to their children, and the film ends with Bubby's new family playing in the yard of their small home located amid a polluted industrial zone. This regenerative ending may feature creativity overcoming disability, but it is not an unironic denouement. Like disability's constant capacity to "pollute" normative society or affect any body, this "happy" ending recalls Bubby's earlier suggestion to Angel that if the whole world is becoming fatally polluted, then everyone is fated to the same end, with no God for salvation. Bubby's mother was partly right: the outside world is toxic — but also toxic with ableism that potentially affects everyone who lives long enough to become disabled — and no amount of regeneration can fully escape that current level of toxicity. Like the chaotically intersecting bodies at his concerts, we are all destined to return to a state of openness and becoming as our corporeal matter disintegrates and recombines.

While Bubby's concerts may provide only a temporary, bounded experience of difference, the same can be said of our experience of watching all three films. Because leisure genres like punk music are voluntarily experienced by small segments of society, their political potential may be contained by their appeal to niche interests, much as these three films have primarily found niche audiences. Only one film offers an ambivalent optimism, yet they all point toward productive moments where distinctions collapse between onstage disability representations and the subcultural non-normativity embraced by audience members. However, subcultural imperatives to deviate from mainstream society by assuming a sense of abnormalcy may make it all the more difficult to sustain those "crip moments"— those moments in which the instability of performing able-bodiedness becomes apparent as disability actually appears (McRuer 157). As I have argued elsewhere, if the visceral affect of liminoid audiovisual phenomena like punk or cinema remains celebrated as socially "subversive" without being acknowledged by participant-viewers as blurring the ableist binaries of normal/abnormal or spectator /"freakish" spectacle, then cinematic depictions of punk performance may remain politically limited ("Freakery"). These limits are narratively reflected in the largely pessimistic endings faced by the characters explored above. These endings essentially contain punk's drive toward aural and corporeal grotesquerie within ritual times/spaces in which the freak can retain his/her liminoid eminence while disability's liminality remains unchallenged. If the seemingly unconventional cinematic premise of a disabled punk musician remains constrained to niche audience — whether by denying punk

rock's increasingly mainstream renown or by denying disability's increasing social prevalence — then we should not be surprised when such premises are resolved through politically
narrow forms of narrative.

Works Cited

Adams, Rachel. *Sideshow U.S.A.: Freaks and the American Cultural Imagination.* Chicago: University of
    Chicago Press, 2001. Print.
Bad Boy Bubby. Dir. Rolf de Heer. Perf. Nicholas Hope, Claire Benito and Ralph Cotterill. Bubby Pro-
    ductions and Fandango, 1993. Film.
Bakhtin, Mikhail. *Rabelais and His World.* Trans. Hélène Iswolsky. Bloomington: Indiana University Press,
    1984. Print.
Brothers of the Head. Dir. Keith Fulton and Louis Pepe. Perf. Luke Treadaway, Harry Treadaway and
    Howard Attfield. IFC Films, 2005.
Brottman, Mikita. *High Theory/Low Culture.* New York: Palgrave Macmillan, 2005. Print.
Chemers, Michael M. *Staging Stigma: A Critical Examination of the American Freak Show.* New York: Pal-
    grave Macmillan, 2008. Print.
Church, David. "Freakery, Cult Films, and the Problem of Ambivalence." *Journal of Film and Video* 63.1
    (2011): 3–17. Print.
_____. "'Welcome to the Atrocity Exhibition': Ian Curtis, Rock Death, and Disability." *Disability Studies
    Quarterly* 26.4 (2006). Web. 8 Apr. 2011.
Control. Dir. Anton Corbijn. Perf. Sam Riley and Samantha Morton. The Weinstein Company and Becker
    Group, 2007. Film.
Curtis, Deborah. *Touching from a Distance: Ian Curtis and Joy Division.* London: Faber and Faber, 1995.
    Print.
Ellis, Katie. *Disabling Diversity: The Social Construction of Disability in 1990s Australian National Cinema.*
    Saarbrücken: VDM Verlag Dr. Müller, 2008. Print.
Fiedler, Leslie. *Freaks: Myths and Images of the Secret Self.* New York: Simon & Schuster, 1978. Print.
Garland-Thomson, Rosemarie. *Extraordinary Bodies: Figuring Physical Disability in American Culture and
    Literature.* New York: Columbia University Press, 1997. Print.
Iocco, Melissa, and Anna Hickey-Moody. "'Christ Kid, You're a Weirdo': The Aural Construction of Sub-
    jectivity in *Bad Boy Bubby.*" *Reel Tracks: Australian Feature Film Music and Cultural Identities.* Ed.
    Rebecca Coyle. Eastleigh: John Libbey, 2005. 122–36. Print.
McKay, George. "'Crippled with Nerves': Popular Music and Polio, with Particular Reference to Ian Dury."
    Popular Music 28.3 (2009): 341–65. Print.
McRuer, Robert. *Crip Theory: Cultural Signs of Queerness and Disability.* New York: New York University
    Press, 2006. Print.
Murphy, Robert F., Jessica Scheer, Yolanda Murphy, and Richard Mack. "Physical Disability and Social
    Liminality: A Study in the Rituals of Adversity." *Social Science and Medicine* 26.2 (1988): 235–42. Print.
Thornton, Sarah. *Club Cultures: Music, Media, and Subcultural Capital.* Middletown, CT: Wesleyan Uni-
    versity Press, 1996. Print.
Turner, Victor. "Liminal to Liminoid, in Play, Flow, and Ritual: An Essay in Comparative Symbology."
    Rice University Studies 60.3 (1974): 53–92. Print.
Waltz, Mitzi, and Martin James. "The (Re)marketing of Disability in Pop: Ian Curtis and Joy Division."
    Popular Music 28.3 (2009): 367–80. Print.
Willett, Jeffrey, and Mary Jo Deegan. "Liminality and Disability: Rites of Passage and Community in
    Hypermodern Society." *Disability Studies Quarterly* 21.3 (2001): 137–52. Web. 3 Apr. 2011.

Acquired Community

Leigh Bowery and *Hail the New Puritan*'s Mise-en-Scène of AIDS

HEATHER WARREN-CROW

Wearing a silver wig and an overblown, double-breasted blazer, Leigh Bowery cuts a drunken path through the city (likely, London). He stumbles — a pratfall — rescues his briefcase, and resumes walking, this time alongside a gentleman who briefly, amicably, puts his arm around him (likely, a member of the band The Fall). Later, we see Bowery talking on the phone in what is presumably an office. He sits next to a secretary with a typewriter. There's something of Lucille Ball's daffiness in him. Perhaps it's his overly lined grin, defined brow, wide laugh. I can't decide whether the silliness of the image is at odds with or exaggerated by the reddish dots that appear to have spread from his yellow shirt and jacket to his face, or vice versa.[1]

Four dancers alternate between pugilistic arm movements and balletic turns on a stage set completely covered in red spots. Three of the four wear yellow blouses with star appliqués, men's briefs, knee socks, and short curled wigs, all decorated with the same polka dots. A fourth sports a sheer peignoir stolen from a soft-core slumber party. Michael Clark, the choreographer of the piece, prances across the dotted floor swinging a bag of bread. He throws handfuls of bread at the camera, giving us a good look at the dotted make-up he shares with two of his peers. Eventually, the raucous soundtrack, a song by The Fall, *ends suddenly. All four dancers adopt defiant poses for the camera.*

These two accounts — the first, my description of English post-punk band The Fall's 1986 music video for their cover of "Mr. Pharmacist," and the second, my summary of a key scene from the film *Hail the New Puritan* (dir. Charles Atlas), which aired on television a year later — are linked by the presence of Leigh Bowery's (1961–1994) iconic costumes. The London-based designer, musician, and dancer had an extraordinary career that moved between different modalities of media and performance, influencing the work of a wide range of creative practitioners, from Alexander McQueen to Boy George. Aptly described by Gary Glitter as a "walking art form," Bowery danced from the club to the stage, the art gallery to the TV studio, Tokyo Fashion Week to New York's *Wigstock* drag festival, the pages of the British fashion rag *i-D* to the canvases of Lucian Freud (Leigh). He exhibited the same collection — blouses and ass-revealing tights worn by models high on mushrooms and poppers — at London's Institute of Contemporary Art and Manchester's Hacienda nightclub. He won a Bessie award for designing costumes for Michael Clark's dance piece *No Fire Escape in Hell*, was the face of a line of greeting cards, and appeared alongside Tilda Swinton in his friend Cerith Wyn Evans's video *Degrees of Blindness* (1988).

Bowery is best known for designing garments that dramatically reshape the body of the wearer through elaborate padding and for using textiles with exaggerated patterns, such as polka dots. Although these spotted looks are not as beautiful as some of his more outrageous creations, they are certainly his most dynamic. Indeed, they are as mobile as their creator. They have appeared in high and low art, films and live performances, ballet choreography and nightclub improvisations; they were passed from the designer to his friends in the Michael Clark Dance Company, his roommates, and lovers, and from flesh to fabric to wall to floor (and back again). They were worn by Bowery in a photograph published in the December 1987/January 1988 issue of *i-D* and another on a Get Well Soon sympathy card, in several images taken later by photographer Fergus Greer, and in Bowery's celebrated solo performance-installation at the Anthony D'Offay gallery in London. The dots' circulation through time, space, and media continued even after his death. British recording artist Boy George (who wore some of Bowery's fashions in the 1980s) worked the spotted look when playing the designer in the 2002 musical *Taboo*, a loving portrait of London's queer nightlife in George's heyday. More recently, design team De Angelis and Garner produced an appropriately garish, grotesque, and strangely beautiful homage to Bowery: wallpaper printed with an ellipsoidal dot pattern composed of stylized illustrations of Bowery's face.

A transmedia celebrity, Bowery danced in clubs and designed extraordinary outfits for himself and other British queers from his arrival in London from Australia in 1980 until his death in 1994 from complications related to AIDS. His colorful tenure coincided with one of the most turbulent and tragic eras in the history of public health in the U.K. 1981 saw the first case history of so-called "Gay Compromise Syndrome" published in the British press. Also briefly known as "Community-Acquired Immune Deficiency Syndrome" (CAIDS), Community-Acquired Immune Dysfunction (CAID), "Acquired Community Immune Deficiency Syndrome" (ACIDS), "Gay Related Immune Deficiency" (GRID), and, more colloquially, "the Gay Plague" and "Gay Cancer," what was later identified as AIDS was initially understood as a lifestyle disease brought on by "immune overload."[2] As Virginia Berridge summarizes, "This [theory] proposed that the high incidence of sexually transmitted disease among gay men, the regular use of antibiotics to deal with them, might in fact lead the immune system to wear out." In addition, late hours, promiscuous sexual behavior, and recreational drugs such as poppers — all associated with dance clubs and queer nightlife — were believed to compromise the immune system irrevocably (Berridge 28–9).

The remedicalization of homosexuality initiated by the appearance of HIV/AIDS continued well beyond the discovery of the virus in 1983–1984 and the recognition of infection through heterosexual contact. As late as 1988, *The* [London] *Times* reported that "some doctors favour compulsory screening, making homosexual acts criminal offences, and identity cards for people carrying the virus," despite, as the article notes, the rejection of such measures by the World Health Organization and the U.K. government (Prentice). The title of a 1985 medical briefing in *The Times* invokes a telling metaphor for the spread of the virus among and beyond various so-called risk groups. "Is the deadly net spreading wider?" the article asks, linking the metaphor of the net to the image of the GRID in readers' imaginations ("Medical Briefing"). As Gay Cancer revealed itself to be neither Gay nor, ultimately, Cancer — in other words, as it became less gay and more queer, less GRID and more AIDS — it also became more threatening to heteronormativity and compulsory able-bodiedness. Not only gay communities, but also the notion of community, itself, were under assault by a disease whose reach was growing faster than attempts to contain it within easily identifiable corporeal milieux. The more AIDS it became, the more GRID heteronormative institutions wanted it to be.

I propose that Leigh Bowery's polka dots performed an aesthetic of community acquisition as a counterforce to attempts within this broader cultural context to fracture and dissolve queer networks. Worn by queers in certain music, dance, and art scenes of 1980s and '90s London, his traveling, transmedia polka dots literalized the metaphor of the "deadly net" of contactual relations amongst acquired communities. Not only did Bowery's dotty looks stage the hypervisibility of the gay male body by aestheticizing facial spots suggestive of Kaposi's sarcoma (a cancer associated with AIDS and, alongside dramatic weight loss, the most visible marker of the illness in the early 1980s), but even more significantly, his designs emphasized the dissident mobility of queers in the age of (C)AIDS.

While a few commentators on Bowery's work have made passing reference to splotches as visual signs of illness, there has been no substantial analysis of his oeuvre in relation to HIV/(C)AIDS and concomitant anxieties concerning queer communities. In part, this is because there is little scholarly work on Bowery. The vast majority of writing on the designer is hagiographic and/or anecdotal, focusing on his flamboyant biography as retold by collaborators and friends.[3] While these accounts are essential to understanding the immediate material circumstances of his practice, they don't adequately address the broader socio-cultural conditions of queer London and beyond. By definition, all patterns — such as polka dots or grids — concretize associations between a single unit and a group; in other words, a dot pattern is only legible as such if an individual dot can be put in relation to a collective of like dots, and a grid can only be a grid if the meeting of orthogonal lines is repeated across scale. Likewise, the sophisticated ways in which Bowery's spot patterns were created, transformed, and deployed invite us to connect the dots, to draw transverse lines of analysis between the one and the many, between Bowery's designs and the widespread pathologisation of queer sociality and mobility in the 1980s and '90s.

Hail the New Puritan's pairing of choreography and costume makes the film a key locus of enquiry within Bowery's network of design relations. A cheeky hybrid of screen-dance, documentary, and fiction filmmaking, *Hail the New Puritan* follows "a fake twenty-four hours" in the life of the very real young Scottish choreographer and dance celebrity Michael Clark (played by himself). It was co-produced by Channel 4 in the U.K. and the New Television Workshop in the U.S., and takes its title from the lyrics of a song by The Fall, a Clark and Bowery favorite. Its depiction of youthful exuberance, effrontery, and boredom create an image of Clark as the wayward prince of the British ballet world and of Bowery as its subversive court jester. Despite its stylish levity, however, *Hail the New Puritan* is not just a portrait of London's arty scenesters. It is also a visual argument for the power of communities of desire, despite the continuing influence of CAIDS. The film's mise-en-scène, and Bowery's oeuvre more broadly, embodies the patterns of visibility, invisibility, mobility, and restriction that affected people living with HIV and AIDS—and people assumed to be dying from GRID or ACIDS—in the 1980s.

———————

Hail the New Puritan begins with what we later discover is a dream sequence. Several dancers rehearse a piece, while another arranges domestic furniture, assembling parts of the set. Leigh Bowery and his friends Sue Tilley and Trojan (née Guy Barnes) sit at the back of the stage in front of a television. They are uninterested in whatever is on TV, as they spend their time chatting, drinking booze, and periodically ambling through the dancers' trajectory to reach a table of food. A performer with lederhosen painted on his naked body plays patty cake with an imaginary partner, and Clark, wearing a white tutu and T-shirt with breasts printed on it, kisses dancer Gaby Agis (who we later learn is his roommate). At one point, Bowery deep throats a banana. He twice removes things from his mouth (gum? gristle?) and places them on the table. Finally, he regards a bowl of stripped turkey bones, complains that there's nothing left to eat, and opens his mouth to consume the camera. The considerable negative space between his lips is replaced by an image of television static, a pattern of white and black spots crawling over and around each other like hyperactive electronic ants seen from far away.

When Bowery moves closer to the lens, we get a better look at his attire: blond wig, ill-fitting coat, red-dotted cravat, blue face, corpse-like. Emphasizing his already pillowy cheeks is a reddish splotch of makeup with a faux swollen center. Later in the film, we see similar lesions on dancers. One wears a loose-fitting pink coat with a low neck that frames the sores applied to his face and décolletage (Bowery wears this same coat near the end of the film). Another accessorizes his monkish robe with a sash and a large sore on his cheek. In time, Clark and his dance partner enter the scene with purplish blotches and vigorous, Rockette-style high kicks. Bowery describes his spotted makeup as "a cross between polka dots and skin rash ... simulating disease" (Tilley 103).[4]

At no point in *Hail the New Puritan* are AIDS, HIV, or Gay Compromise Syndrome mentioned. Nobody is identified as a person living with HIV or AIDS. Perhaps nobody in the film was at the time of its production. Perhaps not. What matters is not the HIV status of the participants—including Bowery, who kept his own a private matter—but broader issues of disability, visibility, and movement that affected their communities-at-large. Bowery's spotted designs, while indelibly associated with his extraordinary persona, present these dynamics as *extrapersonalized*. The very excessiveness, artificiality, and promiscuity of his looks destabilize the mechanism that seeks to contain queer sexuality by attaching a specific body to a compromised lifestyle, a deficient immune system, or an imminent death. Moreover, the dancing in *Hail the New Puritan* accentuates the dynamism of the dot pattern through its semantic instability. Clark's choreography—sometimes coolly formal, considering his idiosyncratic take on both ballet and traditional Scottish dancing—gestures towards CAIDS without making it completely legible. In other words, when *Hail the New Puritan* gestures, it doesn't point a rigid index finger in imitation of the State; it points a very flexible toe. Bowery and Clark make a scene out of CAIDS without putting it literally *in* the scene.

"Scene" is an interesting word, and certainly apt in relation to Bowery and his cohort of artists, musicians, designers, dancers, club kids, and other hipsters. In a general sense, "scene" means "place" or "milieu." This can be material (such as a stage for performance, the scenery on that stage, a curtain or a screen), fictional (where a play or novel is set), textual (a play or section of a play), or social (a community with shared interests). A scene can be an action (an event, disturbance, or freak-out) or an image (a vista), a thing or an activity, something to be made, seen, read, rehearsed, walked on, checked out, or admired. In French, "scène," as part of the term "mise-en-scène," refers to what is put in front of a camera — that is, the costumes, sets and props, lighting, performers, acting, and choreography. The mise-en-scène of *Hail the New Puritan* includes Clark's choreography (taken, in part, from his live stage production *New Puritans*), Bowery's costume designs (assless pants, platform shoes, floppy military jackets, various frilly things, and, of course, spots and faux sores), the dotted stage floor and walls, the streets of London (overcast, somewhat depressing), and the underground club scene, bristling with seedy, creative energy.

Most viewers of *Hail the New Puritan* in the 1980s were all too aware of the scene of (C)AIDS. Initial published reports of the "gay plague" came to the U.K. from the United States in 1981. As Virginia Berridge explains in her study *AIDS in the UK*, the first British case history identifies the patient as a gay man who holidayed in Miami (14–15). As late as 1985, *The Times* is still portraying HIV/AIDS as "the American Nightmare" (Thompson). The following year, *The Times* states that "599 AIDS cases have been reported in Britain, 296 of whom have died. Compared with the United States, this is still a fleabite, albeit a deadly one" (Jones). Despite the prevailing view of the epidemic as a threat located elsewhere (the U.S., Haiti, parts of Africa, etc.), London's Terrence Higgins Trust was established in 1982 to promote awareness of GRID within the U.K. medical community and the public-at-large, notably through events at pubs and clubs (Terrence Higgins Trust). Keith Alcorn, founder of the British LGBT activist group OutRage, argues for the role of discos in mobilizing queer collective action in the 1990s (although, equally applicable to the time of *Hail the New Puritan*): "Dance clubs ... provide a sense of community which is quite different from the political community. These are communities of the body rather than the imagination, and they probably provide more powerful collective experiences (for young gay men) than anything else in our society." These "communities of the night," as Alcorn also calls them, "encompass the genuine diversity which political activists seek to represent" (qtd. in Watney 71).

Bowery was not an activist, but he was a central figure in communities of the body and communities of the night. He founded the short-lived but infamous club Taboo, known for a highly selective door policy that ensured creatively dressed clientele.[5] Bowery and his friends Trojan and designer David Walls were given the reverential moniker "The Three Kings" (Smith 70). Although Bowery regularly styled his friends (and occasionally sold clothes at boutiques in London and abroad), the designer, himself, was the most fantastically attired of them all. He managed to dance all night in dangerously tall platform shoes, full body stockings, restrictive corsets that remodeled his flesh into alternate forms, taped genitalia preventing him from urinating or otherwise handling his penis, a thick layer of makeup and wax, and hoods limiting his vision and leaving him soaked in sweat.

Many of his outfits embody an insolent aesthetic of prophylactics, wryly commenting on desires to protect the self or others from contamination, while, quite literally, impeding skin-to-skin contact with himself and other club kids. These prophylactic looks evoke certain aspects of (C)AIDS's mise-en-scène — namely, the plastic bags, gloves, hoods, and other protective gear that were featured costumes and props in contemporary media coverage. In 1985, a British journalist remarks that his dentist now wears masks and gloves, what the author calls "'Star Trek' garb"—something very familiar to us today, but clearly foreign at the time. He also notes, with a certain snide humor, that "punch — and even cocaine bowls — are ignored in favour of the now commonplace waiter wearing disposable plastic-lined white gloves, pouring drinks from a-just-seen-to-be-opened bottle of wine, spirits or soda" (Thompson). The same year, a British prisoner was put in isolation because of a swelling on his body, assumed (but not proven) to be related to AIDS. Attending police officers in court wore masks and hoods in his presence (Berridge 61).

Such bodily containers are designed not only to reassure the wearer of an able-bodied near future, but also to evince a catastrophic recent past. As Virginia Berridge recounts an anecdote from a virologist who studied HIV: "I had a prick with a needle from a syringe, and reported it to the safety officer. I didn't expect it to be broadcast ... I went to the bar to a lunchtime leaving party. One staff member said, 'Oh, he has AIDS, put him in a plastic bag'" (Berridge 61–2). This statement has two meanings: the plastic bag is protective Star Trek garb as well as a body bag for corpses. By the same token, the idea of "Gay cancer" combined temporalities, eliciting both terror of the future and a feeling that the queer body is always already gone. As Robert McRuer reminds us, glossing John Nguyet Erni, there is a powerful cultural belief that people living with HIV/AIDS and people with other disabilities "are in some ways better off dead or already dead" (20). The plastic bag materializes "the two ruling structures of fantasies of AIDS in our culture" (in 1994 and, I would argue, even today)—"the fantasy structure of morbidity" and "the fantasy structure of containment" (36).

Bowery invoked the desire for protective plastic coverings and the fear of body bags through several performances that flaunted his bodily fluids, including vomit, saliva, shit, urine, blood, or materials that mimicked them. One of these acts directly addressed AIDS. Performing at an AIDS benefit, he flagrantly posed the threat of queer contamination by facing his ass to the audience and discharging a mixture of feces and enema water. Even more shocking is his answer to the question of how he wishes to be remembered after his death. In the same interview in which he expresses his "greatest regret" as "unsafe sex with more than 1,000 men" and says that his preferred way to die is "by firing squad at the Theatre Royal, Drury Lane," he insists that he wants to be known "for injecting a syringe full of warm HIV blood into Princess Diana on one [of] her visits to an AIDS ward" (Greenstreet 10). However offensive and misdirected, this statement is best understood as a critique of the government's inadequate response to the HIV epidemic. More to our discussion, Bowery imagines an act of terrorism drawing focus to the inextricability, in heteronormative discourse, of AIDS, imminent death, and proximity to queer bodies.

Bowery created many garments that materialize the fantasy structures of morbidity and containment through fabric sheaths combining full-body stockings and elaborate hoods. The simplest, most direct of these (if not the most visually appealing) is a puke green, mascot-style outfit that looks like a condom designed by Dr. Seuss. Playfully commenting on the homophobic epidemiology of the queer body, Bowery prevents any contact with his flesh, while turning his entire body into a mascot of a penis. He is, in a sense, giving his homophobic viewers what they want — a completely contained queer body — and what they fear — a big, grotesque, swollen gay dick. Indeed, there appears to be a growth on the shaft that is either Bowery's belly pushing against the velvet or extra padding around his torso. Even worse, this giant velvet penis has outstretched arms and grasping fingers. It's here, it's queer, and it wants YOU.

Another of Bowery's velvet creations adopts a more serious approach to this aesthetic of prophylactics: a luxurious brown sheath that constricts his body and swirls glamorously around his feet. His head and décolletage are covered in a white hood. Holes reveal clownish red lips and orbits blackened with makeup. His gaze is transverse, distant. Surrounding his open mouth is the painted-on frown of an unhappy clown. The hood's entry points produce a different kind of body than the one we see in the last look, which completely encloses Bowery's form in an unassailable velvet membrane. Now, his lips are visible, open, accessible. He has the willing expression of a sex doll.[6]

Despite this dramatic performance of self-immobilization, Bowery's open mouth emphasizes the threat that queer bodies were (and still are) believed to pose. Even the most isolated and restricted body contains within it the possibility for queer connections, the power to create patterns linking the individual and the group. While Bowery's mouth in this look is directed towards future possibility, the splotches on *Hail the New Puritan*'s dancers, sets, and costumes show us what happens when that potential energy becomes kinetic — when the promise of an open mouth is transformed into a sure sign of queer contact between people and between flesh and matter.

———

According to "Maculate Conceptions," Steven Connor's brief but brilliant history of Western attitudes towards dotted textiles and blotchy skin, spots have long been associated with the unhygienic, the impure, the ill and dying, and the sexually promiscuous. "Desdemona's strawberry-spotted handkerchief which leads to such disaster in *Othello*," he reminds us, "joins together the associations of disease, deception, lust and corruption"— evoking the bloody tissue as an index of tuberculosis and the bloody undergarments that indicate early miscarriage (or, I would add, menstruation, another kind of defilement) (1). In medieval Europe, splotches were considered to be evidence of various fevers and were featured in visual representations of the leprous beggar, shielding his or her red dotted face with a large brimmed hat. Later, dots became fashionable: women and some men used black fabric circles (and sometimes other shapes) to cover up facial pimples, scars, and sores. The association between dots and disease continued, however, as they were used to mask signs of illness, especially among prostitutes. The French called these beauty marks *mouches* or *moucherons*, equating glamour (or at least, vanity) with flies that swarm trash and rotting flesh.

The *Book of Leviticus* has a number of injunctions against spotted fabric and various unholy comminglings (Connor 2). *Leviticus* 19:19 gathers several crimes under one umbrella: don't crossbreed cattle, sow fields with different kinds of seed, or wear clothes made of two kinds of material. *Leviticus* 13 moves back and forth between leprous fabric and leprous skin, as if they were one and the same, while *Leviticus* 14 details the appropriate response to leprosy — whether it affects clothing, houses, or people is of no matter. Despite its practical purpose, the marking of quarantined houses with paint may be a holdover from the Levitican belief in the leprosy of architecture.

In the worlds of contemporary Western fashion and the domestic arts, the most high-profile dot pattern is the polka dot. This pattern was named after the 19th century craze for the polka, a rollicking Eastern European dance that lent its name to a large number of now forgotten products attempting to capitalize on its popularity (Connor 15). *Godey's Lady's Book*, a popular 19th century American women's magazine, identifies 1880 as a particularly dotty year:

Some readers may recall that while we were pursuing queer gods in the way of Eastern ideals and fabrics, the same period also gave rise to the dot fad. GODEY'S says in 1880 there were large dots, little dots, polka dots, Japanese dots, French dots, printed dots, brocaded dots, light dots, dark dots; dotted dresses, dotted mantles, plain fabrics trimmed with dotted ditto, and dotted fabrics trimmed with plain ones; dots of every style and of every size; dots forever ["Modes and Manners of Seventy Years"].

Nineteenth century polka dots, though faddish, were considered somewhat elegant; by the mid–20th century, however, polka dots were firmly established as childish and homey, appropriate for nurseries and innocent women. Minnie Mouse's and Lucille Ball's polka dotted dresses, the Itsy Bitsy Teeny Weenie Yellow Polka Dot Bikini, and the long-running comic book character Little Dot (whose only distinguishing characteristic is her love of wearing, drawing, and seeing spots) evince childlike joie de vivre, baby-talk sexuality, and hygienic, synthetic femininity. Syphilitic ladies of the night these are not. For Connor, "The polka dot represents the most conspicuous triumph of the spot over cultural mistrust — or rather, perhaps, the triumph of mistrust over the spot ... the polka-dot defends against the indeterminacy lurking in the spot by its perfect circularity and the clear differentiation it makes against foreground and background" (14). Whether polka dots remain forever classy or girly, they attempt to suppress their own prehistory as the splotchy scars of chickenpox, the leprous wall or face, and the patches used to cover the signs of venereal disease.

Outside the domains of fashion and design, the most well known use of dots is arguably by Roy Lichtenstein, whose signature Ben-Day dot patterns join the supposed childishness of the comic book to surface-level feminine affect and the artificiality of mechanical reproduction. Instead of presenting dots as a revelation of what insidious impurities lie beneath the skin (illness, deception, sexual appetite), Lichtenstein promises us nothing but surface. With the artist's ceramic busts from the 1960s, each head has exactly the same shape, but appears to have different features through changes in the surface application of color and dots. These spots tell us that surface is what matters. Surface creates form. There is nothing to reveal.

From *Leviticus* to Lichtenstein: this is the historical scene in which Bowery's pattern can be recognized. His polka dots, when painted on his and others' skin, partially cover the original coloration of their faces and chests. Like the hooded looks described in the previous section, these designs play with concealing the queer body and masking the face as a site of identification. At the same time, they pretend to reveal what is otherwise hidden, invoking the longstanding relationship between spots and the hermeneutics of disease and sexual defilement. While turning to the Hebrew *Book of Leviticus* may seem like a departure from late–20th century visual culture, it demonstrates the ability of Bowery's work to prompt viewers to see patterns across bodies, sets, and scenes of history. The power of the pattern helps us make connections between orders of magnitude and put individuals in relation to larger and larger collectivities. Bowery's patterns show a keen awareness of not only contemporary issues affecting queer club kids, but also the collective historical significance of textiles and silhouettes. The dotted looks — from the true polka dots to the faux sores — return to the now sanitized dot its maculate history. Surface and depth are joined.

Indeed, Bowery's spots ask us to think about the domesticity of polka dots (their association with childhood and non-threatening femininity) alongside their history of revealing otherwise hidden sexual promiscuity. After all, the home — the ultimate incubator of able-bodiedness — is the place where most queer fashion designers learn to sew or knit. The closet holds their first attempts at needlework, conceals their sexuality, and for some, their HIV status. One of the perceived threats of promiscuity is the defiling of the home, bringing the traces of others into the family unit or preventing oneself from settling down, from deserving a (heteronormative) home in the first place. Co-present with fears of contaminating the family home are desires to keep the disabled and/or queer body hidden inside. In 1985, residents of Queens, New York objected to the city's plan to relocate 10 AIDS patients to a local nursing home; one protestor made the following rallying cry: "'They will be ambulatory!' ... 'They will be walking our streets!'" (Rimer). I am reminded of the designer's dotty, stumbling walk through urban space in The Fall's music video. Bowery's work combines the protected domestic surface ("interior" design that's really one Mobius plane folded in on itself), the impossible depths of the closet designed to prevent queers from becoming streetwalkers, and the freedom/exposure of public space.[7]

History tells us that the dot is exceptionally good at multiplying — in other words, the dot wants to become pattern. The red splotches that indicate leprosy in medieval visual culture easily spread from houses to skin to clothing to the pages of illustrated manuscripts. The little black flies on the face of a glamorous but supposedly immoral woman threaten to swarm the face of an impressionable virgin. Even the silliest dots have the power to generate more of the same. Many of the storylines featuring comic book character Little Dot portray her love of her namesake mark through her obsessive creation of more dots. Always wearing spotted clothing, she is often shown holding a brush and painting dots on others, both animate and inanimate — a doghouse, a cat, a snowman, the shoes of a hippie sleeping on a bench, and a light bulb, which projects colored dots onto the floor and walls. Other times, she has more inventive ways of producing dots: she gives her dog a bath, sending perfectly round soap bubbles into the air; uses stilts to make holes in deep snow; leaves a ring of colorful spots around the tub after a bath; and snips the ends off of three-dimensional music notes, using the cherry-like spheres to decorate a cake. The August 1965 cover of *Little Dot's Uncles and Aunts* is particularly appropriate to our discussion. Dot is inside a spacecraft that's a dead ringer for the Mercury or Gemini capsules, but covered in clownish red dots. She peers out into deep space filled with shapes that mimic the spots on her dress and hair bow: circular meteorites, a pink planet and dotted yellow moon, and that round rock in space called Earth. Throughout forty-five years of Dot comics, Little Dot emerges as an artist who both creates and sees patterns of spots across scale, from the circles that appear on her heart in an X-ray to planetary spheres. More accurately, Little Dot seems to be the medium through which dots can multiply themselves.

As ridiculous as Little Dot comics are, they demonstrate something essential about Bowery's prints (which may appear equally ridiculous to some viewers): spots gain significance through accumulation and multiplication, the gathering of dots to make a pattern and patterns to make a series. They are, like General Idea's infamous project *Imagevirus* (1987–94), what Gregg Bordowitz calls an "accretion." Bordowitz bases his reading of *Imagevirus* on repetition and seriality in the poetry of Gertrude Stein: "She forces the reader to look at the accretion of word upon word, sentence upon sentence, sentiment upon sentiment. All these accretions always sum up into one as a matter of regularity and regulation — one body of literature. Imagevirus is an accretion like that" (91–2). General Idea's *Imagevirus* has certain affinities with Bowery's work in both form and content. It mobilizes a critique of the pathologisation of queer bodies by animating a pattern across media, mediums, and materials.

General Idea's project began with one painting of the letters A-I-D-S arranged in a square, a deliberate quotation and metamorphosis of Robert Indiana's LOVE graphic from 1966 (which itself morphed into a steel sculpture in 1970 and then multiplied into numerous objects exhibited around the world). Between the first instantiation of *Imagevirus* and the AIDS-related deaths of Jorge Zontal and Feliz Partz (two of the three members of the collective) in 1994, General Idea produced wallpaper, paintings, lottery tickets, stamps, an image for the Times Square electronic billboard, a ring, T-shirts, scarves, sculptures, a fabric piece, a video, a cover of the official journal for the Ontario Dental Association, and numerous posters pasted on subways, streetcars, and the walls of buildings in North America and Europe — all with their A-I-D-S graphic. *Imagevirus* performs the process of accretion by which letters become words, words become images, images become patterns, and patterns go global. General Idea first transformed L-O-V-E into A-I-D-S at a time in which the acronym was fresh, as we know, and previous monikers had been scientifically discredited but not culturally forgotten. The significance of creating a traveling pattern out of letters is lost without an acknowledgment of the names that ghost AIDS (ACIDS, GRID, etc.), the importance of shifting the illness from Gay Related and Acquired Community to simply Acquired, and the fear of queer, mobile love (or at least, sex).

Imagevirus angered some AIDS activists at the time for what they thought was a flippant or at least grossly ineffectual attempt to intervene in the crisis. As a call to arms, the collective Gran Fury responded with the painting RIOT (1988), a transformation of the letters A-I-D-S into another four-letter word, evidence of their radically different political methodology. However, more recently, the politics of *Imagevirus* have been re-evaluated by Bordowitz and others. The power of accretion, the role of humor and irony, the productive ambiguity of the project (Is this an advertisement, public service image, or art project on the outside of my tram?), and General Idea's commitment to collaboration have been reclaimed as political gestures. Additionally, I would add, the artists' insertion of *Imagevirus* into the public transportation systems of various cities draws attention to the widespread fear of AIDS's mobility while marking the choreographic patterns of insistently mobile urban queers. I am reminded of Vito Russo's impassioned commentary on the complex politics of queer mobility:

> A friend of mine in New York City has a half-fare transit card, which means that you get on buses and subways for half price. And the other day, when he showed his card to the token attendant, the attendant asked what his disability was and he said, "I have AIDS." And the attendant said, "No you don't, if you had AIDS, you'd be home dying" [Queer Rhetoric Project].

The term "gay plague," with its concomitant mental images of dead bodies and quarantined houses, served to neutralize panic surrounding something even more destabilizing to normativity — the fact that most people living with AIDS were and are neither dying nor stuck at home. They are riding subways and cable cars. They are dancing.

Imagevirus, unlike Bowery's work, is about nothing but AIDS. In other words, the spread of *Imagevirus*'s logo is explicitly about AIDS in ways that Bowery's dot patterns are not. The latter's designs respond more broadly to the pathologisation of queer bodies as well as the fear of their communities and mobility — of which AIDS, ACIDS, CAIDS, etc. were pivotal but not exclusive contributing factors. Despite the differences between these bodies of work, both speak to the ability of pattern to gather and hold together a "we" in the face of powers that seek to individuate. After all, the three-person General Idea brought their working methods into the content of their art through pieces exploring the political and aesthetic potential of the ménage-a-trois. Bowery, Clark, and their friends had a messier, more fluid but nonetheless viable collective of artists, musicians, and designers working with and alongside the Michael Clark Dance Company. Additionally, like *Imagevirus*, Bowery's dots move from apparent triviality to broad significance through the accretion of dots into patterns and patterns into intermedial configurations.

The traveling AIDS logo maps where General Idea had been (Manhattan, San Francisco, Hamburg, Ontario, etc.) or appeared to have been. Whether or not the group really did fly to the sites of their street art and gallery shows, *Imagevirus*, like graffiti, says "I" was here — or rather, "we" were. Likewise, Bowery's dots inscribe a trajectory of movement between and among bodies and objects, art forms and sites. They hold a fragile "we" together, just barely, in a simple but provocative way: we wear his clothes.

While *Imagevirus* is largely about the movement of the AIDS pattern through public space, the geography of Bowery's dotted designs brings the home into intimate relation with dance clubs, stages, and the street. Indeed, a pivotal scene near the end of the film is set within the actual apartment shared by Bowery and Trojan. Their performance of getting dressed within the home is just as important as any performance within the club, and by some accounts, even more so. The designer and his roommate/former lover try on elaborate outfits (created by Bowery, of course), stare questioningly at themselves in the mirror, and drink, while Bowery critiques the looks that parade in and out of the living room and Trojan mopes around the apartment. The two men and their good friend Rachel Auburn, who spends much of the scene volleying insults from her relaxed perch on a chair against the wall (incidentally, covered in the most extraordinary Star Trek-patterned wallpaper), are *Three's Company* on acid — or rather, straight vodka and downers. While their love for each other is unmistakable, they are not a family forged through hugs and compliments.[8]

The support of alternative modes of domesticity is central to the missions of both LGBT and disability activism. While Bowery wasn't an activist, he did make a lifestyle out of such alternative modes. On a Friday the 13th in 1994, he married his friend, collaborator, and assistant Nicola Bateman. She took his last name and performed in the band Minty, alongside Bowery, Richard Torry, and Matthew Glamorre. Her most significant contribution to the group is the now infamous act in which Bowery conceals her underneath his dress, sings and dances with her hidden inside his costume (no mean feat for either of them), and then gives birth to her. In a version of this performance filmed for the documentary concert film *Wigstock: The Movie* (1995, dir. Barry Shils), Bowery wears a mask mimicking facial prostheses, a dress combining garish flowers and a white grid pattern that loses its right angles as it stretches across his exaggerated girth, contrasting plaid sleeves, and white pantyhose. Late in the show, he lies down on a table with his knees up and his crotch facing the audience. Bateman pushes herself headfirst through the pantyhose, ripping them open, and emerges, naked, bald, "covered with red body paint and KY Jelly and wrapped with a string of sausages" (qtd. in Tilley 204). She appears disoriented. "Oh my God, Wigstock's first baby!" Bowery cries out in his campy way, and suddenly tears the faux umbilical cord with his teeth.

This performance and others undoubtedly provoked — and continue to provoke — anxieties pertaining to the difficulty of containing the queer body, and by extension, the "gay plague." Bowery's queerness spread out in all directions and media. He identified as a man but often dressed as a woman, married a woman, slept with men and, infrequently, women. In doing so, Bowery literally embodied the most dangerous threat to hetero/able-bodied sexuality and the normative home: the HIV-positive, multiply partnered bisexual man married to a straight woman. While the marriage and his HIV status were not widely known, his high-profile performance of birthing a bloody woman from underneath a grotesque yet mumsy housedress — as well as the strangely eroticized display of biting an umbilical cord and later feeding his new baby — invoked contemporary fears of mothers passing HIV to fetuses and babies as well as the horror of queer fluids on display without shame. Moreover, this performance mocked the heteronormative rhetoric of "and baby makes three" while insisting on the palpable, material connection between a queer transvestite and his wife.

Ultimately, Bowery and his longtime collaborators, lovers, and friends modeled a form of belonging that both countered and responded to Margaret Thatcher's regime of privatization in the 1980s. Thatcher, who took office two years before the first article about Gay Compromise Syndrome appeared in the British press, was quoted in a 1987 issue of *Women's Own* magazine as saying:

> I think we have gone through a period when too many children and people have been given to understand "I have a problem, it is the Government's job to cope with it!" or "I have a problem, I will go and get a grant to cope with it!" "I am homeless, the Government must house me!" and so they are casting their problems on society and who is society? There is no such thing! There are individual men and women and there are families and no government can do anything except through people and people look to *themselves first* [Keay].

Her limitation of collectivity to the procrustean bed of the biological family unit confirms compulsory able-bodiedness by rejecting the interdependence of subjects and institutions outside of the (heteronormative) home. At the same time, the State's inadequate response to HIV/AIDS required activists and people living with HIV to "look to themselves" and other queers for help, motivating communities of the night to provide "housing" for vulnerable bodies.

The connection made in *Hail the New Puritan* between Bowery's fashions, communities of the night, and the spaces that house them solidifies in a series of key scenes at the end of the film. Let us return now to Bowery and Trojan — drinking, laughing, whining, and getting ready in their apartment. As they prepare for the club, Michael Clark arrives. He immediately frets about his outfit, which is nothing compared to Bowery's maxi dress with an extra pair of vestigial sleeves or his frilly pink backless coat. We recognize this latter garment from one of the previous dance scenes, although the designer pairs it with ruffled panties instead of men's briefs and omits the raised sores. Bowery is also dissatisfied with his look ("Is it today?" he asks rhetorically) and returns in a short blonde wig, heavily padded black overcoat, and red dotted face, hands, and cravat. Clark, who needs to leave to meet his lover, makes a move to kiss Bowery goodbye. "Will I catch anything?" he asks, choosing not to make contact with Bowery's splotchy face.

The tense moment between the men does more than perpetuate the bitchy attitude of the group; it draws attention to the kissing that has gone on throughout the scene and continues into the next. Indeed, the potential energy of Clark's almost-kiss becomes kinetic, carrying him into and through subsequent spaces. Before exiting Bowery and Trojan's apartment, he kisses Rachel; then, he has sex with his male lover (filmed in Bowery's real-life mirrored bedroom); and finally, he goes to a nightclub, kissing his many friends and huffing a popper as he negotiates the crowded, humid space of the disco. He licks the ear of woman who pushes him away. He kisses a gloriously attired transvestite, getting her lipstick on his lips, and then erotically sips from a friend's straw. He is always in motion — spinning, licking, spanking, and of course, kissing. Clark is not only flaunting the swapping of spit and other bodily fluids believed to pose such a threat at a time in which "everyday social moments like a kiss on the cheek become taboo," punch bowls are ignored, and dentists start wearing Star Trek garb (Thompson). His animated dance of contactual relations carries him from men to women and back again: it is the "deadly net spreading wider" in choreographic form. In other words, Clark's circuitous path through the nightclub mocks the panic evoked when GRID became AIDS and gay becomes queer.

Finally, Clark leads the other clubbers, including Bowery, in a simple dance. Everybody does the same moves at the same time in choreographed solidarity. Their synchronicity is politically complex. The dancers' gesture-based movement, which begins with overhead clapping, includes a peace hand sign that flips around into a sign for vagina, a move that is best described as the sexy teapot, a beckoning gesture followed by fingers rubbing against the thumb to indicate "give me money," and a "Heil Hitler" arm with the other hand flat under the nose to suggest Hitler's moustache. This part of the dance is accompanied by loud, synchronized marching. The routine ends with a solo in which Clark glides into the men's restroom (presumably to do drugs or have another sexual encounter).

The invocation of fascism in club culture is especially shocking considering Clark's Aryan features and the Third Reich's policies on homosexuality, disability, and, of course, Jewishness. This component of the dance can be read as another example of Clark, Bowery, and his friends' embrace of the taboo and offensive. Bowery did exactly that with many of his creations. After paying a textile factory to produce the fabric worn in the "Mr. Pharmacist" video — a homey yellow gingham marred by red spots — he had another version made with swastikas printed on the same base fabric, juxtaposing the horror of fascism with cloying domesticity, childishness, and, by extension, queer icon Judy Garland, who wore a gingham pinafore throughout *The Wizard of Oz* ("There's no place like home," she repeats). We can compare this aspect of Clark's and Bowery's work to Genesis Breyer P-Orridge's Eva Adolf Braun Hitler persona and, according to Michael Bracewell, the theories of George Bataille, whose ideas on transgression influenced London-based artists of the early 1980s (Bracewell).[9] Alternatively, or perhaps additionally, we can read the dance within Clark's choreography, more generally, as its exploring of the tensions between the individual subject and the group. Catherine Wood describes Clark's aesthetic as "haunted by the ranked ghosts of fascist militarism ... and injected with the energy of music video and the period's flamboyant androgyny" (399). In the case of the club dance in *Hail the New Puritan*, synchrony is both empowering and, briefly, frightening. The dance performs the togetherness of this community of the body, and yet also warns us of another kind of togetherness — the solidarity of fascist body culture.

Most importantly, the rehearsed choreography, unlike looser and more realistic club dancing, is performed for the camera — in other words, not for them, the performers, but for us, the viewers. This dance is not about queers insisting on having a good time despite their pathologisation by medical discourse; it is about queers self-consciously performing the process of an individual becoming a pattern. The spread of Clark's movement throughout an acquired community, the sharing of bodily fluids among men and women on the dance floor, the kinetic energy of one dot generating another and then another — these all materialize the power of the pattern both to threaten and enable. Patterns can pathologize a community or make queer connections across scale and difference; they can be lines of Fascist goosesteppers or a trio of red-spotted dancers with pointed toes, periodically collapsing to the dotted floor (in the scene from *Hail the New Puritan* that I described at the beginning of this article). In other words, a pattern can be a GRID or polka dots.

Bowery and the Michael Clark Company were part of an acquired community. They were held together, just barely, by love of transgression, fear of fascistic control over the subject, faith in the transformative power of fashion and sex, and commitment to movement as political articulation. *Hail the New Puritan* makes a scene of their so-called "deadly net" of queer relationality. The clubbing sequence, in particular, reminds us that this community was sustained by shared looks (both glances and costumes) and intimate contact. The mobility of Bowery's spots throughout and across this film performs Community Acquisition in order to destabilize the lingering patterns of GRID and CAIDS discourse.

Conclusion: *After the Ellipses*

The number of websites, blogs, and YouTube channels with documentation of Leigh Bowery's looks is impressive. Images of his patterns, especially his dots, continue to accrete long after his death. They circulate among fans, friends, musicians, and designers. Whether fashionistas or fiber artists, Bowery's cultish followers usually emphasize his radical commitment to individual expression. There is nobody like Bowery. At the same time, they demonstrate the generativity of his look by dressing up like him, doing their make-up like him, playing him in the musical *Taboo*, or making garments deemed "so Leigh Bowery."

One of the most unusual tributes to the designer/performer is the video *Leigh Bowery* (2006), from The Disabled Avant-Garde (artists Aaron Williamson and Katherine Araniello). It features the artists watching documentation of Bowery's performance at the Anthony D'Offay gallery in 1988. Araniello, in a wheelchair, wears garish club gear. The left cheek of her mask is painted with an outline of lips, reminiscent of Bowery and Trojan's Picasso-inspired makeup. Her right cheek has black spots. Williamson has a jaundiced appearance, with a huge phallic nose, pink wig, cheap tiara, and red facial blotches. Periodically, the artists imitate Bowery's movements (which, despite his oversized persona, are quite subtle in this performance). They also dance and make grunting noises. The camera moves nervously between medium shots of the duo from behind to close-ups of their accessories and Araniello's wheelchair. Images of the artists are superimposed atop swirling backgrounds (e.g., psychedelic handcuffs, close-ups of threadbare pink fur, layered collages incorporating their faces). The greenscreening occasionally makes a pattern out of the artists' self-consciously tatty attire multiplied throughout the frame (The Disabled Avant-Garde).

This video makes a clear, queer connection between two contemporary performance artists who identify as disability activists and Bowery, the designer/artist who claimed not to identify. The camera's skittish close-ups invite viewers to compare cosmetic accessories, such as masks and plastic tiaras, with the life-sustaining plastic and rubber attachments to Araniello's wheelchair. While these aren't the same, of course, the figure of Bowery gloriously preening on the television in the background suggests that there is more to the comparison than we might think. Bowery designed mobile, plastic assemblages of skin, metal, fur, foam, rubber, make-up, and other people. He transformed one of history's most iconic stigmas — which means, etymologically, puncture marks on the skin — into a dot, the dot into a pattern, and then placed this pattern into dynamic configurations of flesh and other designed materials. By aestheticizing and re-materializing the stigma, Bowery questioned its nature. Indeed, his work persists in reminding us that the marks affecting both queers and people with disabilities are not stable and natural but mobile and cultural — in this case, trashy, magnificent, (low) culture. His marks are open mouths, ready to make queer connections with dicks, dildos, and other objects.

As Bowery explains in the *Sunday Times* magazine, "My body is capable of innumerable shapes and forms. The idea of transforming oneself gives courage and vigour" (qtd. in Tilley 112). The polymorphous perversity of Bowery's intimacy with matter and media continues to enable strangely beautiful ways to challenge the so-called natural body. Through artists like Araniello and Williamson, Bowery can keep on dancing with others across the bounds of time and space. By dancing and dressing with Bowery, as it were, Araniello and Williamson mark alternative choreographies of metal and makeup, fabric and plastic, and always already maculate flesh.

Notes

1. Although the background of the print looks to be light yellow in the video, it is most likely yellow and white gingham. Sue Tilley, Bowery's biographer and good friend, remembers that Bowery had a factory on Brick Lane print burgundy dots on this traditional textile (102).
2. A May 11, 1982, *New York Times* article reporting on the rare cancers and infections seen "among some heterosexual women and bisexual and heterosexual men" nonetheless bears the headline "New Homosexual Disorder Worries Health Officials" (Altman).
3. Another reason for the paucity of scholarly writing on Bowery is the fact that fashion studies has only recently been taken seriously by the academy, while costumes are all too often neglected by film studies and dance studies.
4. According to Tilley, "One of his most popular looks [in 1985] was a short pleated skirt with a glittery, denim, Chanel-style jacket teamed with scab make-up and a cheap, plastic, souvenir policeman's hat" (57).
5. As Sue Tilley recalls, Taboo's door policy was "Dress as though your life depends on it, or don't bother" (53).
6. This look and the one previously described were documented by photographer Fergus Greer as part of a series of photographs taken between 1988 and 1994.
7. Explicitly connecting fashion and interior design, Bowery had a job making garments out of curtains for a woman who ran a clothing store (Tilley 97–8).
8. Bowery later became the godfather of Auburn's son, Jack (Tilley 87).
9. Bracewell explains that a revival of interest in Bataille's theories in early 1980s London culminated in the festival *Violence Silence*, a series of events dealing with ritual and evil as understood through very basic interpretations of Bataille's writings.

Works Cited

Altman, Lawrence K. "New Homosexual Disorder Worries Health Officials." *The New York Times.* 11 May 1982. Web. 1 Nov. 2011.
Atlas, Charles, as told to David Velasco. "Charles Atlas Reflects on Michael Clark." *Artforum.* Sept. 2008. Web. 1 Nov. 2011.
Berridge, Virginia. *AIDS in the UK: The Making of Policy, 1981–1994.* Oxford: Oxford University Press, 1996. Print.
Bordowitz, Gregg. *Imagevirus.* London: Afterall Books, 2010. Print.
Bracewell, Michael. "Leigh Bowery's Immaculate Conception." *Frieze* 19 (Nov.–Dec. 1994). Web. 1 Nov. 2011.
Connor, Steven. "Maculate Conceptions." *Stevenconnor.* Web. 1 Nov. 2011.
The Disabled Avant-Garde. "Leigh Bowery." *YouTube.* 16 Mar. 2008. Web. 1 Nov. 2011.
Erni, John Nguyet. *Unstable Frontiers: Technomedicine and the Cultural Politics of "Curing" AIDS.* Minneapolis: University of Minnesota Press, 1994. Print.

Greenstreet, Rosanna. Interview with Leigh Bowery. *Leigh Bowery*. Ed. Robert Violette. London: Violette Editions, 1998. 9–10. Print.

Hail the New Puritan. Dir. Charles Atlas. Electronic Arts Intermix, 1985–6. Film.

Jones, Michael. "Preaching to the Infected: James Anderton on AIDS." *The Times* (London). 14 Dec. 1986. Web. 1 Nov. 2011.

Little Dot's Uncles and Aunts 1.14 (Aug. 1965).

Keay, Douglas. "AIDS, Education, and the year 2000!" Interview with Margaret Thatcher. *Women's Own*. Margaret Thatcher Foundation. 31 Oct. 1987. Web. 1 Nov. 2011.

"Leigh Bowery Interview Gary Glitter." *YouTube*. 17 Mar. 2011. Web. 1 Nov. 2011.

McRuer, Robert. *Crip Theory: Cultural Signs of Queerness and Disability*. New York: New York University Press, 2006. Print.

"Medical Briefing: Is the deadly net spreading wider? / Social groups vulnerable for AIDS." *The Times* (London). 2 Aug. 1985. Web. 1 Nov. 2011.

"Modes and Manners of Seventy Years." *Godey's Lady's Book*. Mar. 1897. *American Periodicals*. ProQuest. Web. 1 Nov. 2011.

Russo, Vito. "Why We Fight." *Queer Rhetoric Project: An Archive of Gay and Lesbian Political Speech*. 21 May 2010. Web. 1 Nov. 2011.

Prentice, Thomson. "GPs 'ignorant and prejudiced about AIDS.'" *The Times* (London). 19 Feb. 1988. Web. 1 Nov. 2011.

Rimer, Sara. "Fear of AIDS Grows Among Heterosexuals." *New York Times*. 30 Aug. 1985: A1. Web. 1 Nov. 2011.

Smith, Raven, ed. *Club Kids: From Speakeasies to Boombox and Beyond*. London: Black Dog, 2008. Print.

Terrence Higgins Trust. "Our History." Web. 1 Nov. 2011.

Thompson, Douglas. "AIDS: The American nightmare / Killer virus breeds US paranoia." *The Times* (London). 12 Aug. 1985. Web. 1 Nov. 2011.

Tilley, Sue. *Leigh Bowery: The Life and Times of an Icon*. London: Hodder and Stoughton, 1997. Print.

Watney, Simon. *Imagine Hope: AIDS and Gay Identity*. London: Routledge, 2000. Print.

Wood, Catherine, et al. "Because We Must: The Art of Michael Clark." *Artforum*. Sept. 2008: 396–411. Print.

Razzle-Dazzle Heartbreak

Disability Promotion and Glorious Abjection in Guy Maddin's *The Saddest Music in the World*[1]

Nicole Markotić

We don't know if he's in a coma or just very, very sad.
—Contest Announcer, *The Saddest Music in the World*

What is it about sadness that is so very, very funny? Director Guy Maddin purportedly explores this question in his "big production"[2] film, *The Saddest Music in the World*. In this essay, I shall examine the contrast Maddin establishes between the commercial exploitation of human suffering and the unruly joy of the fragmented and disabled body, which capitalism stages and displays. More than simply titular sadness, his film develops and exploits notions of grief, melodrama, and the commodification and marketing of emotions as ways of exploring how these characters enact agency and embody representations of a persuasive market ideology. Maddin's characters display a striking variety of disabilities, at times feeding a contemporary audience's desire for post–Freudian, psycho-biographical explanations for behavior, often decontextualized from a larger socio-cultural rhetoric. Within a familiar narrative of the capitalist exploitation of emotion for profit, *The Saddest Music in the World* singularly depicts disabled characters as protagonists who exhibit their disabilities on their own terms, while paradoxically acknowledging that one cannot stage disability without at the same time enabling its excess. Ultimately, I argue, Maddin's film articulates a new positioning for disability in contemporary film and mass culture: commodified and packaged in a film that both invokes and mocks deliberately convoluted and layered disability tropes.

Identity and Disability in Maddin's World

Celebrated Canadian director Guy Maddin occupies a strange position — both marginalized and central — in the Canadian film scene. He has a tendency to engage obsolete (for lack of an accurate word to define an artistic strategy that invokes dated technology at the same time as it revels in contemporary tools to manipulate and break apart that technology) cinematic styles that give him new (old) ways to represent and contest main-stream narrative investments in the normative body. David Church writes that Maddin "layers his low-budget tableaux with the grain and grime of decades long gone" (2). And Mark Peranson says of Maddin's films that they are "culturally toxic, and the past that he presents is one that we'd never want to live in" (11). Other critics write about his films as being in "a dream world which operates by dream logic" (Diehl 4), that they "wallow in feelings of yearning and humiliation" while all being "extremely funny" (Steven Shaviro in Church, 70), that the "most hackneyed of plot-twists are made to creak with the weight of divine purpose" (Will Straw in Church, 61), that they visualize the postmodern, with a sense of "bargain basement artifice" (Geoff Pevere in Church, 49), and that they exist in a "perpetual state of crisis and hysteria" (William Beard in Church, 81).

Part musical, part melodrama, part cinematic tribute to early sound-era films, *The Saddest Music in the World* relies on hand-held cameras, black-and-white shots, two-strip color shots, 1930s cameras and film,[3] and a soundtrack reliant on the 1932 hit, "This Song Is You" to convey a retro sense of time. Maddin creates this retro past not simply by embracing nostalgia for the pre–World War II film era; rather, he employs nostalgic effects in his film in order to project, and then critique the commodification of time and place and the aesthetics of its affect. Rewriting (with George Toles) Kazuo Ishigaro's original screenplay that was set in 1980s London, Maddin sets *The Saddest Music in the World* in the Canadian prairie town Winnipeg in 1933 during the Great Depression. Indeed, the film's account of Depression-era Winnipeg (the "world's capital of sorrow") both romanticizes and fablizes that city, reveling in its small-town friendliness, extremely frigid temperatures, excessive amounts of snow, and hockey-focused culture. By presenting Winnipeg as a "centre" of cultural capital (even if that capital is negatively defined), *The Saddest Music* brings together a motley collection of characters, related, intertwined or co-dependent in order to define and express their multifaceted bodies. As he introduces a critique of national zeal (the film revolves around a music contest between competing nations), artistic objectives, and the complicated layers of promotion and endorsement in a heartbreak-fascinated culture, Maddin turns to filmic nostalgia to demonstrate how codified notions of bodily exhibition, place, and time structure any performance of sadness or joy. Here, in particular, Maddin locates disability in the context of the logic of capitalism. The film ultimately insists that — paradoxically — one cannot stage disability without placing the disabled body itself on stage with all its potential to exceed or undermine the culturally designated, carefully controlled and commodified meanings assigned to it.

The *Saddest Music* offers the premise that beer-baroness Lady Helen Port-Huntley (Isabella Rossellini) finances a song contest to determine the saddest music in the world, open to all countries with a prize purse of 25,000 "depression dollars."[4] A contest, then, invented to heal national war wounds while perpetuating emotional gratification through extreme national identity. The Eurovision-style contest encourages first the commodification and staging of individually or collectively expressed suffering, then its promotion as an ideal of national unity, all within a carnivalesque box-office aesthetic. The competition will exhibit and commemorate the music of anguish, which the film aligns with disability through the performative spectacle of sorrow, as embodied through various characters, not the least Lady Helen herself who is a double amputee. Maddin's film ostensibly depicts the greed-driven side of the Great Depression as Lady Helen profiteers by organizing her international radio music contest. As host of the contest, Lady Helen anticipates a legal alcohol market that will soon emerge once the U.S. Congress calls an end to prohibition: "If you're sad, and like beer, I'm your lady," she mugs to a (not-yet-invented television) camera. Her interest in music, then, stems only from a business angle: she wants listeners around the world, but especially south of the Canadian border, to think of her product when they wish to indulge in (or need) a drink.

In Maddin's plot, Chester Kent (Mark McKinney), prodigal down-on-his-luck son and neglectful brother, returns to Winnipeg from New York, where he makes his living as a musicals producer. As the Canadian son who embraces a United States his father detests, Chester proclaims himself "American Ambassador of Sadness" and determines to win the prize money, even if he has to spend all of it buying singers, dancers, writers, performers, and "ethnic" extras[5] to join in his excessively extravagant musical production. Alternatively, he plans to take up with Lady Helen, his former lover, and thus "win" the contest money on behalf of the United States through back-door influence. Fyodor (David Fox), father to Chester and also a former lover to Lady Helen, wishes to do his country proud by representing Canada in the song contest, and to reinsert himself as Lady Helen's lover by building her an aesthetically perfect prosthetic. Meanwhile Roderick (Ross McMillan), brother to Chester and son to Fyodor, returns to Winnipeg from Europe after his young son dies and his wife Narcissa[6] (Maria de Medeiros) disappears in a wide-eyed haze of grief-induced amnesia.

Roderick arrives as Gavrillo the Great, entering the radio competition on behalf of Serbia. (These divisive nation-claims within one family gesture towards the multiple cultural backgrounds most Canadians embody, but also make clear the impossibility in North America of binding the diverse and varied body onto one uncontested nation-based identity.) Roderick's skin is so sensitive that he feels pain if someone touches him, and he wears a baroque hat and veil ensemble to protect him from light. In a Maddin-style coincidence, Roderick discovers that his brother Chester's current lover is his own long-lost Narcissa. In its playful mix of disabilities and national stereotypes, the film self-consciously caters to various stock images of Canada as underplayed but proud, the United States as exaggerated and exploitative, and the troubled relations each has with other countries and their national music. Announcers claim various entries as "a cavalcade of misery" and "a frightening contest of human despair," and after each musical round (the end signaled by a hockey match buzzer) the crowd cheers, drinks wildly, and the round winners (at times joyously and at times with trepidation) slide into a jacuzzi-sized vat filled with Port-Huntley beer.

Lady Helen presents her contest of sorrow as a prize opportunity to focus attention away from the Depression. And who better, according to her own assessment of her recent past, to judge misery? Years previously, Lady Helen had one leg amputated by mistake and the other amputated because of injury incurred as a result of a car accident involving two of her rival lovers: father and son characters Fyodor and Chester Kent. In a flashback scene, Lady Helen rides illicitly with Chester in his car. When Fyodor steps onto the road to stop them, Chester's vision is obscured by Lady Helen, who leans over him to perform oral sex. They crash and one of her legs is pinned under the car. Having been driven to drink by Lady Helen's affair with his son, Fyodor, a doctor, is drunk when he begins an emergency amputation, and he thus saws off the "wrong leg." The "right leg," irreparably crushed, was subsequently amputated as well. Years have passed since the incident, and when Chester reappears in Lady Helen's life, she launches into her tale of woe and loss to incite pity in him, as well as to remind him of the guilt he should carry for her truncated dancing career. All within minutes of the opening credits.

David Mitchell and Sharon Snyder argue that in traditional narratives secondary or tertiary characters act as foils for the protagonists and that when such characters are disabled, they tend to embody the protagonists' (usually tragic) flaws through "disability as a narrative device." Disability thus acts as the "crutch upon which literary narratives lean for their representational power, disruptive potentiality, and analytical insight" (49). Indeed Mitchell and Snyder's teasing out of the central role of disabled characters as "narrative prostheses" has shaped much current disability theory. This function of disability in narrative shapes its representation such that rarely in the history of film are disabled characters represented as happy with their own bodies, let alone as having enviable bodies.[7] Instead, the disabled body is typically a trigger for, among other things, pathos of the kind that Lady Helen expects hers to elicit. Conveying and triggering emotion, especially heartbreak, is such an over-coded film ambition that "hankies" were once a movie marker for how much an audience will appreciate any particular film.[8] Yet Guy Maddin's film troubles this paradigm. *The Saddest Music in the World* portrays disabled characters as happy *and* fraught, full of malaise and yet decidedly upbeat. Maddin's film is one step beyond the traditional filmic usage of disability criticized by Mitchell and Snyder. Not only do *all* the major characters embody an assortment of disabilities, but it is the apparently nondisabled Chester's striking affective deficit — his utter *lack* of ability to experience the kind of melancholy that disability is so often used to generate — that drives the narrative of the film forward.

Staging Pity for the Disabled

When the film audience first views Lady Helen Port-Huntley, she is seated at a boardroom table, apparently nondisabled, commanding a meeting, while wearing a platinum blond wig and glittering tiara. But when Chester arrives to see her, she has arranged to be seated at a grand piano, gigolo at her side. At Chester's refusal to take her angry words seriously, Lady Helen pounds on the piano keys and pushes off the piano bench so that he and the film audience must witness her wheeling over the fur-covered floor. The shot gives us Chester's viewpoint, inviting the viewer to indulge in what Rosemary Garland Thomson critiques as the stare: "Staring offers an occasion to rethink the status quo," Garland Thomson says in her book analyzing the action, passivity, violence, celebration, and acceptability of staring. "Seeing startling stareable people challenges our assumptions by interrupting complacent visual business-as-usual. Who we are can shift into focus by staring at who we think we are not," says Garland Thomson (6): namely, disabled. Rather than present the stereotypical disability trope of the "angelically pure invalid" (20), described by Lois Keith in her groundbreaking book on disability and illness in classic girls' fiction, Maddin gives us a self-aggrandizing and unlikable Lady Helen who does not incite pity in audience members any more than she does in Chester. In doing so Maddin achieves exactly the opposite of a conventional pitying reaction. Lady Helen herself, however, regards the sight of her body as (to again invoke a Garland Thomson title) "extraordinary," a body that will incite particular emotions in particular audiences. She both resents the customary reaction to her body and uses it to her advantage, abjectifying it in order to produce the reactions she demands, specifically that Chester recognize and acknowledge her loss. Placing herself in a physically "lowly" position to invoke pity, Lady Helen wheels out to shock viewers outside the diegesis, who hadn't known until this point that she is an amputee, and to distress Chester within it, who presumably *must* already know this fact about his former lover, but who has yet to respond on camera. Lady Helen wishes him to acknowledge her utter calamity in *not* being that young performer *now*. But Chester, true to form and in contrast to a predictable film viewer's reaction, responds to her mobility with a cheerful "You got a new dolly!" admiring the plank with wheels upon which she seats herself. His jauntiness and delight at seeing her again serve to reject valuing Lady Helen's body as categorically "less" than that it was before her accident (and letting audiences in on the punch-line that he not only knows about her amputation, but already knows her method of ambulation).

In addition to a focus on her mobility, as she either wheels herself in an awkward and graceless manner reminiscent of horror movies' antagonists or she has her gigolo, Teddy, lift and carry her, Lady Helen attempts to further compel Chester to acknowledge and bemoan her loss. She plays the embittered ex-"star" who has had to abandon a promising career prematurely, surrounding her office with black-and-white stills of her dancing on stage, or performing various gymnastic moves. In all the photos, her legs are prominently displayed. Although Lady Helen is now a rich capitalist succeeding in a traditionally male occupation, such success does not much please her. Rather, the loss of her biological legs coincides for her with the loss of her allure; she was once the admired woman of multiple lovers, including competing father and son. These days, her "gams" don't garner her an income, but her capitalist wits do. Such achievement does provide her a measure of grim cheer, but paradoxically also undermines her sense of (feminine) self. Bitterly, as a stock has-been stage-star character made even more bitter by the ostensible disfigurement of disability, Lady Helen makes money as if to avenge her former self. Ultimately, she arranges to "fix" the contest for the United States and split the winnings with Chester, thereby guaranteeing that the country with the saddest citizens is also the country with the largest beer market. That she intends to rig the contest is no surprise, but even the obsequious radio announcers sound flabbergasted when she herself appears onstage for the United States finale: "Isn't it rather odd that Lady Port-Huntley is actually in one of these numbers when she's also the judge?" The second announcer's reply — "Well, Mary, I think she looks spectacular!"— puts the emphasis yet again on Lady Helen's striking, prosthetically enhanced appearance onstage, instead of on her power as critic and arbiter. Already rich and steeped in reactive emotion, her participation in the finale number comes across more as a vicious slight against all other (able-bodied) performers rather than as old-fashioned greed.

Unlike Lady Helen, whose attitudes and affective manipulations parody and exceed the figure of the disabled revenger, Roderick re-enacts his grief to keep it fresh, active and present in his body. As a performance, being distraught perpetuates his loss as fundamental to his being. Gavrillo the Great has, after all, arisen not only from Roderick's body, but also from the corpse of his marriage and, ultimately, from the tragedy of the assassination of Archduke Ferdinand of Austria in 1914 that triggered the Great War. As the actor who plays Roderick notes, although Roderick's "tactic is to theatricalize his own grief," *all* the characters' displays of grief are "comically inadequate" (McMillan). For example, Roderick carries his son's heart in a glass jar, preserved with his own tears. Maddin has made a movie not only about sadness but about the eye-catching, ear-harkening *spectacle* of sadness. The manufactured spectacle of sadness that exploits disability, nationality, ethnicity and gender centers around identity boundaries which are cheaply (and secularly) remedied by the consumption of beer. Just as the film is about to topple into the hot tub of maudlin self-pity, it gestures toward the all-encompassing grief of the loss of a child as a quintessential, sublime sadness. For the most part, this film partakes in a double activity of poking fun at the self and national absorptions of heartache and their manipulative, commercial potential, at the same time as it praises opening oneself to tender emotion.

Ultimately, the *problem* for Lady Helen, evident in the dolly scene at the piano, is that Chester seems socially incapable of pity and does not recognize guilt as an emotion. Indeed, viewers learn that — since the moment of his mother's death when he was a child — Chester has never cried, never admitted to personal sadness. Charlene Diehl says of Chester's perpetual buoyancy: "He is a boy suspended forever in the moment of his mother's death; having refused that moment, he has locked himself into it perpetually" (10). But Chester is more than a perpetual boy emotionally disabled by a biographically induced inability to express sorrow. He is representative of a social "problem," one that enables entrepreneurial success and disables human emotion. Chester's refusal (or inability) to pity is depicted in the film as a lack, rather than the result of the potentially liberatory perspective of refusing to see amputation as loss. Because he does not identify disability as pitiful — one of the most iconic identifications film narratives ask us to make — Chester does not come across as a reliable character with whom the audience can relate. Rather, the social intelligibility of disability as anything but tragic works to convince viewers that just as something is "wrong" with Lady Helen physically, so too there is something "wrong" with Chester emotionally. That he cannot pity her may be emotional ailment on Chester's part, but if, as I am suggesting here, one avoids pathologizing his reaction, then Chester operates as a masculine devotee who refuses to objectify the feminine body; an (ostensibly) able-bodied viewer who refuses to "abjectify" the disabled body.

"Doesn't it make you sad?" Lady Helen demands of Chester. "Well, life's full of surprises," is his chirpy reply. Chester — charlatan, impostor, and opportunist — refuses the expected narrative of pity and awe regarding Helen's "lost" legs. He seems, in fact, unable to cling to any past, whether for his emotions for Helen, for his father, or for his emotionally-distraught brother, Roderick.

Staging Capitalism

Despite being unable to emotionally move Chester by reminding him of her "plight," Lady Helen eagerly listens to his plans for the contest she is to judge. "Here's an angle for you, Helen," he pronounces. "America versus Canada: a brash son comes home to duke it out musically with his war-vet pop. The old man's drowning his sorrow; the son wants no part of this. In order to win the dough, that Yank's gotta find his tear ducts in a hurry." Chester outlines the plot to come, and also analyzes his own situation without pity or sentiment. Helen responds with a ready "You've got something there," demonstrating a world view that would allow, even insist, that she strive to trade her own narrative of misery for capitalist success and fortune. Chester's plan is already working: this story of misery and distress sells tickets, sells a lot of beer, and wins the game. Heartbreak — in its most wretched state — is a marketable commodity, valuable for the listening pleasure it will bring to contest listeners. Says one of the contest announcers: "As far as [the crowd is] concerned, sadness isn't hurt one bit by a little razzle-dazzle showmanship." To Chester, performing sadness requires no emotional weight. Performing sadness for him has the opposite effect that it does for his brother: it's a matter of staginess, rather than authenticity, showmanship rather than experiential sensation.

The film appears to position Chester's inability to feel or to express emotion as a typically repressed masculine character or as a pathology, or both. His uplifting attitude is projected as either unfortunate (were he able to cry, he would be able to properly mourn his mother's death), crass (by exploiting other countries' losses, Chester appropriates and absorbs their talents and skills), or simply dishonest (he is "faking" his cheerful outlook). But Chester also dislodges viewers from the easy emotional reactions and interpretive conclusions familiar to "hankie" films. By *not* wallowing in pity about what are basic life-related corporeal shifts, Maddin offers a Chester who models a viable alternative to a self-indulgent response to misfortune: the more Chester ignores his feelings, the film suggests, the more creative he becomes. Creativity has often been associated with struggle or distress. See, for example, Freud's essay, "Creative Writers and Daydreaming," in which he outlines the artistic impulse as a characteristic of an "unsatisfied" person (146) or Jean Tobin's argument about Freud and the post–Romantic perception of creative artists: "Poets were seen, among other things, to be impoverished, in poor health, alcohol and drug abusing, prone to early death, associated with suicide, mentally and emotionally unstable, unfortunate in love, sexually licentious, often scandalous, politically rebellious, and social outcasts" (19). In contrast, Maddin shapes a more complicated character in Chester Kent. He may not have cried since his mother's sudden death, but he has devoted his life-work to producing music theatre. The show, necessarily, cruelly, goes on.

There is yet another way to look at Chester. In his "Course in Melancholy," which Alan Davies led in the fall of 2011 at the University of Windsor, Davies said that the seventeenth-century English scholar and author of the classic *The Anatomy of Melancholy* Robert Burton "both suffered from melancholy, and flourished creatively in the midst of it" (seminar discussion). Publishing in 1621, Burton designates melancholy as both a passion (of the heart) and a perturbation (of the mind). The cause, for him, could also be artistic endeavor (his writing), and the treatment (for him) was writing; melancholy, then, serves as a pharmakon, simultaneously toxin and cure. Burton vacillates over whether melancholy is "disease or symptom" (148), but distinguishes it from "ordinary passions of *Fear* and *Sorrow*," describing it as an "anguish of the mind" (149). For Burton, melancholy is deeply connected to romantic love as well as to art, and he inventively argues that the force of the imagination greatly contributes to its cause (220). In *The Saddest Music*, Chester's inability to experience sadness is tied not only to the loss of his mother in the past, but also to his inability to fully commit to romantic love in the present. Indeed, Chester cannot release romantic love from its roots in family tenderness; even as he taunts and dismisses his brother's anguish over personal loss, Chester's main love interests in the film remain his brother's wife and his father's sweetheart. So for Chester, coupled love always connects to a triangular and familial rivalry, and thus to a blissful nostalgia he refuses to endorse.

Meanwhile the father, Fyodor, aspires to win back his erstwhile sweetheart Lady Helen and reestablish himself as the benevolent patriarch. Motivated by grief, guilt, and love, he reveals to Roderick a pair of prosthetic legs he has made out of glass and filled with Port-Huntley Muskeg Beer. He aims to replace what he has taken from Lady Helen, and he fashions these glass legs for her because she cannot physically tolerate the wood or plastic models available. Once she tries them on, Lady Helen is ecstatic with her new legs, which she considers aesthetically superior to her original ones, flaunting them and caressing them. The fact that Lady Helen is overjoyed by the beer-filled legs suggests that the nature of her resentment has not been, in fact, the loss of physical limbs, but derives from a loss of a normalcy sustained through a male-defined and commodified image of the desirable female body. Throughout the film, Lady Helen radiates abjection and objectification; for her, the one arouses the other. She takes advantage of them in tandem to enable her to meet emotional and economic needs for profit, attention, desire, and — most of all — control.

Lady Helen's embittered character as the powerful and bitter magnate who presents herself through photography and radio voices all but disappears when she assumes the beer-filled prosthetic legs as her own, reconfiguring her — and the film audience's — notion of subjectivity. She is no longer a woman-without-legs, nor has she become the original "whole" she held on to so fiercely. Through prosthetic remedy, she transforms into Helen, a woman who dances, a woman who admires her body for the relationship she has with it, not for what she wishes it could be, or could offer. To perform in this way, Lady Helen does not need a return to her "lost" body; rather, she rejoices in her consummate, new, sleek, artificial legs. In his autobiography about his near-complete paralysis, *The Diving Bell and the Butterfly*, Jean-Dominique Bauby writes, "Oddly enough, the shock of the wheelchair was helpful" (11), in that his friends could stop pretending about, and relying on, his recovery. Indeed, when Lady Helen first tries on the glass legs, she admires how they glitter (the result of light hitting the beer) and how smooth they are, exclaiming, "I'll never have to shave." Just as Bauby embraced his wheelchair for both the mobility and signage it gave him, so too does Lady Helen embrace her new abilities and aesthetics enabled by these extraordinary legs. Ultimately, Lady Helen is both the embodiment of capitalistic consumption and its casualty: she produces the most sought-after consumer product of prohibition — alcohol. Her prosthetic legs are full of sparkling beer while her biological legs were lost to her own consumption of semen while riding in the second most fetishized consumer product of prohibition — the automobile. But more than a botched operation, what makes Lady Helen the casualty of capitalism is her constant ache for a past embodiment; she makes money, it would seem, out of spite. Yet unlike Chester, Lady Helen accepts the intense emotions that accompany physical change. Her unbridled joy at this newfound vanity contrasts with his ongoing inability to experience passion as anything but emotion-for-sake of promotion.

Conclusion: Staging Disability as Finance Capitalism

The contest finale enacts a predictable showdown between the siblings: Chester and his huge ensemble for America and solo cellist Roderick for Serbia, each brother embracing a country "blamed" for global misery and destruction. Chester is a parody of corporate United States as much as his brother, Roderick, is a parody of nostalgia for a pre-finance-era imperialism. The two brothers fight for the love of the same woman, for the attention of their father, and to win a contest that will justify their emotional choices. They love the same woman, they share the same childhood memories, and they have both chosen substitute nationalities. Chester wishes to prove that sorrow is no more than a useful commodity; Roderick is determined to prove that great sorrow leads to great art. Roderick has always possessed the saddest song — a cello melody he last performed at his son's funeral — but has resolved not to include it in the contest since he wants to play it again only upon reuniting with his wife. Once in Narcissa's physical presence, Roderick is able to launch this captivating tune in a haunting dénouement that demonstrates the power of unmitigated grief, far outweighing Helen's lament over lost limbs. His grief, though, is portrayed with such farcical overtones that it fits Linda Williams' definition of melodrama, as one of three film categories, along with horror and pornography, that relies on a "system of excess" that "stands in contrast to more 'dominant' modes of realistic, goal-oriented narrative" (25).

During the finale, Gavrillo's high cello note — the rarefied sound signifying the very saddest music — shatters Lady Port Huntley's glittering prosthetic legs. This time round, it is the reverberation of an elegiac melody, rather than a speeding consumer product (Chester's car), that functions as the destructive force that denies Lady Helen her legs, and destroys them. Standing on shards of glass, she can no longer negotiate the fluid subjectivity she must display in order to live in the music-beer-tragi-comedy world she herself has created. "You can be fixed," Chester attempts to reassure her, at last demonstrating some portion of the sympathy she has longed for, "Anything that's built can be rebuilt." But Helen is not swayed by his optimism; she stabs him to death with a piece of the glass. Glibly, Chester retorts with: "Well, now you've given me something to laugh about," refusing to grieve at even his own demise. Then both he and Helen do laugh, at the downfall of the contest, at their destructive plottings, and at the carnivalesque absurdity of their tragic love affair.

Roderick fares little better. Though his grief is genuine, it has become a talisman he carries with him everywhere. Such excess cannot sustain itself; like Lady Helen's fetishized legs, the glass jar in which he carries his son's heart has also shattered. Roderick, and what he allegorically represents (the lost generation of World War I, the inciting event of which, in the heart of Europe, was emotional genuineness), loses *because* he comes across as excessively and not sufficiently capitalist, and because he is unable to embrace the rapacious capitalism that demands one's own sorrows and defects be repackaged as cultural commodity. Chester, even though he loses his own life at the end of the film, wins: he's an allegory of United States finance capitalism, which triumphed in the West in the wake of the collapse of the 19th-century monarchies that World War I swept away. Both Lady Helen and Chester Kent embrace capitalism and through the economic appropriation of art have learned to profitably perform and exploit their own emotions.

A parody of melodrama in Linda Williams's terms, *The Saddest Music in the World* ends by bringing private and national affective excesses to the fore. Chester plays the piano as a life-threatening fire rages through the theatre, but not helping anyone escape, not even himself. Roderick and Narcissa leave grasping each other's arms, while Lady Helen disappears in Teddy's arms, whisked off-screen by wealth, not love. Given how many of the film's characters have physical or emotional flaws, the film does not simply position Chester's "problem" as its melodramatic crux nor it does not suggest that his lack of empathy for others constitutes a character arc. By the end of the film, Chester doesn't "learn" to be more empathetic or to put others' needs before his own. There is no emotional "cure" for any of the film's depicted mental disabilities (although the tapeworm that possesses Narcissa does die). Chester's lack of demonstrable sadness underlines his arrogance and pretension. Unwilling to own such a faulty character trait, and unwilling to give it up, he constructs his own *lack* as a *capability.* Despite finally producing a tear as his world combusts around him, Chester remains dedicated to the stage till the end, even as all other characters close to him, contestants, and audience members flee the destructive fire. He dies, stabbed with glass and engulfed in magnificent flames, having completed playing and singing "This Song Is You," and the film ends with his final words as a voice-over: "I ask you, is there anybody here as happy as I am?"

Notes

1. I would like to thank Louis Cabri, Sally Chivers, Eunjung Kim — and especially Marja Mogk — for excellent critical feedback.

2. Although modest for some films, Maddin swoons about this film that it was to be made with: "a $3.5 million budget, a 24-day schedule, and real movie stars" (*The Village Voice*).

3. Maddin filmed *The Saddest Music in the World* entirely with a combination of handheld cameras, including Super 8, Super 16, and with many of his actors receiving camera credit. Maddin also relied on push processing to increase the grain, iris shots to evoke silent-film techniques, and two-strip Technicolor (or "Melancolour," as he terms it). Maddin eschewed using contemporary special effects (for example, when filming Lady Port-Huntley's amputated legs), because he regards such "digital effects as grotesque artifacts of the present" (*The Village Voice*).

4. The film's portrayal of the music contest parodies the Eurovision Song Contest, a long-running annual competition among countries of the European Broadcasting Union, in which each country may submit a single song that will be performed on live television. Commencing in 1956, it is one of the longest-running television shows in the world, and is also one of the most-watched programs in the world, according to Matthew Murray, "viewed by 600 million people in 35 countries" (quoted in Raykoff and Tobin, xvii). The contest commands a series of components, say Raykoff and Tobin, including "fast pace and catchy

rhythms," an "appealing dance routine," and costumes (xviii), all major elements in *The Saddest Music*'s finale number. In contrast to Maddin's film, where Canada loses after only one round, the inaugural 1956 contest was won by Switzerland, the host nation for that year. Even though audience members cannot vote for their own nation's efforts, the inaugural contest evoked the ideals of national allegiance inflamed at a moment when people still grieved war losses and held nation-centered grudges amplified over two world wars.

5. Lee Easton and Kelly Hewson succinctly describe and analyze the casting of the various national musicians: "Maddin cast his national musicians from actual groups who were in Winnipeg performing at the folk music festival. What this means is that the stereotypical quality of the national groups' musical numbers is not as parodic as we might think, and/or the groups think they have to be parodic to distinguish and make a spectacle of themselves" (235). The levels of staging are multiple: Maddin casts "real" folk musicians to satirize a musical contest in which a "director" such as Chester Kent exploits and restages nationality as both central (he constantly highlights music from identifiable ethnic origins) and unimportant (in his finale he has the contest entrants from India performing as Eskimos).

6. Narcissa has no memory of Roderick or of their son, and first appears as Chester's paramour. When she first speaks, it is in response to Fyodor demanding to know if she's an American. Lee and Hewson point out that her reply: "I'm not an American, I'm a nymphomaniac," aligns notions of nation, feminine (excessive) sexuality, and the pathologized body (229–230). In addition to her amnesia, she also claims to follow the counsel of her tapeworm, suggesting she experiences mental, emotion, and physical malaise.

7. One exception in such mass media portrayals is the 2007 ad by SoBe drinks, that shows a young athletic man removing part of his leg and inserting cans of Arush into a prosthetic slot, as if replacing batteries; the product was discontinued as of 2009.

8. In her pivotal article on the role of gendered bodies in genre film, Linda Williams makes note of the "long-standing tradition of women's films measuring their success in terms of one-, two-, or three-handkerchief movies" (27).

Works Cited

Bauby, Jean-Dominique. *The Diving Bell and the Butterfly*. Trans. Jeremy Leggatt. New York: Knopf, 1997. Print.

Burton, Robert. *The Anatomy of Melancholy*. Eds. Floyd Dell and Paul Jordan-Smith. New York: Tudor, 1938. Print.

Church, David. "Introduction." *Playing with Memories: Essays on Guy Maddin*. Ed. David Church. Winnipeg: University of Manitoba Press, 2009: 1–25. Print.

Davies, Alan. "A Course in Melancholy." University of Windsor: 19 Sept. 2011. Seminar discussion.

Diehl, Charlene. "Making a Problem of the Problem Body: Guy Maddin's *The Saddest Music in the World*." Film and the Problem Body Conference. University of Calgary: 28–30 Jan. 2005. Conference paper.

Easton, Lee, and Kelly Hewson. "'I'm not an American, I'm a Nymphomaniac': Perverting the Nation in Guy Maddin's *The Saddest Music in the World*." *Playing with Memories: Essays on Guy Maddin*. Ed. David Church. Winnipeg: University of Manitoba Press, 2009: 224–238. Print.

Freud, Sigmund. "Creative Writers and Daydreaming." *The Standard Edition of the Complete Psychological Works of Sigmund Freud: Introductory lectures on psycho-analysis (Parts I and II)*. Trans. James Strachey and Anna Freud. London: Hogarth, 1962. Print.

Garland Thomson, Rosemarie. *Staring: How We Look*. Oxford: Oxford University Press, 2009. Print.

Keith, Lois. *Take Up Thy Bed and Walk: Death, Disability and Cure in Classic Fiction for Girls*. New York: Routledge, 2001. Print.

Maddin, Guy. *From the Atelier Tovar: Selected Writings*. Toronto: Coach House, 2003. 9–13. Print.

_____. "Sad Songs Say So Much: A Shooting Journal." *The Village Voice*. 6 May 2003. Web. 1 Aug. 2012.

McMillan, Ross. Personal interview in *The Saddest Characters in the World: The Cast of The Saddest Music in the World*. Dir. Caelum Vatnsdal and Matthew Holm. 2003. DVD extra.

Mitchell, David, and Sharon Snyder. *Narrative Prosthesis: Disability and the Dependence of Discourse*. Ann Arbor: University of Michigan Press, 2000. Print.

Raykoff, Ivan and Robert Deam Tobin, eds. *A Song for Europe: Popular Music and Politics in the Eurovision Song Contest*. Hampshire: Ashgate, 2007. Print.

SoBe drinks advertisement. Web. 22 June 2007.

The Saddest Music in the World. Dir. Guy Maddin. Perf. Isabella Rossellini, Mark McKinney, and Maria de Medeiros. IFC, 2003. Film.

Tobin, Jean. *Creativity and the Poetic Mind*. New York: Peter Lang, 2004. Print.

Williams, Linda. "Film Bodies: Gender, Genre, and Excess." *Genre, Gender, Race, and World Cinema*. Ed. Julie Codell. Malden, MA: Blackwell, 2007: 23–37. Print.

Seeing the Apricot

A Disability Perspective on Alzheimer's in Lee Chang-dong's *Poetry*

SALLY CHIVERS

The proportion of the post–65 population is on course to double within the next 25 years in most of the developed world. Media reports describe doctors as swamped by their caseloads despite years of notice that this change would come and ample public alarm about what it would mean for health care systems. Popular media also portrays policy makers as scrambling to create adequate care and living provisions for a population that is expected to redefine independence. Newspapers feature alarmist series about this "silver /aging / gray tsunami," a troubling metaphor (given the devastating effects of actual tsunamis in the early 21st century) mostly meant to evoke waves of dementia patients whose needs will flood already overtaxed medical systems. Lee Sung-Hee, president of the South Korean Alzheimer's Association, puts it this way: "I feel like a tsunami's coming ... sometimes I think I want to run away" (quoted in Belluck A1). Similarly, Philip Longman indicates the scope of this panic in his subtitles for an article in *Foreign Policy*: "A gray tsunami is sweeping the planet — and not just in the places you expect. How did the world get so old so fast?" (52). The idea that the globe will be drowned as the result of demographic changes rests on assumptions that aging only results in declines in health and ability, which threaten to overrun the vitality of younger generations.

Similar to print media, cinema has shown an increasing interest in dementia, particularly in portraying in great detail the experience of Alzheimer's,[1] largely from a caregiver's perspective. In *Forget Memory: Creating Better Lives for People with Dementia*, Anne Davis Basting offers an impressive discussion of films about memory and memory loss. Alongside films about youthful memory loss (examples include *The Vow* [Michael Sucsy, 2012], *Fifty First Dates* [Peter Segal, 2004], the Bourne series [Doug Liman, 2002; Paul Greengrass, 2004, 2007; Tony Gilroy, 2012], *The Majestic* [Frank Darabont, 2001], *Memento* [Christopher Nolan, 2000], *A Moment to Remember* [*Nae meorisokui jiwoogae* John H. Lee, 2004]), there is also an unwieldy and growing collection of films specifically on dementia featuring some middle-aged and some old-aged characters (*Away from Her* [Sarah Polley, 2006], *Iris* [Richard Eyre, 2001], *Son of the Bride* [*El hijo de la novia* Juan José Campanella, 2001], *A*

Song for Martin [*En sång för Martin* Bille August, 2001], *The Savages* [Tamara Jenkins, 2007]). Such dementia films typically reinforce a set of troubling assumptions about an aging process gone wrong: especially that dementia is only a worst-case scenario of growing old, that care is an individual rather than a social concern, and that caregivers are more important than those they care for. They often dwell upon a deep and abiding love that they propose ought to be able to nourish both the care-receiver and the caregiver. But the films also support, in variably subtle and obvious ways, the eventual institutionalization of dementia patients.

Pulitzer Prize–winning film critic Roger Ebert facetiously coined the term "movie Alzheimer's": "the form of the disease where the victim has perfectly timed lucid moments to deliver crucial speeches, and then relapses." Although he was writing about *Friends with Benefits* (Will Gluck, 2011), he could just as well have been referring to *The Notebook* (Nick Cassavetes, 2004) in which Anne Hamilton (Joan Allen) remembers her past romance just long enough to share a brief passionate embrace with her long-time husband. Or even the more sophisticated *Away from Her* in which Fiona Anderson's (Julie Christie) last-minute lucidity confounds her husband Grant's (Gordon Pinsent) attempt at self-sacrifice. Pointing out this feature is not an attempt to argue that movie depictions of Alzheimer's aren't realistic nor that they ought to be. Rather, the ubiquity of the plot device illustrates what purpose Alzheimer's serves in standard cinema narrative. Naming it demonstrates its prevalence as what disability studies scholars David T. Mitchell and Sharon L. Snyder might call narrative prosthesis. That is, the plots rely upon a confused character to demonstrate the seeming wholeness of the apparently lucid characters as well as the potential wholeness of the dementia patient in her moment of lucidity. The startling moments of lucidity add to the grief experienced by the loved ones who surround the dementia patient because they enhance what is portrayed as loss of self.

Typical Alzheimer's plots offer a difficult choice about location of care as the central conflict. The brief moments of lucidity become more poignant when they call into question the caregiver's perspective which has usually been based, until that point of the film, on a vain hope of recovery or a resignation to bereavement. The U.K.-U.S. coproduction *Iris* features writer and philosopher Iris Murdoch's (Judi Dench) dementia as both a betrayal and an extension of her past creative brilliance. However, the focus is on her devoted spouse, John Bayley (Jim Broadbent), who does what he can for her. The Canadian film *Away from Her* presents Fiona Anderson (Julie Christie) grappling with the diagnosis of early-onset Alzheimer's through her resolve to move herself into an institution. But once she makes that move, the focus shifts to the difficulties Grant has accepting the changes it brings. The German film *Song for Martin* portrays an aging composer in the first stages of Alzheimer's, which progresses rapidly. But the main concern becomes that of his new wife and the effect his illness threatens to have on her career. These examples in particular demonstrate that a romanticization of Alzheimer's pervades narrative film and cannot simply be attributed to the reductive tendencies of the Hollywood machine, though there are also multiple Hollywood examples.[2]

Cultural scholarship on dementia focuses on ideas of the self, defying the popular notion that dementia obliterates the self and promising that a new self might be possible within or even because of changes to memory (Eakin; Basting *Forget Memory*). Similarly, North American and U.K. disability studies are preoccupied with identity and with pushing beyond identity as a key critical framework (Asch; Garland-Thomson; Hughes, Russell and Paterson; McRuer; Siebers; Davidson). Both of these approaches offer ways to think about the significance of "movie Alzheimer's" and counter narratives that might appear in its wake. In this essay, I draw on them collectively to look at the ways in which one South Korean film about dementia provokes critical thought about aging, while relying on stale views of disability in order to do so.

Poetry's *Alzheimer's*

In 2010, Lee Chang-dong's *Poetry* (*Shi*) drew accolades and multiple awards from European and Asian film festivals.[3] The film presents a central character with Alzheimer's but differs in almost every way from the contemporaneous habits of presenting dementia as a worst-case late life scenario. *Poetry* offers a dementia counter-narrative in which, as Canadian novelist David Chariandry writes in his novel about a son returning home to his mother (who has dementia), "forgetting can sometimes be the most creative and life-sustaining thing that we can ever hope to accomplish" (32). Neither Chariandry's nor my point is flippant, fantasist or dismissive of the potentially devastating effects of dementia and the many other symptoms alongside memory loss that it can entail. *Poetry* (2010) offers an alternate view of Alzheimer's, one that does not imagine within the story world of the film that institutional care is possible, let alone necessary, and one that does not portray Alzheimer's as a symbol of old age gone wrong. Instead, due to the early stage onset of her illness, the engaging central character Mija (Yun Jeong-hie) gains a moment of blissful forgetfulness accompanied by new skills of commemoration. She gradually coaxes viewers towards a new understanding of both memory and reconciliation.

Unlike so many other films about dementia, in *Poetry* the actress (Yun) playing a character with Alzheimer's (Mija) is the only lead. In this film, the character with dementia has no devoted partner for the film to focus upon and the topic of care for the person with Alzheimer's is never raised; instead, she is portrayed as a caregiver in her professional and personal lives. The film shows her typical day as drudgery filled with care for an impressively ungrateful teenage grandson. In order to demonstrate Mija's transformation in consciousness, *Poetry* presents another disabled character, Mr. Kang (Kim Hira), a gruff miserly stroke survivor for whom she also provides laborious care and who functions to demonstrate her subtle resistance to normative views of her as a foolish "old lady." She navigates this drudgery with an increasing sense of moral purpose, demonstrating a moving poise amidst what might have become a chaotic existence.

Critics praise *Poetry*'s slow pace and its poetic qualities, particularly in contrast to what film critic Manohla Dargis calls "the prosaic qualities of its world, its ordinariness." Most English-language reviews of *Poetry* also praise Yun, a 1960s screen star who returned to work for the role (Woong-ki). Specifically, Kenneth Turan refers to her "surpassing delicacy," and commends her nuanced emotional performance, as do others. Similarly, Dargis describes "a tour de force of emotional complexity that builds through restraint." Bill Goodykoontz attributes much of the success of the film to these skills on the actress's part: "Writer and director Lee Chang-dong's film is moving without ever stooping to melodrama; Yun is the main reason why." She gives Mija, he claims, "an almost heartbreaking dignity." Rob White comments the ways in which this characteristic reflects a difference in *Poetry* from Lee's earlier work: "Whereas [Lee's] previous films are dominated by harrowing psychic and linguistic breakdowns, *Poetry* involves emotional restraint and a profoundly moving emphasis on eloquence" (4). The combination of ordinariness and a subtle emotional appeal offers a representation of Alzheimer's that is neither sensationalist nor sappy. Rather than draw on traditions of horror or melodrama, Chang-dong intriguingly uses a pastoral frame to convey an urban experience of dementia.

Poetry opens and closes with a scenic shot of water flowing near a bridge. As the film's understated horrifying plot lines unfold, viewers come to understand the site to be one of both death and choice. The opening shot tracks from the water to a bucolic shore populated by young boys playing happily with the grass and sand, backed by mountain scenery. The camera follows a curious young boy's gaze back to the water, where it rests close-up on a girl's body, floating face down. Yet, more jarring than the corpse is an abrupt shift to a noisy urban scene, including a busy hospital waiting room where Mija waits to see her doctor. After Mija leaves her medical appointment, she comes across the girl's grieving mother as the distraught woman collapses, prostrate with grief in the hospital parking lot. The sight distracts Mija from the comments her doctor has just made about her memory loss. Neither she nor viewers yet realize the disturbing connections between these two plots — that of her illness and that of the girl's death.

Yun's skill in portraying powerful yet muted emotions is remarkable not only because she effectively expresses the subtleties of Mija's early stages of dementia but mostly because she must convey Mija coming to terms with the trauma of her grandson's participation in the gang rape of a schoolgirl Park Heejin, whose "Christian name" is Agnes, which led to the girl's suicide — the floating corpse from the opening scene. When Mija first witnesses that girl's mother's grief in a hospital parking lot, it shakes her to the extent that she tries to talk about it to almost everyone she passes. But when she subsequently learns that her grandson played a role in the rapes that provoked the suicide, she ceases to bring it up, and Yun conveys her inner turmoil through the delicate emotional expressions praised by the critics. Agnes's mother's grief and her own family's disgrace are never far from Mija's mind, however fragmented Mija's thinking may seem. Her thoughts guide her actions rather than her words, affecting the plot as much if not more than characterization.

Language of Poetry

Most characters disregard or at least dismiss Mija, neither listening nor speaking to her. Her employer's daughter-in-law, a cashier, feigns interest but actually laughs over her head at the next person in line. The medical specialist who diagnoses Mija with Alzheimer's expressly states that she would rather talk to someone else rather than tell Mija herself about her own medical categorization. Mija's surly grandson Wook (Lee David) offers the most obvious example of this disdain. He grunts at her, turns the television louder seemingly to block out even her physical presence, ignores her except to complain about the food she has served him, and speaks to her only in the most perfunctory manner, usually including an abbreviated expression of his resentment towards her. Even his band of trouble-making friends is more respectful; they are silent with her, but offer requisite bows in her general direction. This pervasive disregard cannot, however, be interpreted as a rejection of a dementing senior since Mija keeps her diagnosis secret throughout the film. Rather it shows the social position that Mija finds herself locked into — caring for a teenager who will almost certainly never care for her.

Wook's treatment is especially galling because Mija takes on enormous social shame and financial burden in caring for him. Her worries over paying the electricity bills he racks up by turning on every appliance in her flat pale in comparison to the cost of the bribe for Agnes' family proposed by the fathers of Wook's accomplices. The men want Mija to contribute to buying the dead girl's mother's (Park Myeong-shin) silence about the boys' crime, thereby protecting them from intervention by their school or the police. But Mija never seems annoyed by how Wook treats her; rather, she is frustrated by his refusal to treat their home with respect and by his seeming inability to feel remorse for his participation in the rape. This failure, and not the "failure" of Mija's memory, pervades the film. The dual focus on Wook's lack of emotional response and failed communication resonates against Mija's efforts to come to terms with her emotions and to articulate them in poetic form. This contrast in characterization treads heavily upon a more typical view of the youthful generation as signifying hope for a future while the older generation poses only a burden to that hope.

The widespread refusal to listen or meaningfully talk to Mija stands out in *Poetry*. Rather than focus on Mija's physical care, the film considers Alzheimer's in terms of its effect on language and its relationship to memory. Thus, *Poetry* avoids the seemingly simple melodrama of a once capable aging grandparent "losing it." The other characters tend to treat her as a dotty old woman to whom they must offer gestures of respect that need not extend beyond surface convention. In fact, only Mija's doctor suspects that she is anything more than as scatterbrained as always. Mija's doctor is not at all worried about the "prickly" sensation in her arm that prompted her visit. Instead, he is concerned that she cannot find language to describe the banal symptom. At a subsequent appointment, the specialist who diagnoses her with Alzheimer's explains her condition in terms of language loss: "You're occasionally forgetting words for now, but gradually your memory loss will worsen. At first you won't recall nouns and then verbs." While her forgetfulness does not seem to have any immediate effect on any other characters in the film, Mija's own awareness of it changes her determination towards the world around her, particularly when it comes to finding a form of expression that is meaningful to her and adequate to her circumstances as a grandmother whose grandson has caused extraordinary grief and suffering.

Mija's interpretation of the specialist's discussion of the progressive loss of nouns and verbs is "The doctor also told me to write poetry a lot," as she tells her absent daughter. She remains acutely aware of parts of speech and is eager to reinterpret her doctor's advice as language-focused. When asked if she understands what the doctor means by verbs, Mija responds, "Of course I know verbs, but nouns are the most important." Having recently enrolled in a poetry writing class, Mija struggles even more than the other students in the class with the concepts she learns from her poetry teacher. However, her struggle comes not from her Alzheimer's, but from the structure of her everyday life. Having been told "You've never seen an apple before," Mija tries hard in her kitchen to comprehend an apple in a new (poetic) way. But, as is usually the case in her domestic setting, she has just had one of many unpleasant encounters with Wook, so she sighs, takes a bite, and says, "Apples are better for eating than for looking at," focusing on the verb rather than the noun. The idea that she should look for beauty in her everyday life, in everything she sees (as her poetry teacher explains) intrigues but baffles her, even though she considers herself to have a "poet's vein" because she "like[s] flowers and say[s] odd things."

Anne David Basting explains, "To people with dementia, the arts bring tools that enable them to express themselves and their vision of the world and are particularly powerful for this group because the arts operate on an emotional level. One needn't have control of rational language to write a poem, create a dance, or take a photograph" ("The Arts" 17). Despite her inability to view the apple in a new light, Mija remains committed to finding poetic inspiration and especially to writing a poem. That poem comes to her in snippets that she collects in her notebook, usually tied to her contemplation of the results of Wook's actions. Immediately after the fathers tell Mija about the crime, they call her a "clueless old lady," while she kneels to contemplate a flower and scribbles, "Blood ... a flower as red as blood." Watching seemingly innocent young boys kick around a soccer ball, she writes, "The sound of birds singing. What are they singing?" On her way to ask one of the fathers to loan her Wook's portion of the bribe money, she writes, "Time passes and flowers fade." When she visits the site of the young girl's suicide, she opens her notebook to write but only records the raindrops. Her focus shifts to the nouns, and the final scene of the poem reveals that those nouns — and the related figures of speech and actions — become means for her to express an emotional connection to Agnes.

The film mostly avoids portraying obvious memory lapses and other clear signs of dementia. However, in a pivotal scene, Mija's failing memory does provide her with brief respite from the pain of her everyday life, illustrating the opposite dynamic of Ebert's "movie Alzheimer's." In effect, she is briefly freed from her lucidity. After the fathers reach an impasse with the dead girl's mother, they decide that the "silly old woman's" words might actually be useful to them. Their leader drives Mija to the countryside to meet with Agnes's mother who refuses their efforts to compensate her through money. Not finding the mother at home, Mija ventures out to find her at work in the fields. Enraptured by the bucolic sur- roundings, and particularly taken by the fallen apricots, Mija crouches to fully "see" them and scratches a few more lines into her notebook. This attempt to find beauty in the everyday world, as instructed by her poetry teacher, seems to push her into a blissful lapse (rather than Ebert's remarkable lucidity) from memories of her grandson's treachery. While she is still in this reverie, Mija finds the girl's mother, hard at work harvesting a crop. The two women chat amiably and Mija bursts forth with her new lines, reading them to the mother: "The apricot throws itself to the ground. It is crushed and trampled for the next life." As Mija turns away, she appears to regain the memory she had previously been spared, and an expression of pure agony flits across her face. Perhaps she realizes not only that she had for- gotten to speak with the woman about compensation and about the awful role her grandson has played, but also that these lines offer an apt metaphor for Agnes. Mija's return to lucidity, though perhaps giving poetic meaning, offers no respite and little hope. Rather than turn back and explain her presence to Agnes's mother, she continues to walk away and returns to her mundane worldly tasks knowing that she has failed Agnes's mother (by failing to reveal herself or enable just compensation) as well as the group of fathers (by failing to rep- resent them or eliminate their collective culpability).

Disability in Poetry

Without considering the film's Mr. Kang subplot, Mija comes across as a burdened but quietly elegant and whimsical grandmother facing new challenges that threaten a past gentle existence. But while Mija appears elegant in comparison with Agnes's mother in the field, she also appears in the film dressed in scruffy clothes engaged in difficult physical labor caring for a disabled older man and his flat. Poetry effectively upends the usual care- giving narrative structure of the Alzheimer's film by punctuating depictions of Mija's daily life with her labor for the worthless Wook and for Mr. Kang as the burdensome disabled figure, who thereby functions as a useful narrative prosthetic rather than as a meaningful three-dimensional figure within the world of the story. Like Wook, Kang treats Mija roughly, but he offers a begrudging recognition of her value in the form of minuscule monetary tips. He also pays some close attention to her behavior, and he attempts to seduce her, or at least to convince her to give him sexual pleasure (the film seems to assume that as a disabled man, Kang could only hope to have sex with a hired partner).

Largely because of his physical disabilities which make him appear dependent upon care for activities of daily living and render his communication difficult, Kang comes across as a symbol of aging gone wrong as well as of masculinity clinging to remnants of power. He is not a fleshed-out character but rather a character in place mostly because of his fleshly failings. His role in the film is largely to illustrate Mija's social position and the transformation of her thinking. For example, a series of bathtub scenes between Mija and Mr. Kang illustrates the change that Mija undergoes throughout the film. In the first scene, Mr. Kang hits Mija; in the second scene, Mija is silent (and, unlike the other characters in the film, Mr. Kang notices her silence); in the third scene, Mija's recoils in horror because Mr. Kang has arranged to have a Viagra-induced erection; and in the fourth scene, she joins him in the bathtub to fulfill his sexual desires, having previously adamantly refused to do so. In this way, encounters with Kang show Mija to be tolerant of or at least accustomed to abuse, chastened by Wook's disgraceful actions, still horrified by male sexual aggression, and finally either resigned or empowered into a sexual act.

The final sex scene between Mija and Kang offers a perplexing view of perceptions of disabled masculinity and an intriguing opportunity for the interpretation of Mija's state of mind. Although she had been very angry about his manipulation, Mija does later choose to offer herself to Kang sexually, and this offering is portrayed as a gift from her in response to his begging her to let him "be a man." The motivation for this action appears to be tied to Agnes, but there is ambiguity as to how. Immediately before Mija returns to Kang's apartment for sex, she visits the site of Agnes's suicide. As she watches the river flowing below, Mija's hat falls into the water where Agnes had drowned, and the older woman imagines a deep connection to the young girl. This perceived bond seems to spur her to return to Kang's flat. It could be that her increased empathy for Agnes compels her to also experience sexual exploitation in order to gain greater understanding or as some form of compensation or self-inflicted punishment. It is also possible that her increased sense of connection to Agnes clarifies her desire to find a way to raise her share of the money to pay Agnes's mother, regardless of the desperate actions that might be required to make that possible. Whatever her motivation, the film portrays Mija's mounting Kang as a form of pity for him, even if it implies she might find sexual satisfaction (or some form of fulfilling affection) with him, despite his loutish personality. His disabled body becomes the site of her redemption.

Mija's redemption takes the form of independence. Subsequent to their final bathtub encounter, Mija extorts from Kang the large sum of money she requires (putting his past paltry gratuities into perspective) to pay her debt to the cabal of fathers. While she appears to have capitulated to their social power, she refuses to bear any further moral responsibility for Wook or to align herself with the fathers' self-righteous agenda to protect their families by shifting blame to the victim, heaping more grief on her family and reputation. That is, Mija does not use this bribe to alleviate Wook from responsibility for his role in the rape. Instead, she turns her grandson over to the police to meet whatever punishment would be decided according to law.

The film closes with scenes steeped in nature similar to those of the opening, accompanied by a voice-over reading of Mija's poem, "Agnes's Song," an ode to the dead girl. In the narration, the older woman's voice is joined by a young girl's voice that eventually narrates the remainder of the poem alone. In this way, Mija's voice gives way to Agnes's, further demonstrating that she has chosen a connection with the young schoolgirl over all others. Whether she chooses to follow Agnes over the bridge railing (that is whether she commits suicide) remains ambiguous. But the film does close with her leaning over that railing, contemplating the running water below where Agnes's body was found floating at the opening of the film. Mija's departure at the end of the film occurs deliberately, not in a fog of memory loss, and is not a move into institutional care as is so often the case in films about Alzheimer's.

Conclusion

South Korea has one of the most rapidly aging populations globally. The country is at the forefront of addressing what an aging population might mean for the nation's economy and well-being as major cuts to the public pension scheme threaten to strain the purse strings of adults who will need to support their aging parents. Added to those individual financial responsibilities, national health care premiums have increased to support the already growing number of dementia patients in nursing home care, and the number of South Koreans with dementia is expected to rise exponentially. Drawing on a portion of that increased revenue, the South Korean government has openly declared a "War on Dementia" and enlisted "dementia supporters of all ages" (Belluck). Rather than focusing on cure through scientific research, they are focusing on developing an interactive and intergenerational social program. The Korean strategy mainstreams rather than segregates older adults with dementia from the general population. That is, they enlist children to work directly with older adults. Younger children play with people with dementia. Older children go through simulation exercises to better understand the experience of dementia. They can subsequently gain credit for engaging in community service conducted with dementia patients. In this manner, people with dementia receive support through direct engagement and younger generations contribute actively to the welfare of their elders and their own socialization. Popular representations and alarmist news stories will not be the only source of knowledge these children receive about dementia in late life.

The depiction of Mija does not address the strong social need to develop clear plans to care for an aging population, which may well include unprecedented numbers of people with dementia. Her example does little to stem the fear of the projected gray tidal wave imagined to be upon the globe due to population aging. The film, which was released when South Korea began its intergenerational war on dementia, does not depict the country's progressive educational and social program. Certainly, the depiction of intergenerational relationships in the film does not even hint at Mija being offered a dementia supporter. However, in relation to its historical context, the film offers avenues to question the role disability depictions play in emphasizing the elements of old age that resonate loudest within popular culture. And it is those elements that the South Korean battle aims to conquer, along with the hopes for reduced costs of care.

Poetry offers a clear counter narrative to Ebert's "movie Alzheimer's," one that imagines memory as a mixed blessing. The treatment of Mija's dementia in *Poetry* invites disability analysis and cultural age scholarship because it resists both a valorization of the coherent self and a simplistic assertion of Mija's new identity once she knows she is experiencing symptoms of Alzheimer's. In another context or another film, Mija's enrollment in the poetry class might simply have been a form of leisurely middle-class late life self-development, but she uses the class to absorb herself in a deep imaginative connection with Agnes, a moving form of commemoration, that ultimately strengthens her resolve to no longer submit herself to the present-day needs and wants of Wook and Mr. Kang.

As Hannah Zeilig explains, "Narratives of age ... represent one of the most interesting ways of provoking critical thought about ageing" (17). In *Poetry*, Alzheimer's does not impair Mija in either a medical, social, or cultural way, except through the condescension of the specialist who diagnoses her. While the diagnosis does seem to worry Mija moderately and momentarily, she does not seek a cure or a solution to problems the illness might bring to her practical life. Rather, the doctor's identification of Mija's new relationship with language pushes her to follow through on a childhood wish to write poetry. A memory lapse infuses the film as a respite, not just as a loss of self. Yet, Mija's determination that Agnes not be forgotten, even as Mija may no longer be able to remember details, exceeds a simple interpretation of the film as equating creativity with a disordered mind. Thus, it is not just Mija's touching poem that demonstrates her creative power but also her ability to orchestrate a devious solution to Wook's dilemma, wherein Agnes's family gets the money and Wook still faces punishment. Importantly, Mija is the oldest member of her poetry class, and she is the only student to complete the class assignment of writing one poem. Though she may never have really seen an apple, her ability to see the crushed and trampled apricot in Agnes' mother's presence offers Mija a way out of the moral and practical dilemmas that face her. Her story provokes critical thought about the subversive power of creative aging.

Notes

1. Dementia refers to a range of conditions that entail cognitive decline. Alzheimer's is just one type, but it has become a symbol for a full spectrum of conditions even though symptoms and medical etiology of different forms of dementia are actually quite different. Because it is the form that is most dominant within popular culture and because it is what is portrayed in the film I focus on, I mostly discuss Alzheimer's in this essay.

2. Examples include *The Notebook, One Special Night* (Roger Young, 1999), *The Savages, I Never Sang for My Father* (Gilbert Cates, 1970), *Aurora Borealis* (James C. E. Burke, 2005), and *Friends with Benefits*.

3. The film won awards for Best Screen Play at Cannes; Best Picture, Screen Play, Actress, and Supporting Actor at the Grand Bell Awards; Best Picture and Screenplay from the Korean critics awards; Best Actress at the Blue Dragon Film Awards; and Best Achievement in Direction and Performance by an Actress at the Asia Pacific Screen Awards. *Poetry* was only considered at the Blue Moon Dragon awards for its actors since Director Lee Chang-dong chose to boycott the ceremony.

Works Cited

Asch, Adrienne. "Critical Race Theory, Feminism, and Disability: Reflections on Social Justice and Personal Identity." *Gendering Disability*. Eds. Bonnie G. Smith and Beth Hutchison. Rutgers, NJ: Rutgers University Press, 2004. 9–44. Print.

Basting, Anne Davis. "The Arts and Dementia Care." *Generations* 30.1 Spring (2006): 16–20. Print.

_____. *Forget Memory: Creating Better Lives for People with Dementia*. Baltimore: Johns Hopkins University Press, 2009. Print.

_____. "Looking Back from Loss: Views of the Self in Alzheimer's Disease." *Journal of Aging Studies* 17 (2003): 87. Print.

Belluck, Pam. "In a Land of the Aging, Children Counter Alzheimer's." *New York Times* 25 Nov. 2010: A1. Print.

Chariandry, David. *Soucouyant*. Vancouver: Arsenal Pulp Press, 2007. Print.

Dargis, Manohla. "Consider an Apple, Consider the World." Rev. of Poetry. Dir. Lee Chang-dong. *New York Times* 11 Feb. 2011: 1. Print.

Davidson, Michael. *Concerto for the Left Hand: Disability and the Defamiliar Body*. Corporealities. Ann Arbor: University of Michigan Press, 2008. Print.

Eakin, Paul John. "What Are We Reading When We Read Autobiography?" *Narrative* 12.2 (2004): 121–32. Print.

Ebert, Roger. "Friends with Benefits (Review)." Review. *Chicago Sun-Times* July 20, 2011. Print.

Garland-Thomson, Rosemarie. "Integrating Disability, Transforming Feminist Theory." *NWSA Journal* 14.3 (2002): 1–32. Print.

Goodykoontz, Bill. "Poetry, 4.5 Stars." *The Arizona Public* 19 May 2011. Print.

Hughes, Bill, Rachel Russell, and Kevin Paterson. "Nothing to Be Had 'Off the Peg': Consumption, Identity and the Immobilization of Young Disabled People." *Disability & Society* 20.1 (2005): 3. Print.

Longman, Phillip. "Global Aging. (Cover Story)." *Foreign Policy* 182 (2010): 52–58. Print.

McRuer, Robert. *Crip Theory: Cultural Signs of Queerness and Disability.* Cultural Front. New York: New York University Press, 2006. Print.

Mitchell, David T., and Sharon L. Snyder. *Narrative Prosthesis: Disability and the Dependencies of Discourse.* Ann Arbor: University of Michigan Press, 2001. Print.

Poetry. Dir. Lee Chang-dong. Perf. Yun Jeong-hie, Lee Da-wit, Kim Hira. Kino International, 2010.

Siebers, Tobin. *Disability Theory.* Corporealities. Ann Arbor: University of Michigan Press, 2008. Print.

Turan, Kenneth. "Movie Review: Poetry." *Los Angeles Times* 6 May 2011. Print.

White, Rob. "Into the Past." *Film Quarterly* 64.4 (2011): 4–5. Print.

Woong-ki, Song. "Sixties Era Cinema Icon Returns to the Big Screen." *The Korean Herald* 14 April 2010. Print.

Zeilig, Hannah. "The Critical Use of Narrative and Literature in Gerontology." *International Journal of Ageing and Later Life* (2012): 1–31. Print.

Breaking the Silence?

Deafness, Education and Identity in Two Post-Cultural Revolution Chinese Films[1]

Sarah Dauncey

Research is revealing that one of the most interesting manifestations of social and political change in twentieth-century China is the way in which disability and difference have been represented in film and other media (Dauncey "Screening Disability"). How to understand these cultural transformations, however, is proving to be a challenge on several fronts. Disability Studies already provides an established and multifarious foundation for the exploration of such issues, but this has been developed almost exclusively in the Western context with relatively little consideration of possible differences elsewhere. Most problematically for this investigation into Chinese experiences is the fact that, in order to better interrogate definitions of disability and de-stigmatize bodily and mental difference, Disability Studies scholars have often focused on foregrounding ideals that will ultimately challenge actual circumstances. The mechanical application of these contemporary Western ideals would only serve to put real-life, late twentieth-century China (a greatly modernized, but still developing, country) into even further relief. Chinese Studies scholars certainly have a greater understanding of this local context; however, the enduring influence of Sinology means that they, for their part, may be sometimes too ready to suggest China's uniqueness and, as a consequence, too quick to abandon Western-oriented theories. This has the potential to compound the China situation by magnifying to the outside world the perceived alterity of people already traditionally viewed as "other" in their own country. A balance between the two is clearly needed.

Through an examination of two dramas from established Chinese film directors — Sun Zhou's *Breaking the Silence* (*Piaoliang mama*, 2000) and Ning Jingwu's *Silent River* (*Wu sheng de he*, 2000) — this essay begins the process of finding that balance. It combines in-depth understandings of the Chinese social and cultural landscape with congruent understandings of disability and difference developed in the West to reveal perceptions of the educational experiences of young deaf people at the turn of the twenty-first century and the ways in which such experiences may play a role in shaping deaf and disabled identities from a young age. The two films have been selected specifically for their exploration of

75

mainstream and special schooling, contrasting forms of education that were, theoretically at least, available to deaf and disabled children following a decade of substantial reform and development in Chinese education and law-making. This focus on education, still universally recognized as one of the most important factors determining opportunities and equality for disabled people (UNESCO 181–184), enables me to analyze in greater depth the significance of different educational experiences in the construction and negotiation of personal and social identities, as well as the potential impact this was perceived to have on access to opportunities in later life. Local attitudes towards disability and difference very much frame and fashion the portrayals of deafness in *Breaking the Silence* and *Silent River*, yet many narratives and tropes, such as the melodramatic potential of deafness and the "supercrip," will also be familiar to Western audiences. The two films appear to simultaneously embrace and challenge both Chinese and Western stereotypes, all of which reflects the interplay of contemporary political initiatives, popular beliefs, personal concerns and artistic sensibilities. The findings of this essay will, therefore, not only provide new evidence of the interaction between concepts of disability, deafness, education and identity as they were broadly understood in China at the end of the twentieth century; it will also demonstrate that while there may be some resonances with Western theoretical articulations and expectations, there is also considerable variance in how such concepts are actually discussed and experienced in China itself, much of which is simply the result of an inevitable divergence between a general model and *any* specific situation.

Understanding Disability in Chinese Film

As I have shown elsewhere (Dauncey "Screening Disability"), the representation of disability in Chinese film follows quite a unique trajectory. Although there were strong similarities to Western cinema at the beginning of the twentieth century as the nascent film industry drew heavily on Hollywood stereotypes and combined these with home-grown negative views of physical and mental difference, the representation of disability actually became sparse through 1950s and 1960s as socialist ideals of personhood began to focus increasingly on normative minds and bodies. So strict were the guidelines on this issue that by the Cultural Revolution (1966–1976) images of disability had practically disappeared from film with just a few notable exceptions.[2] The end of the Cultural Revolution, however, immediately liberated film from many of these restrictions, which consequently opened up the possibility of exploring personal, rather than collective, experiences, and allowed the inclusion of characters that did not necessarily conform to socialist ideals of fitness. This was to have a profound effect on disability representation. Almost overnight, films started to reveal the traumas experienced by disabled people during the previous decade and, moving into the 1980s, began to explore issues faced by disabled people as the country entered a new period of reform and opening up. International campaigns, such as the UN's International Decade of Disabled Persons (1983–92), also had an impact by prompting the establishment in 1988 of the influential Chinese Disabled Persons' Federation (hereafter CDPF) which was tasked, among other things, with developing new cultural projects to raise awareness of disability. As a result, numerous state-sponsored films were produced that focused on exposing prejudice, and encouraging a more caring social mentality towards disabled people; additionally, such films frequently illustrated the "superhuman" potential of disabled people in line with prevailing self-sufficiency and self-improvement campaigns. Disability representation became more prominent through the 1990s when increasing exposure of the film industry to market forces saw the "added interest" provided by disability in terms of potential melodrama or exoticism that could enhance both the domestic *and* international marketability of such films, many of which were directed by prominent filmmakers and were lauded by critics and audiences alike.[3]

Despite such a dramatic transformation in disability representation, there are few academic works that discuss the implications of this. Where relevant films are mentioned, disability tends to take a back seat even when major characters are disabled or plot development revolves around an impairment. Sheldon H. Lu's study of the trajectory of the body in modern Chinese culture, for example, makes only limited reference to the disabled body despite its subject matter. Where he does so, he simply asserts that the "mentally retarded" younger brother, Erming (Wu Jiang), in Zhang Yang's bittersweet *Shower* (*Xizao*, 1999) stands as a metaphor for the "mentally challenged" Chinese citizens unwilling to adapt to modernity (172–174), a reading that disregards the fact that Erming is a well-developed and purposeful character who is loved by his family and valued by the community. By contrast, Deirdre Sabina Knight's sophisticated examination of two docudramas from the 1990s — *Sons* (*Erzi*, 1996, dir. Zhang Yuan) and *The Common People* (*Guanyu ai de gushi*, 1998, dir. Zhou Xiaowen) — reveals how the depiction of madness and cerebral palsy in these works presents unique moral dialogues on mental and physical anguish, highlighting the way in which the families concerned must navigate the disjuncture between traditional Confucian values and modern biomedical ethics. Steven L. Riep's paper similarly draws on cross-cultural understandings to show how *Colors of the Blind* (*Hei yanjing*, 1997, dir. Chen Guoxing) and *Happy Times* (*Xingfu shiguang*, 2000, dir. Zhang Yimou) both reinforce and challenge existing Western cinematic conventions *and* Chinese social stereotypes of blindness, a conclusion that resonates with the findings of this essay.

With such gaps in Chinese Studies research, Disability Studies offers a natural point of reference, particularly with regard to its exploration of the power of film to shape popular perceptions of deafness and disability. Hollywood, argues John S. Schuchman, has been "a substantial contributor to the public's misunderstanding of deafness and to the perpetuation of attitudes that permit discrimination against deaf citizens" (x). Paul Darke goes further to suggest that the medical model "has almost total hegemony over the modern definition of disability on film" (97), which, he argues, sustains negative stereotyping by characterizing disabled people as ill, isolated, dependent, and infantilized (104). While both evidence the way in which such images are defined by the interplay of Western social, cultural and political factors, Darke asserts that the nature of disability representation is so static that the same conclusions would probably apply regardless of impairment, country, era or genre (106). What I propose here, however, is that ignoring the implications of a specific cultural context to apply too generic a Disability Studies approach can result in a one-dimensional outcome that encourages us to simply label images as negative without knowing whether they signify the same things in the culture that produced them (a point I will return to in more detail later). Such an idea already finds strong support elsewhere, as Clare Barker and Stuart Murray have shown in their fascinating exploration into the ways in which Disability Studies could respond to postcolonial locations of disability, where metaphors may then "be meaningful not just as 'crutch[es]' (Mitchell and Snyder 49) in the telling of some 'other' tale of postcolonial experience, but as part of foundational cultural and historical *disability* narratives" (Barker and Murray 233).

Chinese Constructions of Deafness and the Implications for Education

There are many reasons why we should be wary of transposing cultural constructions formed in one society onto another without due consideration. We only have to look at Western societies to see how issues of deaf identity and culture and their relationship to broader discourses of disability reveal a complex and fluid dynamic in which even terminology defies totalizing definitions (Corker; Brueggeman; Branson and Miller). Yet, for some time, a growing proportion of Sign Language users in the West have identified themselves as a distinct linguistic and cultural Deaf minority and contend that while they have long been subjected to disabling and "normalizing" practices they do not consider themselves disabled. By contrast, if we look back to the 1990s when the two films under study here were produced, the vast majority of deaf people in China, sign language users or not, still considered themselves "disabled" (Callaway *Deaf Children* 17), undoubtedly due to the strong influence of the biomedically informed state narrative of disability promulgated by the CDPF (Kohrman 61). It is only more recently that these Western understandings of Deaf empowerment have begun to permeate into China as international agencies and foreign institutions have worked to support development in the country (Johnson, Lytle and Yang 20–22). Even so, awareness of the d/Deaf distinction remains relatively limited and there is much debate in government, academic and popular circles about what it means to be deaf in China today.

It is important to recognize, therefore, that issues of deaf identity from late twentieth-century China frequently reflect issues related to the construction of disabled identities in general, and vice versa, although there are clearly some features that, by their very nature, are unique to deafness, and many of these are not limited to China alone. Callaway's research throws light on how Chinese understandings of deafness could have a substantial impact on children and their educational experiences. From interviews with parents at a Nanjing deaf rehabilitation clinic in 1994, as well as letters from those parents to the head of the clinic, Callaway discovered what seemed to be a "consistent set of images of deafness," all of which had a strong influence on a parent's responses to their child's impairment and, consequently, their attitude towards their child's education. First was the fact that deafness was regularly referred to as an "illness" (*bing*) for which a cure should be sought. Second was the notion that deafness and muteness were semantically linked through the use of the term "deaf-mute" (*longya*). Thirdly, deaf people were said to exist in a "soundless/silent world" (*wu sheng de shijie*) separate from the society of hearing people. And, finally, was the desire for their children to be "normal" (*zhengchang*). These factors, argues Callaway, resulted in an overwhelming urgency among parents to train their child to speak so that they could be accepted into mainstream education ("Constructing Deafness" 68–9). What is more, she suggests, this desire was intensified further in urban areas because of the "One Child Policy" as, in the same way parents of daughters were putting more effort into protecting their only child's rights and interests, parents of deaf children were also concentrating more resources and time on their child to ensure a positive educational outcome, as well as putting more pressure on authorities to have the child accepted in mainstream school (Callaway *Deaf Children* 33–34).[4]

One of the main developments emerging from the flurry of activity in the 1990s aimed at enhancing the legal rights of disabled people and improving educational support for disabled children was, in fact, a move towards promoting the integration and inclusion of deaf students in mainstream classrooms.[5] However, as Johnson, Lytle and Yang (21) indicate, with few extra support mechanisms or sign language interpreters at that time, there was not a high level of success for deaf students in such environments. The expectation was that the majority of children would be educated in special deaf schools where "hearing rehabilitation" could be conducted most effectively alongside a general curriculum delivered in sign-supported Chinese, although pupils were known to revert to a natural Chinese sign language with their peers and elsewhere (Callaway *Deaf Children* 71–72).[6] But this, too, would come with its own problems. The many hours devoted to oral language training were made all the more complex by the tonal nature of the Chinese language, which made for an extremely frustrating experience for pupils (Biggs 8–9). It also resulted in the watering-down of an already highly vocational curriculum, which meant that only small numbers of students were able to attain functional speech and many were leaving school with a substantially lower level of academic achievement than their hearing peers (Johnson, Lytle and Yang 24). The restrictions this then placed on post-secondary options and job opportunities would have, according to Biggs, further perpetuated negative assumptions about the potential of deaf people and their perceived ability to contribute to society, and consequently reinforced the urgency of parents to "normalize" their child by encouraging them to act "as 'hearing' as possible" (7).

Breaking the Silence

Chinese cultural constructions of deafness, their relationship to broader conceptions of disability, and the approaches to deaf education resulting from these, provide a complex and dynamic context for the two very different films analyzed here. *Breaking the Silence* (also known by the more literal translations *Beautiful Mama* or *Pretty Mother*), was the first major critical success for its director Sun Zhou. The recipient of national and international awards, particularly for lead actress Gong Li as Sun Liying, the film also received praise from various state organizations, including the CDPF and All-China Women's Federation (ACWF). The film follows a single mother, Sun Liying, as she struggles to prepare her son Zheng Da (Xin Gao), who has a significant degree of hearing loss, for the test that will determine whether he has sufficient hearing and speaking abilities to be accepted into mainstream school. To achieve a sense of realism, specialists at the China Rehabilitation Center for the Deaf and the Guangzhou School for the Deaf were consulted in the making of the film; Gong Li also spent some time with mothers and their deaf children as part of her preparation for the role (Lao). The film's gritty realism is further intensified by its atmospheric cinematography: scenes are shot in dark underpasses, poorly lit rooms and freezing weather conditions, all of which provide for a melancholic exploration of the ways in which a divorced woman who, with unreliable child support and no welfare assistance, makes the decision to give up regular employment so that she can spend time developing her son's speaking ability. Such was the impact of Gong Li's portrayal that the term "pretty mother" is now regularly used in a wide variety of media to describe any woman who has gone out of her way to care for her own or other disabled children.

Despite the fact that Sun Zhou had intended that Sun Liying be the focal point of the story, it was soon apparent that his inclusion of an "added interest" in the form of a deaf son had become the *sole* point of interest for audiences (Xu 18). This dynamic possibly led to the most commonly used translation of the film's title (which foregrounds the "silent world" of deafness) over the original Chinese title (which emphasizes the caring role of the mother). The unanticipated shift in audience reception possibly also goes some way to explaining why critics in more recent times have criticized the film for its lack of concentrated attention to Deaf issues and have alleged that Zheng Da is a mere "emotional foil" to Sun Liying and the "root of her torment" (Zhang 161). The suggestion that Zheng Da functions as little more than a "narrative prosthesis" (Mitchell and Snyder), however, overlooks what I argue is actually one of the core themes of the film — Zheng Da's identity. Society at large has already categorized him; from the teachers at the mainstream school to the local children on the street, his impairment makes him different, "other," and it is what defines him in their eyes. By contrast, both his parents, and consequently Zheng Da himself, struggle with his identity, which provides for a fascinating observation of the way in which perceptions of deafness were represented in late 1990s China.

From the very outset we are told by Sun Liying that her son is "a child with an illness" (*you bing de haizi*). She also overhears, to her distress, her former classmates talking commiseratively about the fact that Zheng Da's deafness is not "curable" while engaging in animated discussion of the achievements of their own children, which only serves to put Zheng Da's alterity into further relief. Because she is so busy at work Sun Liying blames herself for his failure to pass the entrance test first time around and so she decides to get more flexible employment. As she reflects: "That way I could teach him to talk and help him learn all the sounds that fill our world. I was afraid that if I waited my kid would never stand a chance." She whispers her aspirations for him into his hearing aid while he is asleep and it becomes clear that she sees that the only way to secure a good future for him is to give him the opportunity to get a full education: "Be a good boy. Go to primary school. Go to middle school. Go to university." Her desire to get him into "normal" school at all costs, intensified by her husband's departure which she blames on the fact that she couldn't give him a "normal child" (*zhengchang de haizi*), sees her attempting to convince the head teacher that he can cope:

SUN LIYING

He's just a little hard to understand. Other than that he is totally normal, really smart. He always gets things first time around.

HEAD JIAO

Why haven't you sent him to a deaf rehabilitation centre? Wouldn't that be better for him?

SUN LIYING

He did go, but his level wasn't the same as the kids there. So I thought it over and decided to bring him here so he could be together with normal kids. It'll make a big difference when he grows up.

Even the sympathetic teacher, Mr. Fang, cannot understand why she would insist upon her son receiving the same mainstream schooling as "normal kids," to which she retorts: "Zheng Da is a normal kid. A piece of plastic behind his ear and he's not normal all of a sudden. Are people who wear glasses not normal?"

Zheng Da's speaking difficulties and apparent inability to use sign language substantially limit his communication and interaction with those around him, with the exception of his mother who tends to speak loudly and clearly to his face, often concluding with the phrase "Listen to what I say/your mum says" (*ting wo/mama shuo*) to further emphasize the importance of the hearing and speaking world to his development. Yet, there are moments when he reveals his own understanding of his identity, primarily that he is "not the same as everyone else" (*wo he bieren bu yiyang*). Although he has a friend in his neighbor, Yanzi, and is invited by a group of children to go ice-skating, he is more frequently shown as an outsider who is subjected to bullying by other children on account of his hearing impairment. In the first instance, he gets into a fight that revolves around his hearing aids and leaves one in pieces as we listen to the bullies jeering "Deafie! Deafie! Dumb kid!" (*Long'er! Long'er! Yaba!*). In the second, he is picked out for the fake red uniform his mother bought at his bequest at the market, which at the time had simultaneously satisfied his own desire to fit in with his peers as well as Sun Liying's ultimate dream for her son. Although the uniform issue is the spark that lights the bullies' interest, attention soon turns to his impairment as they taunt him: "He's deaf! Look, he really is a deafie!"

Sun Liying ends up resorting to low paid and illegal jobs to raise the massive 5,000 *yuan* for a new hearing aid. Assaulted by a man she cleans for, she takes his money and buys a new hearing aid only for Zheng Da to refuse to wear it, knowing that it singles him out from the crowd:

ZHENG DA

How come I'm the only one who has to wear hearing aids?

SUN LIYING

Because you're deaf; you're different.

ZHENG DA

I'm scared.

SUN LIYING

Don't be scared. You have me. There's nothing to be scared of. You can't hear so it is even more important for you to go to school and do your best. Someday, we'll be the same as everyone else.

The final scene sees Zheng Da going into school for another test. He is now determined to succeed, but equally and understandably fearful of failure, a feeling commonly articulated by Chinese children who are forced to undergo constant oral training (Biggs 9). Sun Liying ponders his fate as he waves her goodbye: "I always thought that Zheng Da was my failure. I never wanted to admit it. But that night his question [about being different] made me realize that he was stronger than me."

Zheng Da's identity, therefore, is predicated on his deafness. This reflects Schuchman's evidence from the Western context that films draw on the pathological view that a deaf person is "defective, not normal," someone to be pitied or cured or both (3–6). Equally, it reflects Callaway's findings, mentioned earlier, of the parental assumptions about the nature of deafness in China at the time. This difference not only implies he should be schooled in a way that differs from his hearing peers, but also suggests he is so substantially different that he is not part of mainstream society. He is, as Schuchman has argued, a stereotypically isolated and vulnerable figure (61). To his mother, therefore, mainstream education is seen as a way of "normalizing" him despite the fact that evidence from China in the 1990s suggested that such a strategy would actually diminish the child's potential levels of achievement. Her desperate attempts to teach him "all the sounds of this world" so that he can speak sufficiently well to be accepted into the local school mirrors the urgency of the parents in Callaway's study for whom the idea of attending a school for the deaf fill them "with dread and definitively crushes their hopes of their child leading a normal life as they see it" ("Constructing Deafness" 69). On the surface, Zheng Da himself also appears to conform to what Davis and Watson (159) argue has become an essentialized or homogenized nature of discourse about disabled children in which they are frequently presented as "sad and despairing," in need of financial support or a cure.

Closer readings of the film, though, in fact suggest that Zheng Da is stronger and more assertive than we are initially led to believe (Galeeazi 43–44). This reading stems particularly from the fact that he understands and questions the way in which society perceives him as "different," and makes a stand against the bullies who so easily use his "difference" as a weapon. This demonstrates the subtle ways in which *Breaking the Silence* begins to nuance assumptions about the ability for disabled individuals to assert their own identity, albeit in a manner that draws heavily on the melodramatic potential of deafness. We can also see how the film has captured in a very vivid way the emotional experiences of the parents and children who are trying to make sense of a world that is changing rapidly but also continues to label people who have impairments as "other."

Silent River

Less well-known in the West, *Silent River*'s overt sentimentalism provides a notable juxtaposition to *Breaking the Silence*'s realism; it also differs substantially in the fact that the main setting is a special school where the predominant form of communication is Chinese Sign Language.[7] Winner of several domestic film awards, the plot revolves around life at the Dayan School for the Deaf where the protagonist, Wen Zhi, is forced to undertake his teacher training because of his own impending "disability" through voice loss. The film's director Ning Jingwu creates what he describes as a lyrical atmosphere using scenes set in quiet Beijing *hutong*, well-ordered traditional courtyards or with the famously picturesque backdrops of Lugou Bridge and the Great Wall, all combined with invariably good weather, where even the rain is turned into an appreciation of the aesthetically beautiful nature of raindrops on lotus leaves (59–60). But this romanticism, which extends to certain aspects of the plot, has left the film open to some accusations that it is merely a "main melody film"[8] due to its apparent uncritical support for the state's reforms and social progress achieved therein (Zhang 158).

Like Sun Zhou, Ning Jingwu has been questioned on the rationale for making a movie on such a topic. His answers, however, reveal a very different motivation and approach:

> Many reporters ask me the same question — why choose this topic? What I want to say is, why not? I wanted to show the greatness of human nature and so I naturally chose this group of people who are overlooked and disadvantaged in our society. I decided to use real deaf people in the main roles because I believed that the film would discover that they have a beauty that is greater than that of even healthy, able-bodied people. I wanted to show that people are equal and so I had to select a special group of people who are not considered equal and are often subject to discrimination. I wanted to show communion and compassion, and so I chose a story in which a group of deaf kids help their healthy, able-bodied teacher to regain his sense of hope [Ning 60].

As Ning mentions, close to twenty of the actors are actually non-professionals, many of whom he met while substituting as a Chinese teacher in a deaf school. This in itself is quite remarkable as Hollywood films rarely involve more than one deaf character and have tended to ignore the existence of an "active, healthy deaf community" (Schuchman 3). In *Silent River*, Wen Zhi is actually the outsider who enters a vibrant and supportive deaf environment having left a world where his music career has been thwarted by his gradual voice loss. Ironically, too, Wen Zhi's inability to sign means that *he* becomes the student the minute he walks into the classroom, much to the amusement of the pupils when he mistakenly signs "shit" instead of "three." The use of sign language as the predominant form of communication among the pupils is perhaps the most innovative aspect of this film as it reveals for the first time in Chinese cinema the viability of sign language as a mode of communication between deaf *and* hearing people.

In the Dayan School for the Deaf, no questions are raised about the appropriateness of sign language or the educational methods more generally; quite the opposite, in fact, as here the utopian nature of the school suggests that this is a natural and enabling environment where pupils are not "ill" and do not need to be "cured," thus putting the film in stark contrast to *Breaking the Silence* and the evidence from sociological research. Once Wen Zhi has become more proficient at signing, this is the only form of communication in the classroom and, even more surprising given the nature of deaf education at the time, there is a complete absence of any form of speech rehabilitation. Furthermore, the pupils are given encouragement to explore technology to enhance non-verbal dissemination of information and communication with their peers. Two particular examples are the signed news broadcasts within the school and a laptop computer bought by Wen Zhi as a parting gift for the class. In what turns out to be a somewhat prophetic statement, he says to them: "Computers and the Internet are good things for us. They don't require us to hear or speak and we can make friends. In one sense it's the most level playing field we have today." Indeed, within just a few years, the Internet was reported as having become "the mode of communication for the Deaf community, with chat rooms, blogs and Web sites that promote dialogue and discussion on these issues" (Johnson, Lytle, and Yang 23).

Outside the school, however, it is a very different matter and several scenes are used to illustrate some of the problems and prejudices faced by deaf people. The opening sequence is a prime example as one of the students Zhang Che (Shan Renbing), unable to hear an approaching car, is berated as a "Deafo!" The main concerns articulated by the students in the film are all related to their transition to higher education or employment in the world beyond the school gates. In the case of Zhang Che, his determination to become a policeman and have-a-go-hero approach constantly gets him into trouble. His father, who doesn't use sign language himself, is frustrated by his son's refusal to take up a place in an acrobatics training program and insists that he "stop daydreaming." The police, too, see his actions as dangerous and argue that they "have to make extra efforts to protect him," echoing the state view that disabled people require extra protection. Despite this Wen Zhi encourages him to study hard to achieve his ambition, although Zhang Che is skeptical: "I really don't think that I can ever be a policeman." Later, however, he is visibly inspired by the real-life case of "China's first deaf detective" Xu Zeming (Xu Zeming),[9] who provides him with an incentive to focus on school work: "Do you know what my biggest obstacle is now? It is not my mouth or my ears; it is the fact that I don't have an education." And in a later visit, Xu offers additional words of inspiration: "The hearing-impaired can't hear or speak well, but we have very keen eyesight. More importantly we can't think of ourselves as disabled." The contrasting views of the father (who wants his son to grasp what he sees as the only viable route to security) on the one hand and the teacher/policeman (who emphasize the importance of education and the potential for individuals to achieve their dreams) on the other, throw up some interesting considerations about the ways in which perceptions about careers for deaf people were changing in late 1990s China and also reveal how the promotion of educative model citizens such as Xu Zeming might have facilitated these changes. Second, the policeman's articulation of the notion that deafness should not be considered a disability, I believe, is one of the first expressions in Chinese cinema of what would become more common in time as Western understandings of deaf consciousness were gradually received in China.

Another student, Xue Tiannan, is similarly frustrated by the lack of equal opportunity after school. While Zhang Che is played by a student at Shanghai Arts High School for the Deaf, Xue Tiannan, a student at Nanjing School for the Deaf, plays herself in the film. She, like her on-screen persona, has been deaf since birth and also has a degenerative eye condition. Her dream in the film is go on to art college; but, towards the end, she finds out that her application has been rejected specifically on account of her impairments:

> I don't know why they won't accept me. The teacher said it would be too hard to teach me with everyone else ... I don't understand why they won't let me study art. Is it because I can't hear and can't speak? Although I can't hear, I can concentrate more on my work. Although I can't speak, I can observe more carefully. Why can't I study art? Teacher, I don't think it's fair.

Anxieties about post-secondary education for deaf children as noted earlier by Cassie Biggs, and Kathryn Johnson et al. are thus reflected in the film, as even talent is depicted as insufficient to break down long-held prejudices about integrating students who are unable to hear or speak into mainstream classrooms. By contrast, however, we also see further reinforcement of the message that deaf and disabled people may have other skills that more than make up for their impairment—"keen eyesight," better concentration, an ability to "observe more carefully"—and this notion culminates in what has been described by one Chinese writer as a "fairytale" ending that makes *Silent River* "no different to any other film with a focus on disability made by able-bodied people" (Hu 5–6).

The "fairytale" ending in question, in which a group of the girls from the Dayan School for the Deaf enter and win a televised dance competition, appears to play to the "supercrip" narrative as the manner of their victory (revealed below in a report on the school's news channel) meant that they had, according to Wang, "achieved their dream of not just becoming normal people but exceeding them" (18):

> They have brought honor to the school; they have brought honor to those with a hearing impairment. What is even more exciting is ... that throughout the competition, not a single judge or member of the audience realized that they were deaf. This proves that the deaf are absolutely no different to ordinary people [*putong ren*].

Although Hu Ke's comment that the depiction of pride in overcoming one's disability is merely a stereotype perpetuated by the "able-bodied," evidence I have collected from personal writings by Chinese disabled people at the time of the film's production strongly suggests that messages of encouragement to be an exemplary citizen, particularly messages that valorized such behavior for *all* citizens, could be very appealing and positive for disabled people. State-promoted narratives of supreme self-strengthening offered a new-found sense of self-worth, pride, and belonging that was actively embraced on an individual level and perpetuated through the publication and sharing of private experiences (Dauncey, "*Three Days*"). The motivational banner above the blackboard in the Dayan School for the Deaf classroom—"Study diligently and strive tirelessly to improve yourself (*qinfen xuexi, ziqiang buxi*)"—would have been commonplace in similar educational environments across the country and its sentiments may not always have been viewed as cynically as Hu suggests.

A similar purpose is served by the scenes in which the students work to enable Wen Zhi to regain hope in a musical career by buying him a guitar and encouraging him to sing for them. This narrative thread may even, as is posited by Galeeazi (43) and Wang (19), go some way to overturning the "able person as a rescuer" trope common to Western cinema and culture (Morris 102–105). Both of these examples and the case of model citizen Xu Zeming force us to rethink, therefore, how Chinese deaf and disabled identities are represented and negotiated through film. They suggest that understandings of empowerment in the Chinese context varied considerably from current Western understandings, so what would be considered stereotypical and stigmatizing in the West might have been viewed very differently by deaf and disabled people in China at that time.

Implications

In one of the most substantial discussions on *Breaking the Silence* and *Silent River*, Chinese writer Zhang Jin compares and contrasts the depiction of deafness in these two films with Nicolas Philibert's *In the Land of the Deaf* (*Au Pays des Sourds*, 1992), a French documentary-style film that is presented predominantly in French Sign Language. Neither *Silent River* nor *Breaking the Silence* come off well in Zhang's analysis which appears strongly informed by developments in Western discourse: "The difference between the two films rests in whether society is warm and caring or cold and uncaring, but they agree on this — deaf people have something wrong with them, they and their relatives are unlucky" (161). According to Zhang, there are several reasons why *In the Land of the Deaf* is preferable from a Disability Studies perspective. Firstly, the Chinese films both make the distinction between the "deaf world" and the "normal world," whereas the French film makes a distinction between "deaf people" and "hearing people" (161–164). Secondly, *In the Land of the Deaf* takes deaf people as the main narrative thread thus making it a true "Deaf film," whereas the focus on the hearing characters Wen Zhi and Sun Liying diffuses the significance of Deaf issues in the Chinese films (164). Thirdly, the full, natural signing used in *In the Land of the Deaf* demonstrates that this is the language through which deaf people communicate among themselves and with hearing people, whereas the often simplistic signing seen in *Silent River* is frequently interspersed with spoken dialogue and narration and is, therefore, done primarily for narrative effect (165–68). And, finally, many of the apparently positive aspects of the Chinese films discussed earlier in this essay may arguably be mere "tokenism" (168–173).

Taken purely from a Disability Studies perspective it is difficult to argue with many of Zhang's findings. There are indeed vast differences in the ways in which these three films portray deafness. Highlighting what are perceived to be appropriate and inappropriate ways of discussing these issues in China is one important way of de-stigmatizing disability and difference now and in the future. However, putting aside the fact that Zhang is attempting to compare two quite different genres, the conclusion that the Chinese films founder simply because of their inability to match *In the Land of the Deaf*'s affirmative articulation of French Deaf Culture wholly disregards the differences in cultural constructions of disability and deafness between the two countries that existed in the late 1990s and persist today, albeit in increasingly less pronounced ways. It ignores many developments relating to disability in contemporary China, such as the thriving Chinese Sign Language classroom revealed in the films that would have been unthinkable even a few years before. Situating the films firmly within the socio-cultural milieu of their production, as I have done here, reveals this and other hitherto overlooked but important aspects of the way in which deaf and disabled identities were formed and negotiated through Chinese cultural narratives at the turn of the twenty-first century. *Breaking the Silence* and *Silent River* reflect a range of experiences faced by deaf children and their parents as they navigate their way through the school system to the world beyond at a time when Chinese society was being transformed by both internal and external forces. While neither mainstream nor special schooling are depicted as providing all the answers, both films concur on the fact that education was perceived to be a critical point in determining opportunities in later life. Equally importantly, the films challenged, and very much continue to challenge, their audiences to consider not only the implications of different types of schooling for children with special needs but also society's assumptions on the way deaf and disabled people are perceived and treated more generally.[10]

By resisting the temptation to approach these films solely with contemporary understandings developed largely in the Western context, we can begin to unravel the fluidity and complexity of disabled identities through an understanding of the particular social and ideological narratives of deafness and disability that frame them, but are also interrogated by them. There is still some time to go before we see what might be termed a fully "Deaf-centric" big-screen film (Hartzell) in China; however, in the ten or so years since the appearance of the two films analyzed here, developments in the Chinese documentary scene have begun to produce films that reflect a more enhanced awareness of disability consciousness. These too still need to be analyzed carefully with the knowledge that disability can be experienced and lived in a multitude of different ways, not just in different countries, but also within China itself.

Notes

1. I am indebted to Tim Wright and Hugo Dobson for their immensely helpful suggestions, Clara Galeeazi for sharing her unpublished dissertation, and Yang Junhui for her assistance in sourcing a piece of research.
2. These included injuries sustained during war and revolution, as well as miraculous "cures" attributed to the power of Chairman Mao's thought.
3. My article "Screening Disability" includes an annotated index of films produced from 1977 to 2007. For an updated version of the index, see Galeeazi 53–55.
4. The rural situation was considerably different as negative attitudes towards educating girls meant that deaf daughters would have had *even less* access to education (Callaway *Deaf Children* 35).
5. See "Zhongguo long jiaoyu" for a chronological list of significant milestones and events in deaf education.
6. Sign-supported or signed Chinese, which follows the rules of spoken standard Chinese (and is, therefore, also sometimes referred to as grammatical sign language), has been considered the legitimate form of sign language by teachers (the majority of whom have traditionally been hearing, although this is changing), the CDPF and China Association of the Deaf, since attempts were made in the 1990s to unify sign language through the promotion of a lexicon based predominantly on signs taken from the major Beijing and Shanghai sign language dialects. Confusingly, both this *and* the dialects or natural sign languages that continue to be used as the preferred method of communication between deaf people are commonly referred to as Chinese Sign Language (*Zhongguo shouyu*) by their respective proponents. For a brief summary, see Xiao and Yu 44–45.
7. Reminiscent to some extent of Callaway's observations, elements from both natural and grammatical forms are observable.
8. Main melody films are Government-sanctioned films characterized by a strong pedagogical and ideological messages that (re)affirm official narratives.
9. Xu Zeming (who plays himself in the film) came to the attention of the local police in a manner similar to Zhang Che. He was taken on as something resembling a special constable and was subsequently commended as a National Blind/Deaf/Speech-impaired Advanced Worker and National Self-Strengthening Model. Contrary to his appearance in the film, however, sources reveal that, because of his "physical disability," he has never worn an official uniform ("Xu Zeming").
10. *Silent River*, for example, is still listed as recommended viewing for disabled people and those who work with disabled people ("Zuo hao xuanchuan") and was shown on the CCTV Film channel two days prior to the start of the Paralympics in 2008 ("*Wu sheng de he*: tamen zhen de hen mei").

Works Cited

Barker, Clare, and Stuart Murray. "Disabling Postcolonialism: Global Disability Cultures and Democratic Criticism." *Journal of Literary & Cultural Disability Studies* 4.3 (2010): 219–236. Web.

Biggs, Cassie. *A Bilingual and Bicultural Approach to Teaching Deaf Children in China*. Beijing: UNICEF, 2004. Print.

Branson, Jan, and Don Miller. *Damned for Their Difference: The Cultural Construction of Deaf People as Disabled: A Sociological History*. Washington, DC: Gallaudet University Press, 2002. Print.

Brueggemann, Brenda. *Deaf Subjects: Between Identities and Places*. New York: New York University Press, 2009. Print.

Callaway, Alison. "Constructing Deafness in a Different Culture: Perspectives from China." *Deafness and Development: Learning from Projects with Deaf Children and Deaf Adults in Developing Countries*. Ed. Alison Callaway. Bristol: University of Bristol, 2001. 68–73. Print.

_____. *Deaf Children in China*. Washington, DC: Gallaudet University Press, 2000. Print.

CDPF. "Zhongguo canlian da shiji (2000 nian) [Great achievements of the CDPF (2000)]." cdpf.org.cn, no date. Web. 25 August 2011.

Corker, Mairian. *Deaf and Disabled or Deafness Disabled? Towards a Human Rights Perspective*. Buckingham: Open University Press, 1998. Print.

Darke, Paul. "No Life Anyway: Pathologizing Disability on Film." *The Problem Body: Projecting Disability on Film*. Eds. Sally Chivers and Nicole Markotić. Columbus: Ohio State University Press, 2010. 97–107. Print.

Dauncey, Sarah. "Screening Disability in the PRC: The Politics of Looking Good." *China Information* 21.3 (2007): 479–504. Print.

_____. "*Three Days to Walk*: A Personal Story of Life Writing and Disability Consciousness in China." *Disability and Society* 27.3 (2012): 311–323. Print.

Davis, John, and Nick Watson. "Countering Stereotypes of Disability: Disabled Children and Resistance." *Disability/Postmodernity: Embodying Disability Theory*. Eds. Mairian Corker and Tom Shakespeare. London: Continuum, 2002. 159–174. Print.

Galeeazi, Clara. "Refashioning the National Body: Politics, Market and the Representation of Disability in Contemporary Chinese Cinema." MA thesis, School of Oriental and African Studies, 2009. Print.

Hartzell, Adam. "The Deaf Film Festival." *The Film Journal* 5 (2003). Web.

Hu, Ke. "Youyi de tansuo — jianping *Wu sheng de he* de bianju [Beneficial exploration — a brief critique of the writing of *Silent River*]." *Dangdai dianying* [Contemporary Cinema] 102 (2001): 4–7. Web.

Johnson, Kathryn, Richard Lytle, and Jun Hui Yang. "Deaf Education and the Deaf Community in China: Past, Present and Future." *Deaf People Around the World: Educational and Social Perspectives*. Eds. Donald F. Moores and Margery S. Miller. Washington, D.C.: Gallaudet University Press, 2009. 17–32. Print.

Knight, Deirdre Sabina. "Madness and Disability in Contemporary Chinese Film." *Journal of Medical Humanities* 27.2 (2006): 93–103. Web.

Kohrman, Matthew. *Bodies of Difference: Experiences of Disability and Institutional Advocacy in the Making of Modern China*. Berkeley: University of California Press, 2005. Print.

Lao, Ji. "Cong guoji dianyingjie zoulai de piaoliang mama [The beautiful mother from the international film festival]." *Sanyuefeng* [Spring Breezes] (2007). Web.

Lu, Sheldon H. *Chinese Modernity and Global Biopolitics: Studies in Literature and Visual Culture*. Honolulu: University of Hawaii, 2007. Print.

Mitchell, David T., and Sharon L. Snyder. *Narrative Prosthesis: Disability and the Dependencies of Discourse*. Ann Arbor: University of Michigan Press, 2000. Print.

Morris, Jenny. *Pride Against Prejudice: A Personal Politics of Disability*. London: Women's Press, 1991. Print.

Ning, Jingwu. "*Wu sheng de he* huo qita [*Silent River* and others]." *Dianying yishu* [Film Art] 3 (2001): 59–60. Web.

Piaoliang mama [*Breaking the Silence*]. Dir. Sun Zhou. Widesight Entertainment, 2000. DVD.

Riep, Steven L. "Blindness and Insight: Global Views and Local Visions of Visual Disabilities in Recent Chinese Cinema." *Proceedings of the Conference on National, Transnational and International Chinese Cinema and Asian Cinema in the Context of Globalization (Beijing and Shanghai)* vol. I (June 2005): 161–167. Print.

Schuchman, John S. *Hollywood Speaks: Deafness and the Film Entertainment Industry*. Urbana: University of Illinois Press, 1999. Print.

UNESCO. *EFA Global Monitoring Report 2010: Reaching the Marginalised*. Oxford: Oxford University Press, 2010.

Wang, Yichuan. "Feichang ren dui zhengchang ren de wenhua fanzhu [Cultural reverse assistance offered by exceptional people to normal people]." *Dangdai dianying* [Contemporary Cinema] 102 (2001): 17–19. Web.

Wu sheng de he [*Silent River*]. Dir. Ning Jingwu. GZ Beauty, 2000. DVD.

"*Wu sheng de he*: tamen zhen de hen mei! [*Silent River*: They are really wonderful!" insun.com.cn, no date. Web. 30 Aug. 2011.

Xiao, Xiaoling, and Ruiling Yu. "Sign-language Interpreting in China: A Survey." *Interpreting Chinese, Interpreting China*. Ed. Robert Setton. Amsterdam: John Benjamins, 2011. 29–54. Print.

Xu, Jiang. "Canjiren de ticai bu hui guoshi [Disabled people are not an obsolete topic]." *Sanyuefeng* [Spring Breezes] 11 (2005): 18. Web.

"Xu Zeming—longya 'jingcha' de chuanqi rensheng [The amazing story of the deaf 'policeman' Xu Zeming]." news.qq.com, no date. Web. 30 Aug. 2011.

Zhang, Jin."*Wu sheng de he*— zhong wai longren ticai dianying zhong de wenhua yiwei [Cultural meanings in foreign and Chinese films about deaf people —*Silent River*]." *Longren wenhua gailun* [An Introduction to Deaf Culture]. Ed. Zhang Ningsheng. Zhengzhou: Zhengzhou University Press, 2010. 156–173. Print.

"Zhongguo long jiaoyu da shiji—lanbiao (1993–2004) [List of the major achievements in deaf education 1993–2004]." chinadeaf.org, 28 Apr. 2008. Web. 26 July 2011.

"Zuo hao xuanchuan wenhua tiyu gongzuo. Cujin canjiren shiye quanmian fazhan [Advertise cultural and sporting projects. Promote comprehensive development in disability work]." zunyi.gov.cn, 2 Mar. 2009. Web. 30 Aug. 2011.

Modernity's Rescue Mission

Postcolonial Transactions of Disability and Sexuality[1]

EUNJUNG KIM AND MICHELLE JARMAN

This essay considers the unique disability narratives in two contemporary international films, *Princess Mononoke* (USA, 1999; *Mononoke Hime,* Japan, 1997, Miyazaki Hayao), and *The Good Woman of Bangkok* (Australia, 1991, Dennis O'Rourke) to investigate the formation of national identity and the negotiation of international exchange. We explore the intervention of subaltern subjects through a discussion of Mononoke's gender and feralness juxtaposed with the social positioning of prostitutes and lepers in *Princess Mononoke,* as well as through an intersectional analysis of Yaiwalak Chonchanakun's gender, visual impairment, and prostitute status in *Good Woman.* While these narratives are enacted upon different historical stages, both films display a similar logic that positions modern society above nature or any pre-existing civilizations — a logic solidified by specific deployments of disability and other subaltern designations.

Disability studies scholarship has developed strong critiques of many oppressive strategies developed under the auspices of modernity to diagnose, exile, institutionalize, normalize, or rehabilitate people with non-normative bodies and minds.[2] Characterized by a near-obsession with order and progress, people with impairments have been either actual targets or positioned as the symbolic focus of many modernization projects. Drawing from European and U.S. disability history and representations, for example, Lennard Davis's *Enforcing Normalcy* traces various ways in which the very development of the modern concept of normalcy has been based upon contrastive cultural meanings of disability. Modernity, in other words, has depended upon the existence of disability to draw the boundaries between accepted and rejected subjects. Socially positioned outside the parameters of cognitive and physical normalcy, people with disabilities in modern Western contexts almost inevitably have been caught up in systems of charity, rehabilitation, or institutional confinement. Postcolonial scholar Dipesh Chakrabarty makes this clear in *Habitations of Modernity* by asserting that the "origins of modernity" and the historical process of becoming modern were not benign: "The fact that one is often ushered into modernity as much through violence as through persuasion is recognized by European historians and intellectuals. The violence of the discourse of public health in nineteenth-century England directed itself against the poor and the working classes" (30–31). Yet even as disability studies scholars have developed critiques of modernity's oppressive medical, rehabilitative, and normalizing processes — especially those targeting the bodies of people with disabilities — these discussions have primarily focused upon situations in industrialized nations. Bill Hughes, for one, has argued compellingly that modernity has been central to "the transformation of impairment into disability" (155–172). Drawing upon the social model of disability, which distinguishes between the bio-physical nature of impairment and the social oppression of disability, Hughes sees the social rejection of people with impairments as a natural byproduct of modernity. Hughes, however, mainly focuses on the internal colonization of Western disabled people as part of the process of modernity.

In this essay, we want to shift this perspective to a more global context in order to explore the cultural deployment of impairment when two different cultures make contact at the point of disability. Specifically, we argue that Western or modern gestures to rescue people with disabilities in non–Western or "pre-modern" locations strategically function to produce hierarchies between different societies and nations. We are engaging with these admittedly problematic terms for two key reasons: first, to call attention to the highly constructed but powerfully hegemonic power of these concepts; and second, to point to the ways representations of disability tend to reify these binaries within and across national, racial, and ethnic boundaries. In other words, narratives of disability play a critical role in constructing hierarchies of "greater" and "lesser" development within and between nations. Trading upon modernity's mask of benevolence, these hierarchies are often signified by one group's charitable acts scripted as the "selfless" and "generous" rescue of disabled people who have been exploited, mistreated, or expelled by societies defined as "pre-modern" — that is to say, groups automatically coded by a relative "lack" of development.

This narrative trajectory is employed in the Japanese animated film *Princess Mononoke*. Disabled and gendered sexual bodies are used in part as agents in the transition from feudal Japan to a new hegemony that embraces modern social systems such as industrialization, gendered division of labor, institutionalization of people with diseases, and the militarization of men and women. In the context of the film, the community that has risen up against the existent power of the emperor strategically initiates projects to help marginalized populations in order to position itself as more humane than feudal society. Lady Eboshi, the monarch driving this modernizing vision, promises integration and greater equality to previously oppressed groups of lepers and prostitutes in her utopian community. In practice, however, her social structure segregates these people in new ways, in spite of their being central to her enterprise. Using claims of inclusion and cure, she justifies new forms of violence against natural forces, the need for expanded weaponry, and a tacit hierarchy positioning her as the benevolent and protective leader. In effect, her assumption of power is built upon specific groups' differences and supported by their dependence upon her. Although the film concludes with the restoration of harmony between humans and nature, our analysis focuses on the logic of the new community leading up to the conflict between nature and modern industrialization.

The second film we examine, the widely known documentary *The Good Woman of Bangkok,* also deploys the powerful logic of cultural superiority to blur the issues of gender exploitation within the international sex market through the process and promise of "rescuing" the disabled protagonist. In his filmic narrative of Aoi (Yaiwalak Chonchanakun), a disabled Thai prostitute, the Australian director Dennis O'Rourke strategically manipulates Aoi's visual (and visible) impairment to evoke a specific response from his audience as to the "double tragedy" represented by her "imperfect" body and her participation in sexual labor. Even as he attempts to reveal his involvement in her exploitation — both as her paying sexual partner, and as the director who positions her as the subject/object of his "compassionate" film — he invokes her history of disability to hint at an original innocence in Aoi. O'Rourke implies that her unique misfortunes, stemming from childhood social rejection and adult prostitution, render her more sympathetic to (mostly Western) viewers, and perhaps more deserving of rescue. Our point is that *Good Woman* purposefully dramatizes the victimization of its disabled protagonist to blur the exploitation enacted in the process of filmmaking itself, and as a result, the film suggests that Aoi's social structures are more cruel and "uncivilized" than those of its first-world viewers. While these two films differ significantly, they both exemplify powerful ways that narratives of modernity's humanitarianism and charitable rescue — especially of disabled and sexually exploited people of color — serve and cloak modernist imperialist tendencies.

Justifying Development Through "Utopian" Segregation

Miyazaki Hayao's *Princess Mononoke* unfolds in an indeterminate historical moment of medieval Japan, where a troubling tension exists between industrialization, feudal tradition, and the natural order. At the opening of the film, Ashitaka, a young prince from a far eastern community, tries to stop a monster boar from destroying his whole village. Although successful in killing the boar, Ashitaka is wounded and left with a scar, which functions as a fatal curse. However, the village oracle tells Ashitaka that the boar beast came from the far west where calamity has fallen, and that by traveling there he might find a way to lift the curse. She also gives Ashitaka the piece of metal found inside the body of the boar, which had transformed it into a monster. As the audience learns, this piece of metal signals the invention of rifles, the integration of armaments into war, and an imbalanced destruction of the natural world. The transformation of the boar into an almost unconquerable force of devastation, then, signals nature's response to this misuse of power.

In due course, the prince journeys to the west where he discovers the source of the metal in Tataraba, an iron- and weapon-making encampment situated high on a protected plateau and run by Lady Eboshi. When Ashitaka explains his curse to Lady Eboshi, she remains unsympathetic. However, she reveals to him what she refers to as her "secret" in order to justify her continued destruction of nature. As Eboshi leads Ashitaka to her garden, an aerial perspective provides viewers with an understanding of the spatial structure of Tataraba: the outer area is reserved for men bringing supplies and performing peripheral labor; in the middle of the fortress, women who have been rescued from brothels by Eboshi do the grinding work of keeping the smelting furnace running; and in the deepest secluded corner, nestled at the edge of the cliff and guarded by lepers, is Eboshi's secret garden.

In a cloister on the far side of the garden, she shows Ashitaka her new guns designed by lepers — a new technology that will enable them to rule over nature. Eboshi tells them she wants the guns to be small and light enough for the women, so they can become soldiers in her two-pronged struggle against the nature gods and feudal samurai warriors. At this point, her secret remains unclear to Ashitaka, and at the sight of the guns, his burning scar causes him to become enraged: "You stole the boar's woods and made a monster of him. Now will you breed new hatred with those guns?" His cursed arm, now possessed and animated by the boar's rage, becomes infuriated with Eboshi when she admits she was the one who shot the boar, but Ashitaka restrains his right arm with all his strength. To mediate this conflict, the chief leper, Osa, tells Ashitaka not to harm the lady because she has been the only person willing to care for them, and to treat them as human beings. Eboshi's humane rescue of the lepers — who are seen as cursed — is revealed as her secret, and through Osa's identification with Ashitaka as a cursed person, this secret effectively subdues the prince's resentment. Notably, the chief leper's testimony about Eboshi provides the revelation of her benevolence. While her own claims of kindness could be construed as manipulative, Osa's narrative performatively constructs Eboshi's efforts as purely humanitarian and altruistic.

The fact that Eboshi's society establishes itself through discovering, collecting, and rescuing prostitutes and lepers from moral condemnation in feudal society suggests that constructions of disability are foundational to solidifying and promoting her modernizing project. Eboshi embraces an enlightenment reasoning by disregarding ancient laws and curses toward prostitutes and lepers. At the same time, she also exploits the stigma of disability to further her modernist initiatives by using her protection of these vulnerable groups to justify violence against nature, increased industrialized labor, and technological advancement in weaponry to support her war against her pre-modern foes. With this in mind, we would like to consider the following questions: How are we to think through scenes depicting historical transitions where disabled people are enshrined in the deepest seclusion but also considered essential to cultural progress? What value is exchanged in the relocation of disabled people and prostitutes — a process seemingly imperative to new social economic formulations?

We want to point out that the existence and rescue of lepers carries specific cross-cultural meanings. In *Madness and Civilization,* Foucault observes that as a result of segregation and confinement, leprosy ostensibly disappeared from the Western world (and Western consciousness) at the end of the Middle Ages. Historian Zachary Gussow argues that leprosy "re-emerges" in the non–Western world as a result of the political activities which situated leprosy as a disease of inferior others, a designation which invited international intervention. This reformulation, Gussow continues, was directly tied to the "interests of imperialistic movements" (19). The projection of this stigmatized disease onto other cultures works in two directions: it further conceals the disease's existence in the Western world, and lepers in colonized spaces become overly representative of their own cultures, a process which further constructs Western power.

In order for leprosy to disappear from Western thought, Foucault points out, practices of exclusion remained intact. This continuing structure pursued a "rigorous division which is social exclusion"— but this modern exclusion also depended upon the promise of "spiritual reintegration" (7). *Princess Mononoke* demonstrates how salvation by exclusion sustains Eboshi's segregated community. This new female- and disability-centered "utopian" community relies upon, and thus reinforces, the mistreatment of these people in the outside world. Eboshi's cloistered community is constructed around protecting its citizens from the hostilities of the outside world, but for this to be successful, these external threats must be continually remembered and reactivated. In effect, although Eboshi claims benevolence, her segregated community enacts the rationale of modern institutionalization, which promises protection to vulnerable populations, but actually serves a greater mission of protecting "normal" society from contact with its marked others.

This logic of segregation and institutionalization is mirrored by processes of internal colonization and imperialist expansion. The film gestures specifically toward Western imperialism in the figure of Eboshi. In the English-dubbed version distributed in the United

States, Eboshi is the only character with a British accent, an implicit reference to the legacy of European colonization. This cultural translation enacted by U.S. distributors of the film bears testimony to the persistent signification of Western imperialism. In their summarization of postcolonialism, Bill Ashcroft, Gareth Griffiths and Helen Tiffin offer a historical backdrop to the conflicts between East and West, as well as between civilization and nature portrayed in the film: "As European power expanded, this sense of superiority of the present over the past became translated into a sense of superiority over those pre-modern societies and cultures that were 'locked' in the past–primitive and uncivilized peoples whose subjugation and 'introduction' into modernity became the right and obligation of European powers" (145). Ironically, the strong subjects of modernity have been established through systems of "caring" for "weak" colonial and internally segregated populations. Moreover, this separatist society peopled with stigmatized exiles justifies a new economic system dependent upon a massive destruction of nature, which the film sets up as the antithesis of human-centered civilization.

The power dynamic between Lady Eboshi and the lepers is illustrated visually in a scene where Eboshi tests a new gun designed by the leper workers. Eboshi stands on the roof of their building, where she dictates improvements from above through a window in the ceiling. This scene clearly positions Eboshi as the ruler of the community and demonstrates that her power grows from benevolent care, through which she inspires the loyalty of "undeserving" people who otherwise would not survive in the "natural order." This power structure between Eboshi and her protected subjects is complicated by the existence of Mononoke, a feral human princess of the forest who resists Eboshi's violence against nature. Mononoke signifies the inevitable resistance to modernity's rejection of groups who refuse to or cannot be assimilated into its violent logic.

Lady Eboshi reveals this complication when she describes her plans for Mononoke to Ashitaka: "With the forest gone and the wolves with it, this will be a land of riches. That girl will be human.... Mononoke, the wild girl whose soul the wolves stole. It is said the blood of the Deer God will cure disease. It could cure these people and perhaps even lift your curse." Mononoke, who was abandoned by people and raised by wolves, fights with her Wolf God family against Eboshi to protect the forest and nature. Significantly, the name the village people have given her, Mononoke, means evil spirit, an appellation that reflects Eboshi's demonization of her feral nature. More importantly, though, she is perceived as evil for resisting their attempts to civilize her. Mononoke provides an important counternarrative, however, to Eboshi's modernizing project. As a feral girl who resists civilization, she demonstrates Ella Shohat and Robert Stam's idea that tropes of empire are not only repressive: they suggest that because tropes function within a dynamic discourse, "they also constitute an arena of contestation; each is open to perpetuation, rejection, or subversion" (137). By embodying the feral wildness of nature, Mononoke rejects the civilizing mission of Eboshi and attempts to assert the indigenous powers of the animals and the forest itself. In many ways, the feral princess might also be thought of as a figure of disability resistance as well. In resisting the regulations of modernization's bodily norms and embodied functions, she challenges the limits of variation such "progress" demands.

In the end, however, Eboshi's predictions prove to be accurate. Although she learns that partnership with nature will be necessary to her survival, her outright exploitation is replaced by a more systematic consumption. Moreover, the transition to modernity requires Mononoke to relinquish her feral status. She still remains outside the confines of the city, but she lays down her arms against Tataraba. In effect, humanizing the feral girl confirms and expands the project Eboshi begins by rescuing the prostitutes and lepers. Although Ashitaka still endeavors to find a way to live within nature without destroying it, in the end, Eboshi's cloak of benevolence succeeds in seducing Ashitaka into partnering with her to rebuild the community after the landscape has been demolished by human wars and Tataraba's continued battles with the nature gods.

Princess Mononoke reveals the parallel relationship between prostitution and leprosy in their shared taint of moral stigma. In this parallel, we see the closely attached cultural positions of disease, disability, and prostitution. Within Western eugenic histories, prostitutes have often been institutionalized and branded with indeterminate diagnoses of feeble-mindedness. Similarly, in *Princess Mononoke,* a feudal, superstitious morality is inscribed on prostitutes' bodies. Although Eboshi treats the women with respect, the men consider the former prostitutes to be permanently defiled, believing this moral taint will infect the ironworks or the village itself. Although Eboshi claims to be modeling a new kind of society, its hierarchical formation depends in large measure upon reinscribing the stigmas previously imposed upon the bodies of lepers and prostitutes. The men of the village can assume their own superiority based upon prior notions of stigma. At the same time, the women and lepers gain feelings of usefulness and independence through their important labor and "redeemed" social status. But all three groups remain subjected to Eboshi: the men lack her seeming compassion, while the others will always be indebted to her for rescuing them. In this formation, her power becomes naturalized as benevolent, a pervasive cloak of its hegemonic impulse.

Constructing Western Masculinity Through Rescue

Unlike *Princess Mononoke's* juxtaposition of prostitution and disability, *Good Woman* provides an opportunity to explore their combined effects and interplay. Parading the centrality of prostitution within an international sex market — which doesn't only exchange sex, but mediates the exotic, racial, submissive nature of its female laborers — this film also scripts disability as central to the "tragedy" of prostitution. Dennis O'Rourke has referred to his film as "documentary fiction," a term he uses to underscore the impossibility of achieving a pure "objectivity" as a filmmaker. Indeed, O'Rourke disavows claims to objective truth by revealing a complicated relationship between himself and Aoi from the outset: he has hired Aoi as a prostitute, and secured her participation as the subject of his film with the promise of purchasing her a farm.

Linda Williams suggests that by making their relationship an explicit part of the film, O'Rourke attempts to pose "the deeper and more important question of the ethical relation of filmmaker-john to client" (176–189). While we agree with Williams that O'Rourke deserves some credit for his transparency, in his construction of fiction/non-fiction, the filmmaker still carefully manipulates visual images and the chronological arrangement of the film to weave Aoi's story into the overall pattern of his film. In this structured narrative, we look specifically at O'Rourke's gesture to rescue Aoi, and how her intersecting identities of sex worker and "handicapped" person function to individualize the systemic issues of the international sex trade and position viewers (especially those identified with the Western, male filmmaker-john) as helpless to change the myriad problems depicted in the film.

This authoritative framing has been a major concern of many feminist critics of *Good Woman* since its original release. Some critics have traced how the film re-imposes an Orientalist, masculinist reading upon subaltern female bodies (see Williams et al.). As well, theorists have discussed the limitations of both feminist and postcolonial theories in under-standing the unique situations of subaltern women, especially those whose stories (like Aoi's) are mediated by a Western male gaze.[3] Martina Rieker points out that this mediation con-structs specific excesses and absences of understanding: "What is excessive in the film is the camera's voyeuristic gaze of the seedy red-light districts, the bars and the interactions between foreign men and Thai women within them" (116–22). This fascination with the locations of sexual transaction, however, curtails any substantive understanding of the multiple iden-tities of these women and the way they define themselves in relation to their worlds. Building upon Rieker's insight, we suggest that Aoi's visual impairment (she is blind in one eye) is figured excessively in the film. Notably, few of the critiques of *Good Woman* mention the film's preoccupation with disability, when in fact O'Rourke features it as a key cause of Aoi's marginalization in Thai society, and as we argue, exploits the narrative of her "hand-icap" to negotiate (and increase) her value as a cinematic subject.

Disability, in Aoi's case, seems to influence the filmmaker's need to intervene in her life by purchasing her a rice farm — a not-so-subtle symbolic offering to return her to an idealized rural past. Her visible impairment is also used as a filmic marker to distinguish Aoi from the numerous other women working in the sex industry who are scanned repeatedly by the camera. This gesture of rescue by a male Australian filmmaker to a Thai sex worker demonstrates a problematic fantasy of superiority — one directly mirroring the unequal power exchange of prostitution. Interviews with other Western customers throughout the film suggest that a similar mentality of benevolence allows them to frame their own par-ticipation in prostitution as economic "help." As one Australian young man states: "I feel sorry for them because they have to resort to what they do. I think it's best that we do go with them because what we give them is their life. So I suppose if we do this, then it helps them and if it helps them it's not so wrong." The film, on one side, exposes the fraught mentality of Western consumers justifying their participation in a politically and morally charged space. On the other side, what is notable in this framework is that while the director admits a similar motivation, he extends this problematic relationship by attempting actually to fulfill this male fantasy of rescue.

While O'Rourke calls attention to the flawed logic in such "self-reflexivity" — especially by revealing his own role as a "john" — he avoids analyzing the larger systemic inequality of global capitalism embedded in the transnational sex trade industry. Aoi's status as a prostitute with a disability in Bangkok is not defined by itself; it is demarcated within the contexts of the growing market of commercialized sexual services, the state and legal support behind it, and international tourism. Anne McClintock explains that in Thailand "prostitution inhabits a twilight realm of legal ambiguity." Prostitution is criminalized, but the male "tour operators" and "entertainment managers" are sanctioned within the loosely defined "personal service sector." In this intentionally ambiguous legal framework, prostitution benefits the male state and is administered by "a system of international euphemisms: massage parlors, escort agencies, bars, R & R (rest and recreation) resorts, and so on" (70–95). During her participation in O'Rourke's project, Aoi resided and remained in this interstice in which the negotiation, sexual service, and filming were all occurring simultaneously.

In *Feminism Without Borders,* Chandra Mohanty points out that international capitalism produces first-world citizen-consumers and third-world workers. She also formulates several questions pertinent to this discussion: "Who are the workers that make the citizen-consumer possible? What role do the sexual politics play in the ideological creation of this worker? How does global capitalism, in search of ever-increasing profits, utilize gender and racialized ideologies in crafting forms of women's work?" (141). In effect, unequal international and gendered power relationships are reiterated in several forms in the film: by the everyday transaction of prostitution, by a Western ideology of help demonstrated in O'Rourke's gesture of absolute rescue, and by the production of the film itself.

The film opens in Aoi's home village in northeast Thailand, where an overview of her life is narrated by Aoi's "Auntie" (probably a close neighbor, not a relative). The film presents Auntie's first description of Aoi as "handicapped": "From the start, when she was born she was handicapped. At seven, she went to school ... but she wasn't able to stay. She had to look after the younger children and work for her parents." During this monologue, the elder woman draws a portrait of Aoi's life in order to explain her ultimate work as a prostitute. Within the structure of this narrative, Aoi's "handicap" functions as an origin myth of sorts, implying that her ultimate work in prostitution is partly (tragically) a result of the stigma associated with her disability. In this sense, the film presents disability as evidence of her innocence — which contrasts starkly with the baseness (badness) of her fate of prostitution.

Following this introduction to Aoi, Dennis O'Rourke inserts his own perspective on the international sex trade as an anonymous Western man. As if tourists themselves, viewers are presented with images of an arrival board at the airport, views of Bangkok from the backseat of a taxi, followed by a long segment in the red-light district featuring naked women dancing in bars and prostitutes on the streets with foreign clients. At the conclusion of these several scenes, the following text appears on the screen: "The filmmaker was forty-three and his marriage had ended. He was trying to understand how love could be so banal and also profound. He came to Bangkok, the mecca for Western men with fantasies of exotic sex and love without pain. He would meet a Thai prostitute and make a film about that." From here, the film moves to the comparatively quiet space of the hotel room where the filmmaker-john turns the gaze of the camera upon the sleeping, partly covered, naked body of Aoi. This double relationship O'Rourke develops with his subject has a double effect upon their complex association: it allows him to repeatedly exploit the intimacy of their space, but also, even as he visually solidifies Aoi's position as prostitute and film-object, he calls attention to her resistance to these attempts at "salvage" as part of their ongoing transaction. In its depiction of Aoi's life as a sex worker, *Good Woman* captures a new form of imperialism, which occurs on the personal level in the form of commercial exchange, as the basic structure of the Bangkok sex trade.

Near the end of the film, in his first concrete statement (beyond a few prompting interview questions), O'Rourke interrupts Aoi from behind the camera with his formal offer to rescue her from prostitution: "Okay, I'm going to buy this rice farm for you, and I want you to stop working. It's time you started caring about yourself." O'Rourke constructs the film narrative to culminate with his gesture of rescuing Aoi from prostitution with this "generous" offer. However, this chronology is misleading because buying a rice farm for Aoi was part of the original agreement they made before beginning to film the documentary (Williams 182–83). O'Rourke portrays this offer as his spontaneous response to her despair, which functions to suggest that they have established some intimate bond. O'Rourke orchestrates the film in order to bolster the perceived goodwill of his offer by persuading the audience of Aoi's goodness — in other words, by demonstrating that she deserves to be rescued. He achieves this in two ways: he uses her disability as an unjust social stigma that propels her into prostitution; and he distinguishes Aoi from other prostitutes by positioning them as voluntary workers. This binary of forced versus voluntary prostitution is common in sex-worker discourse and filmic representations about prostitution, and perpetuates the idea that one group is more at fault than another. In Aoi's case, her disability is crucial to establishing her innocence, and positions her story as more tragic than those of the other women working alongside her. Thus the filmmaker's highly individualized "intervention" fails to acknowledge the structural injustices and dangers at work in sex tourism. Instead of investigating the cultural, economic, and imperial structure of the Thai sex market, in which the trade of sex is normalized as a major source of national income and actively promoted to foreign tourists, O'Rourke focuses his film on an individual — on Aoi's "tragic" situation and his concern for her health and survival.

After offering to buy the rice farm, he continues, "But Aoi, this life you lead will kill you ... I will do it [buy a rice farm] for you only if you go home ... Aoi, I want you to promise me that you'll stop." His demand and desire for control over Aoi only invites her resistance, if not contempt. Aoi's response reflects her astute awareness of the motivation behind his "kindness": "I don't like anyone to think I need their help. If you want to help me, that's up to you. But don't expect anything from me.... There are some things I cannot do. I am sorry. Don't help me if you want something in return. I don't need that." Interestingly, Aoi's reaction to his offer immediately follows a scene featuring a blind street band, in which one of the members announces with a microphone to passersby, "We are a blind band and we rely on charity." O'Rourke's comparison of the blind band's pursuit of charity and Aoi's blanket rejection of it again demonstrate her strong character, an orchestrated subjectivity which both invites and negates specific forms of Western rescue.

As a means of portraying the extent of her inner conflict, scenes in the hotel room are shot very close, often with a double image of Aoi, either from a mirrored reflection or her own image projected on a television screen next to her body. Within these intimate scenes, Aoi reveals the details of her young life. Although at the time of filming she is only twenty-five, she has much to recount: her husband leaving when she was two months pregnant, her father's gambling and resulting familial debts, her growing hatred of all men, and her dream of somehow leaving Bangkok to return home. The film transitions repeatedly from the raucous sex bars of Bangkok to scenes of Aoi's village — her aunt, mother, and son — to daytime scenes in the city with friends who work with her, then back to intimate interviews with Aoi. The transitions between the city and the countryside contrast the differences of urban versus rural worlds. Through this contrast, O'Rourke represents Aoi's wish to return as overly nostalgic, which implies that her daily life in Bangkok would render the final return impossible (also rendering moot his demand for her to go home).

In addition to providing her personal story, these close-up interviews allow the audience to gaze upon Aoi's eye, despite large glasses she wears to shield herself from this invasive gaze. At the same time, while O'Rourke puts her impairment on display, the fact that she is blind in one eye is revealed slowly. During a continuation of the interview with "Auntie," viewers learn more about her childhood experience of having an impairment: "People would tease her about her eye. She would cry and run home. By seven or eight she was so embarrassed she wouldn't go out to play. Her father asked her if she'd like to see a doctor and she went. But nothing could be done." Immediately following this scene, O'Rourke cuts to a very close shot of Aoi in the hotel room in which she is rubbing her left eye with a tissue, providing a visual close-up of her disfigurement. In fact, Aoi only mentions her impairment once during the film: "I am a woman with only one eye. And a woman who earns money for going with men." This fleeting statement of her identity as a prostitute with a disability comes as a voice-over accompanying a shot of Aoi standing on a Bangkok street in the daylight, looking off into the distance. Exploiting her look of despair, O'Rourke implies that her disability combined with her work in the sex industry represent a reductive "double victimization." Yet the statement might also be read as a self-evident explanation of her intersecting disability, gender, sexual, and cultural identities.

A final textual overlay concludes the film: "I bought a rice farm for Aoi and I left Thailand. One year later I went back but she was not there. I found her working in Bangkok, in a sleazy massage parlor called 'The Happy House.' I asked her why and she said: 'It's my fate.'" After making his gesture of rescuing Aoi from her "fate," O'Rourke transitions from third-person filmmaker to first-person narrator. He now openly resides in the action of the narrative, signifying some transformation within him and his relationship to the audience. Through this sudden shift, O'Rourke conceals his personal process of alteration through the film's singular dedication to Aoi's failed rehabilitation — which would have entailed "escaping" prostitution. Through the process of filmmaking, the director manages to claim a subject position, while his failed rescue abandons Aoi to continued objectification. In other words, his selfhood is established through othering Aoi, a process perpetuated by the film's negation of her agency in the social, familial, and economic negotiations of prostitution. In the end, the film implies that Aoi has ostensibly given up, or perhaps sees herself as too damaged to escape, and this pretense of closure allows the filmmaker to assert his "superiority" (which simultaneously proves to be void), and to confirm Aoi's "inferiority" through his failed rescue.

Conclusion

Within the narratives of *Good Woman* and *Princess Mononoke,* people with disabilities, prostitutes, and feral subjects provide material evidence for the necessity of external intervention in "unhealthy," "pre-modern," or otherwise "underdeveloped" social contexts. Although modernity "promises" a form of integration to stigmatized bodies, in actuality, these subjects are constructed as being in need of rescue from their own culture. In many ways, disabled and stigmatized bodies are strategically positioned to prove the benevolence of modernity, and as such, they provide those in power with the negotiating tools to further their imperialist and colonialist goals.

In a poignant moment, Aoi articulates her own understanding of this insidious power relationship: "My friends tell me that ... even if you have promised to buy me a rice farm, it's not a big thing. Compared with your film, it's not much. I'm sure you'll get much more from your film." Resisting the hierarchy perpetuated by the discourse of rescue, Aoi reframes the transaction as reciprocal by telling him, "I think it's all right; you're doing me a favor, I can help you too." Although constrained by the limits of her circumstances, Aoi's resistance to O'Rourke allows viewers to witness a reappropriation of her subjectivity through remaining in the sex industry. In O'Rourke's simplistic offer to buy Aoi out of prostitution, he obscures the challenges she would face if she left the city to pursue a life running a farm. In the process, the film is unable to portray Aoi's decision to stay in Bangkok as an assertion of agency, and instead implies that by refusing his offer, she is willingly participating in her own exploitation.

In parallel, the fictionalized *Princess Mononoke* situates Eboshi's colony as a protected, internally segregated utopia, but in order for Eboshi to maintain this construct, the threat to her rescued social exiles from pre-modern society outside Tataraba's walls must be continually reasserted from within. Feminist film scholar Poonam Arora argues that films depicting minorities of non–Western cultures, regardless of the cultural background of the film-makers, have often represented the "Third World" merely as Other. Within this context, those marginalized within the "Third World" are "positioned solely as the recipients of the viewer's sympathy, serving as one-dimensional symbols of the degradation rampant within the Third World" (295). Arora's argument has to be contextualized by the textual specificity of her analysis, but her insights into the ways symbols of degradation are deployed remain key to reading representations of disability across cultures. Narratives of disability interplay within an ongoing production of ethnographical Others for uneven global consumption and interpretation.

Martina Rieker interrogates *Good Woman* as the representation of a third-world Other through which the filmmaker seeks to encounter a transcendental experience: love (116). She asks, "What gets sustained and refigured in the attempt to locate a humanist essence within the commodification of human relations?" (117). To answer her own question, she suggests that O'Rourke's obsession with human essence and his uncritical engagement with regard to Enlightenment narratives leads to a reinscription of the legitimating structures of capitalist modernity (118). Problematic binaries such as Western/non–Western, first-world/third-world, modern/pre-modern constructions — which Shohat and Stam have called "tropes of empire"— continue to be deployed in these ongoing transnational constructions. Shohat and Stam point out that within colonialist discourse, familiar tropes of race, ani-malization, infantilization, the primitive, savagery, and the wild have been crucial contrasts to figuring Euro-Western superiority (137–41). Intersecting with these dehumanizing dis-courses, disability is often folded in as a constitutive element of such tropes. As demonstrated by these films, disabled people in "pre-modern" or "non–Western" locations serve to provide reliable ethnographic accounts of individual and collective experience, but these depictions persistently obscure the power relations at work within representation making. Unfamiliar with immediate social contexts, non-local audiences are induced to sympathize with minori-ties within other cultures, but at the same time, to interpret that larger culture as somehow inferior. In the meantime, as the spotlight shines upon the seemingly inherent connection between disabled people's marginalized lives and these locations of "underdevelopment," external audiences are able to displace or ignore the material experiences of disabled people within their own societies, and resolidify their own identities as modern, "first-world" cit-izens.

In both *Princess Mononoke* and *Good Woman,* the female protagonists resist — and thus expose — the violence at the heart of modernity's benevolent gestures of inter- and intra-cultural rescue. Like Aoi, Mononoke rejects assimilation into the structures of modernity. These films also powerfully demonstrate the ways in which disability has been deployed to invoke sentimentality toward marginalized people as a prelude to inviting intervention from Western systems and modern rehabilitation, as well as to mediate the hierarchical relation-ships among cultures and nations. Our essay has attempted to interrogate these often obscured discursive, cultural transactions of disability by calling attention to the exclusion, violence, and dehumanization enacted upon disabled bodies–especially under the guise of mercy, benevolence, or rescue.

As Bill Hughes points out, "When a person with an impairment encounters a discrim-inatory gaze — be it institutional or personal — she encounters — not a pure look — but an act of invalidation" (164). As we have suggested, the superficial inclusion offered by such invalidating gazes is to become recipients of help or aid. In this gesture of rescue, modernity actually reveals its determination to maintain the inassimilable difference of the object of its gaze. Even more to the point, these films reveal an important power dynamic enacted by highly industrialized societies in their relationships to differently developed groups and nations. As disabled people within such contexts become the narrative focus, the larger culture is often positioned as somehow "lacking" as well — as inferior to the contrastive, more civilized, benevolent and caring modern or Western cultures. Transnational narratives of disability often perpetuate this myth of rescue, a myth deserving much greater analysis and critique, from both postcolonial and disability studies perspectives.

Notes

1. We would like to thank Norma Field, who brought *Princess Mononoke* to our attention in her remarks at the University of Chicago. We also thank David Mitchell and Sharon Snyder who first introduced *The Good Woman of Bangkok* to us. We especially thank Nicole Markotić and our anonymous reviewer, whose valuable suggestions greatly improved the content of our piece. An earlier version of this essay was presented at the Film and the Problem Body Conference held at the University of Calgary in January, 2005. This essay was first published in the *Canadian Journal of Film Studies/Revue Canadienne d'Études Cinématographique* 17:1 (2008).

2. See Lennard Davis, *Enforcing Normalcy: Disability, Deafness, and the Body* (New York: Verso, 1995); Sharon L. Snyder and David T. Mitchell, *Cultural Locations of Disability* (Chicago: University of Chicago Press, 2006); Henri-Jacques Stiker, *A History of Disability* (Ann Arbor: University of Michigan Press, 1997); and Rosemarie Garland Thomson, ed., *Freakery: Cultural Spectacles of the Extraordinary Body* (New York: New York University Press, 1996).

3. Shohat, for example, has argued that although critical cinema studies has tended to critique colonialism, too often these analyses have suspended the subaltern woman theoretically between feminist criticism and postcolonial theory. See Ella Shohat, "Imaging Terra Cognita," *Public Culture* 3.2 (1991): 40–71.

Works Cited

Arora, Poonam. "The Production of Third World Subjects for First World Consumption: *Salaam Bombay* and *Parama.*" *Multiple Voices in Feminist Film Criticism.* Eds. Diane Carson, Linda Dittmar and Janice R. Welsch. Minneapolis: University of Minnesota Press, 1994: 295. Print.

Ashcroft, Bill, Gareth Griffiths, and Helen Tiffin. *Post-Colonial Studies: The Key Concepts.* New York: Routledge, 2000. Print.

Chakrabartry, Dipesh. *Habitations of Modernity: Essays in the Wake of Subaltern Studies.* Chicago: University of Chicago Press, 2002: 30–31. Print.

Davis, Lennard. *Enforcing Normalcy: Disability, Deafness, and the Body.* New York: Verso, 1995. Print.

Foucault, Michel. *Madness and Civilization: A History of Insanity in the Age of Reason.* Trans. Richard Howard. New York: Vintage, 1973. Print.

Gussow, Zachary. *Leprosy, Racism and Public Health: Social Policy in Chronic Disease Control.* Boulder, CO: Westview Press, 1989. Print.

Hughes, Bill. "The Constitution of Impairment: Modernity and the Aesthetic of Oppression." *Disability & Society* 14.2 (1999): 155–172. Print.

McClintock, Ann. "Screwing the System: Sexwork, Race, and the Law." *Boundary 2* 19.2 (1992): 70–95. Print.

Mohanty, Chandra. *Feminism Without Borders: Decolonizing Theory, Practicing Solidarity.* Durham: Duke University Press, 2003: 141. Print.

Reiker, Martina. "Narrating the Post-Colonial Everyday: An Interrogation of *The Good Woman of Bangkok.*" *Visual Anthropology Review* 9.1 (1993): 116–22. Print.

Shothat, Ella. "Imaging Terra Cognita." *Public Culture* 3.2 (1991): 40–71.

_____, and Robert Stam. *Unthinking Eurocentrism: Multiculturalism and the Media.* London: Routledge, 1994. Print.

Williams, Linda. "The Ethics of Intervention: Dennis O'Rourke's *The Good Woman of Bangkok.*" *The Visible Evidence Collection.* Eds. Jane Gaines and Michael Renov. Minneapolis: University of Minnesota Press, 1999: 176–189. Print.

Williams, Linda, Chris Berry, Annette Hamilton, and Laleen Jayamanne, eds. *The Filmmaker and the Prostitute: Dennis O'Rourke's The Good Woman of Bangkok.* Sydney: Power, 1997. Print.

Chocolate's *Ass-Kicking Autistic Savant*

Disability, Globalization and the Action Cinema

RUSSELL MEEUF

In the climactic showdown of the Thai action film *Chocolate* (2008), the film's heroine, Zen, a twelve-year-old autistic girl with preternatural martial arts skills, takes on a series of fighters put forth by the Thai mafia, culminating in a battle with a young epileptic whose mastery of the Brazilian martial art *capoeira* is augmented with powerful, unpredictable spasms. In a bizarre battle of different disabilities, Zen bests the youth by observing and then mimicking his moves using her uncanny ability to quickly internalize fighting styles. These kinds of scenes in which the hero, just before getting a chance to confront his primary nemesis or achieve his goal, must demonstrate their fighting versatility by facing a series of opponents with different styles is a staple of action cinema that usually affirms the bodily control and physical endurance of the healthy, able-bodied, typically male hero: the ideal modern, global subject. Zen is a more capable fighter than her epileptic opponent, but the two are also offered up as a "freak show"-inspired spectacle of bodily difference. Indeed, the image of two children with disabilities violently beating each other for the audience's enjoyment only highlights the darkest and most exploitive tendencies of the filmmakers' vision of a capable and powerful disabled person. And yet, the scene's generic disruptions also invite a broader consideration of the larger social exploitation and vulnerability of the body than offered by conventional action cinema.

Arguably the most pervasive and popular genre across national and cultural borders for the past thirty years, action cinema consistently links morality, national identity, and a celebration of ingenuity and individualism to the spectacle of a body accomplishing heroic feats. *Chocolate*'s twist on the genre not only gives us an unconventional hero — underage, female and disabled — but blends the fast-paced violence of the action film with the pathos-laden plot of the maternal melodrama. Balancing the two genres, *Chocolate* unsettles the normative assumptions of the body in action cinema, dramatizes the inequalities of globalism, and brings to the surface of the film the kinds of disability anxieties that are most often repressed underneath the kinetics and muscled mastery of the typical male action

101

hero. In contrast to the film's generic lineage, *Chocolate* envisions the modern, global subject in terms of bodily vulnerability and the social ostracism of non-normative, gendered, and culturally-hybrid bodies. Ultimately though, *Chocolate* contains this ideological rupture and its disability representations by closing with its melodramatic plotline, restoring Zen to her father and presumably her childhood, and confirming the triumph of globalization's humanity over exploitative local cultures.

Exploitation and Ambivalence

Chocolate is prefaced with a director's note stating that the film was inspired by a group of special children with a dream to "unleash the amazing potential of human movement that is not often seen in everyday reality" and to "encourage unconditional love given to the special children of the world." On the one hand, children with disabilities have long been exploited by media as a source of pity, sympathy, and emotional appeals for a variety of purposes, including — ostensibly — their own wellbeing (see Longmore "Conspicuous" Shapiro). On the other hand, *Chocolate*'s unusual focus on disabled children for an action film and its opening tribute potentially connect it to progressive social change within Thailand. In 2007, the year before the film's release, the Thai government approved the Persons with Disabilities Empowerment Act, which replaced a 1991 law and provides more legal rights and funding for people with disabilities. The passing of this law and its 1991 predecessor was supported by Thailand's highly esteemed Princess Royal, Maha Chakri Sirindhorn, who has been a vocal advocate for people with disabilities. In 2001 she accepted the Franklin Delano Roosevelt International Disability Award on behalf of Thailand for its efforts to create innovative policies concerning disability rights ("Thailand Wins"). In this context, the exploitive melodramatic appeal of the film points to very real shifts in material support and perhaps social attitudes, reflecting the complex relationship between melodramatic exploitation and larger cultural progress regarding disability.

The film opens with Masashi, a young boy fascinated and exhilarated by the world's imperfections. When an older Masashi, now a Japanese Yakuza working in Thailand, falls for Zin, a beautiful enforcer for the Thai mafia, they invoke the ire of No. 8, a leading Thai gangster and Zin's other lover. No. 8 discovers their secret love and banishes Masashi back to Japan, leaving Zin in poverty to raise Zen, her love child with Masashi, in a cheap apartment next door to a Muay Thai martial arts school. Zen is later diagnosed with autism, and Zin takes in Moom, a chubby and lovable young boy who helps care for Zen. When Zin is diagnosed with cancer and can't afford treatment, Zen and Moom try to raise money by collecting on debts owed to Zin from her days in the Mafia. At first they simply ask for the money, but when that doesn't work they discover that Zen has been internalizing martial arts for years by simply watching the Muay-Thai students next door (along with some Tony Jaa action films). Beating up several gangs of burly fighters, Zen and Moom start to collect from Zin's debtors. Meanwhile, Zin tries to seek out Masashi for help. His arrival back in Thailand precipitates a final showdown between Zin, Masashi, and Zen, and the thugs of the Thai mafia. Zin is killed in the fight, driving Zen to hunt down and kill No. 8. In the end, Zen is united with her father who will raise her.

Zen is a classic example of the trope of the autistic savant whose extraordinary abilities become an objectified spectacle and source of wonder, precluding any realistic articulation of the lived experience of autism. Within the context of the action genre, though, Zen's autism is effective in the film's attempt to introduce a disabled action heroine: it allows her the kind of intense focus known to be necessary for martial arts, lending her skills a sort of verisimilitude. During her fight sequences, some of her impairments appear to abate, heightening the impression that her autism is a plus rather than a minus — at least when it comes to defeating the bad guys. In this way, Zen is also an example of the stereotype of disability compensation in which people with disabilities are represented as having special powers and skills that make up for their perceived lacks (Longmore "Screening Stereotypes"). Ultimately, Zen's supercrip capacities are central to the film's pleasures, which are focused not just on defeating the bad guy, but on exacting a kind of social justice. Several scenes in *Chocolate* showcase Zen turning the tables on those who would degrade her for her gender, her poverty and her disability.

As Eunjung Kim and Michelle Jarman astutely argue in relation to *Princess Mononoke* (Japan 1997) and *The Good Woman of Bangkok* (Australia 1991), in international cinema "narratives of modernity's humanitarianism and charitable rescue — especially of disabled and sexually exploited people of color — serve and cloak modernist imperialist tendencies" (54). Rhetorics of saving, progress, and disability, have often functioned to draw populations into the structures of modern medical discourse and social policy while positioning "developed" nations as rescuers over "developing" ones in need of rescue. *Chocolate*, however, is largely ambivalent regarding modernity and the forces of globalization. For the majority of the film it depicts the gendered, disabled body as oppressed by the inequalities these forces have generated. In fact, the literal rescue attempt in the film by her father (a transnational figure) fails while the film is in action-film mode, providing a brief spectacle of swordplay before the father is wounded and Zen herself must exact revenge on No. 8 using her martial arts skills. In its final shots, though, the film returns to its narrative of maternal melodrama in which Zen's father does appear as an international savior, ostensibly transporting Zen to an ephemeral "global" world away from local Thai sites of poverty, injustice and social oppression.

Melodrama, Globalism and Social Injustice

Within the film's melodrama, Zen and Zin are constructed as tragic victims, despite Zen's empowered ass kicking. In fact, *Chocolate* exemplifies Linda Williams' claim that the spectacle of the suffering woman is the central vehicle in the generation of emotion in melodrama (270). After Zin's diagnosis, in a montage set to somber yet heartwarming music, we see Zin lovingly soothing Zen's tears and hear a voice-over letter she writes to Masashi describing her willingness to surrender herself to her role as Zen's caretaker. The melodrama of their situation reaches it apotheosis when the exhausted Zin, weakened from chemotherapy, is unable to maintain her usual routine with her daughter. Zen erupts in a tantrum, knocking Zin's wig off. The sight of her mother's long black hair, which Zen had often used as a source of comfort, now reduced to a few thin and mottled clumps, drives Zen into a screaming fit of agony.

Using Williams' concept of the "body genre" — genres such as horror, pornography, or melodrama whose pleasures and cultural relevance are tied to their ability to elicit visceral sensations at the margins of respectability — Sharon Snyder and David Mitchell argue that most body genres employ the disabled or monstrous body to generate such sensations. For example, killers often appear more frightening for their physical or mental disabilities, and threats appear more horrifying when they involve potential illness, impairment or disability. Arguing that disabled bodies effectively function as "delivery vehicles" (162), they posit that, "the extreme sensations paralleled in screen bodies and audience responses rely, to a great extent, on shared cultural scripts of disability as that which must be warded off at all costs. Bodies are subjected to their worst fears of vulnerability and/or the already disabled body is scripted as out of control" (163). Thus the centrality of disability and disease in *Chocolate*— both the sad burden of Zen's autism and the tragic suffering of Zin's cancer — provides the emotional foundation for the film's melodrama, deploying fears of the disabled or diseased body to produce the sensations of pathos on which the narrative relies.

The use of disability to generate fear and pathos links the film's action and melodrama sequences. For example, when the Thai gangster No. 8 learns of Zin's involvement with Masashi, rather than killing them he instead forbids them from seeing one another, banishes Masashi from the country, and then promptly shoots off one of his own toes. His loss of bodily wholeness serves as a constant reminder of Zin's betrayal — as he tells Zin later, he is reminded of the pain when he walks or runs. Later in the film when Zin violates No. 8's decree by reaching out to Masashi in Japan, he cuts off one of Zin's toes, an act of violence intended to both intimidate Zin and remind her of his own suffering. By linking internal, emotional pain with physical disfigurement, the film constructs the "incomplete" body as a literal manifestation of a scarred and traumatized psyche.

For Williams, though, the body genres do not simply affirm the dominant narratives of the body or bodily vulnerability. Instead, the appeal of body genres is rooted in their articulation of sensations that help pose — but do not necessarily resolve — cultural problems regarding the body, gender and identity. Thus Snyder and Mitchell argue that body genres typically use disability to help pose these problems, as *Chocolate* does. For example, the film's reliance on a common melodramatic narrative trope — being too poor to afford vital medical procedures — functions in complex ways regarding constructions of the "healthy" body. While there is no mention in *Chocolate* of actual social policies, such as the fact that Thailand has since the 1990s had in place a system of universal health coverage that should cover the poor, but often doesn't in practice (Suraratdecha et al.). Yet the film's depiction of this situation dramatizes a sense of personal oppression that suggests the perception of unequal access to health care as a fundamentally unjust reality. It does so in a world in which globalization has entailed the export of profit-based health care and rehabilitation services that have facilitated unequal access based on class and social privilege (Davidson 118). While *Chocolate* is a far cry from actual ideological critique, its evocation of vulnerability through raw scenes of Zin's suffering at the hands of cancer, chemotherapy and poverty opens the possibility of acknowledging the embodied tensions and economic injustices of globalization as a system.

Additionally, Zin's struggles to raise Zen are tied to the lack of services for Zen, whose need for supervision limits Zin's employment opportunities. While Moom functions as Zen's loving sitter, he resorts to hawking Zen in a street performance in which she shows off her extraordinary perception by catching balls thrown at her by the crowd, which causes her injury. This situation highlights the lack of educational opportunities or support for families with children with disabilities, which in developing countries may be tied to economic policies of the IMF, World Bank, and industrialized creditor nations. By forcing nations who have received economic development loans to privatize social services and adhere to onerous debt repayments and economic adjustments, they restrict the capacity for local communities to provide for their members. As Michael Davidson points out, "development" is defined only as economic growth, not social improvement, and "access" refers to new markets and economic opportunities, not access to social services (117). The film's focus on a single mother and her young daughter, moreover, reflect the reality that women, children and people with disabilities are typically the most vulnerable populations at the hands of global capitalism (Sampson).

This is not to suggest that *Chocolate* is actively posing a critique of the Thai health system, the state's support for people with disability, or global capital. While these economic and political realities are certainly the broad ideological backdrop that informs *Chocolate's* construction of the material world, this is not an anti-globalization film on an ideological level. Snyder and Mitchell are largely suspicious of the sensational and emotional work of body genres, rightly pointing out how disability often works to elicit fear and anxiety. But the pathos of melodrama can also be used to help express a different set of fears and anxieties, the fears of exploitation, injustice, and exhaustion experienced by the globally dispossessed. How might we understand melodramatic appeals that rely on often-problematic assumptions about disability as a source of pathos if they result in better social policy, reflect a broader cultural acceptance of the social injustices facing people with disabilities, and help articulate the experiences of vulnerability inherent in unjust social systems? While still recognizing the harmful associations between disability and cultural fears of loss and incompleteness, can the sensations of vulnerability elicited by the plight of disability also signal a much broader sense of the embodied exploitation of globalization that impacts and makes vulnerable *all* bodies?

Action, Capitalist Labor and the Production of Disability

The cultural problems and anxieties at the core of the film's melodrama are addressed (though not resolved) through the adrenaline-laced fantasy of its action choreography rather than by a savior from global modernity. Though a victim in the film's maternal melodrama, Zen becomes a heroine who transforms the pathos of her oppression into the motivation for her violent retribution in the film's action narrative. This narrative trope, of course, is standard in the action film, which frequently relies on overwrought, melodramatic narrative devices as the justification for what otherwise might be seen as irrational or immoral violence (for example, see Meeuf). But rather than relying on melodramatic pathos to rationalize the self-righteous violence of a muscled male in a position of social privilege, *Chocolate* instead foregrounds the justified retribution of a cultural outsider against the social oppression that marginalizes her. In doing so, the film's action choreography draws attention to the exploitation of the body in global capitalism.

Like the Classic Hollywood musical, the emotional and ideological core of the contemporary transnational action film lies not in narrative structure or character development but in the elaborate spectacle of choreographed action. Typically, such action sequences rely on a highly stylized mise-en-scène of urban industrialization: skyscrapers, trains or subways, airports, city streets and alleys, nightclubs, factories, construction sites. *Die Hard's* John McClane must navigate and fight his way through a Los Angeles office building still under construction; *The Protector's* Thai action superstar Tony Jaa must battle hordes of anonymous henchmen in a multistory Sydney nightclub as well as in an abandoned warehouse filled with dilapidated streetcars and graffiti-splattered automobiles. Jackie Chan turns modern objects and urban settings into effective tools and elaborate backdrops for his acrobatics in his action films, offering a fantasy of mastery and skill within the spaces of globalization.

Similarly, the spaces of action in *Chocolate* are those of urban capital, labor and manufacturing. Zen faces attackers in an ice cutting and packing plant, a chocolate shipping warehouse, and an open-air meat packing facility. Each sequence foregrounds labor: production, processing, shipping. These are not spaces, though, that offer stylized representations of the exploitive labor practices of global capitalism in the developing world. The chocolate warehouse in particular, which produces a commodity for export, stands out as an apparently well organized, updated, and seemingly safe working environment, emphasized by its cleanliness and high-key lighting. In contrast, the shadowy ice-cutting facility and the dim brown tones of the fly-infested meat station, both of which appear to produce commodities for local consumption, suggesting that substandard conditions are local — not global — ones. On the other hand, this range of labor settings reflects the film's sustained concern with labor and the body. That bright, well-organized international corporate warehouses serve as visually dynamic spaces of labor and action alongside dimly lit, unsanitary, outdoor butcher stations suggests their systemic economic connections, as does their shared association with the Thai mafia. Taken together, they represent conditions of contemporary physical labor.

While the policies of globalization have a direct impact on the experiences of people with disabilities, the inequalities and working conditions of globalization also actively produce disability. From disease and impairment caused by poverty and malnutrition, to the injuries of wars fueled by the international arms trade or caused by industrial equipment, to the health repercussions of environmental pollution, the majority of the world's impairments and disabilities are caused by social factors, not nature or chance (Barnes and Mercer 141). This includes "workplace impairments, chronic lung disease, repetitive stress disorders and psychological damage caused by 'Fordist' modes of production and 'Taylorized' efficiency" (Davidson 118). If the typical action film provides the spectacle of a heroic body overcoming physical pain to tame the spaces of global capitalism, the disability-centric action sequences of *Chocolate* instead foreground the very real bodily vulnerabilities of capitalist labor.

Rather than obscuring such anxieties and realities behind the spectacle of the masculine, muscled, able body wreaking havoc, *Chocolate* instead allows sensations of vulnerability within capitalism to inform the appeal of Zen's martial arts mastery in complex ways. She is the disabled underdog who triumphs in the workspaces from which she is otherwise barred, yet her mastery is demonstrated through visceral images of her attackers' injuries within those same workspaces. These kinds of graphic images are not uncommon in action films — how many times have we seen Jason Statham break someone's arm backwards? — but in *Chocolate* they are suggestive of workplace injury by virtue of where and how they occur. As workers/fighters are crushed under palettes of boxes, diced up by ice-shaping machinery, and suffer innumerable slashes and gashes at the hands of butcher knives, the dangerous realities of capitalist labor to produce disability form the backdrop of our identification with Zen's extraordinary agility and martial arts skills. This dynamic is most prominent at the butcher station where Zen weaves frantically between the equipment uses for processing pork: meat hooks, industrial knives, boiling vats of water. As Zen slashes workers' torsos and limbs, pigs hang nearby, a constant reminder that the slashing and puncturing of flesh in the fight is a version of the everyday labor performed in that same space and its dangers. The film's anxieties of bodily vulnerability are produced in part by exploiting viewers' fears of disability and bodily impairment, much as Snyder and Mitchell argue that body genres typically do. But at the same time, I would argue that Zen's status as hero invites awareness of broader, intersecting realities of disability and inequality within global capitalism, both in her own person and in the spaces in which she fights.

Disability, the National Subject and the Global Subject

The reimagining of the typical global subject in *Chocolate* through the figures of Zin and Zen stands in sharp contrast to the vision of the able body and modernity in other prominent Thai action cinema, particularly the other action films of *Chocolate*'s director, Prachya Pinkaew. Pinkaew's Tony Jaa vehicles *Ong Bak* (2003) and *Tom Yum Goong* (2005), for example, center on the conflict between traditional Thai culture and the pervasive, corrupting presence of global modernity. Both films tell the story of a young man identified with traditional Thai culture (played by Jaa) who must venture into modern, urban spaces to rescue sacred objects from evil capitalist gangsters. In the case of *Ong Bak* a statue sacred to the young man's rural village that was stolen and taken to Bangkok, and in the case of *Tom Yum Goong* an elephant stolen by a Chinese gang syndicate in Sydney, Australia. In both films, the extraordinary abilities of Jaa's body to master the urban spaces of Bangkok and Sydney become affirmations of the health and incorruptibility of traditional Thai culture in the face of unhealthy and sinister global modernity. This theme is made explicit through disability in *Ong Bak* where Komtuan (Suchao Pongwilai), the evil gang boss who facilitated the theft of the statue, uses a wheelchair and only speaks through an electrolarynx. The result in both films is to firmly associate traditional culture and Thai national identity with a dynamic and muscled male body able to overcome the grotesque bodies and bankrupt ethics of the modern underworld.

So while Pinkaew's *Ong Bak* and *The Protector* evince a clear suspicion of globalism and rely on problematic visions of the disabled body to articulate Thai national identity, *Chocolate* places the audience's emotional investment in a motley crew that doesn't fit the national or global ideal. Zen's autism marks her as an outsider to the body politics of modernity, as does Zin's scar, her limp, and her battle with cancer. Even Moom enters the family because of his socially stigmatized body: Zin takes him in after witnessing a gang of boys beating presumably because of his chunky and awkward frame. The gangster No. 8 functions seemingly as the only mouthpiece of nationalism in the film, but this is a nationalism marked by xenophobia and social ostracism. He claims that Zin's cancer and Zen's autism are the result of her ethnic miscegenation with Masashi. No. 8's hateful vision of Thai purity and concomitant stigmatization of the disabled and "unhealthy" body shifts the film's focus away from nationalism as a solution to the excesses and corruption of global modernity and instead privileges the experiences of individual people with multiple affiliations and more fluid ethnic identities.

In the final shots of the film Zen stands on a seaside walkway under a vibrant blue sky with large turbine windmills lining the horizon, the wind blowing through her hair. Her father joins her silently and leads her away. The film offers no sense of where these shots might take place — Thailand, Japan, Australia, Canada, the United States — instead relying on generic images of nature and clean modern technology, positive markers of globalism. Earlier in the film, Masashi had forsaken his ties with the Yakuza in order to seek out Zin and Zen in a scene whose setting and blocking are structured to indicate his rejection of traditional culture and embrace of his multi-ethnic and "imperfect" transnational family. So the surviving father-daughter pair become a kind of a modern, placeless family adrift, blowing in the wind, seeking out a new existence for themselves somewhere amidst the "flows" of global modernity. The images of the clean, white, and environmentally friendly technology contrasts with the gritty, dirty, and dangerous images of industry offered throughout most of the film. So while Zen and Masashi are set adrift, the film leaves us with a sense of promise for the outcasts and the "imperfect" of the world within global capitalism.

With this ending the film works to contain the disruptive anxieties it had previously dramatized, using the resolution of the maternal melodrama — the sacrifice of the mother and the promise of a better future with a benevolent father — to revise its vision of the tensions of global modernity. That such a promise is associated with the father and not the mother reflects, on the one hand, the typical patriarchal bent in the maternal melodrama in which the mother must sacrifice herself for the good of her daughter and, on the other hand, the higher vulnerability of women in the global economy. Ultimately, by displacing the bodily exploitation and anti-disability bigotry onto the local or the national, the film envisions a new transnational family that moves freely through the bright and anonymous spaces of the "global."

Conclusion

In this analysis of *Chocolate*, however, I indicate how disability might function not as a crutch but rather as a transformative force within transnational genre conventions, disrupting the repression of the disabled body and turning the film into a site of contestation where ideas about the body, its exploitation, and its vulnerabilities within global capitalism can be made visible and sensational. In a globalized world in which the body is increasingly subject to a range of definitions, forces, and physically dangerous conditions, transnational cinema such as *Chocolate* brings these anxieties to the surface. While it does not resolve such tensions nor advocate for political change, it does elicit the kinds of emotions and sensations of vulnerability that lay bare modernity's exploitation of disability and the body, even as such disruptions are brought back under control by the structures of melodrama and the fantasy of a progressive globalization.

Works Cited

Davidson, Michael. "Universal Design: The Work of Disability in an Age of Globalization." *The Disability Studies Reader*. Ed. Lennard Davis. New York: Routledge, 2006. 117–28. Print.

Kim, Eunjung, and Michelle Jarman. "Modernity's Rescue Mission: Post-Colonial Transactions of Disability and Sexuality." *Canadian Journal of Film Studies* 17: 1 (2008): 52–68. Print.

Longmore, Paul K. "Conspicuous Contribution and American Cultural Dilemmas: Telethon Rituals of Cleansing and Renewal." *The Body and Physical Difference: Discourses of Disability*. Eds. David T. Mitchell and Sharon L. Snyder. Ann Arbor: University of Michigan Press, 1997. 134–159. Print.

_____. "Screening Stereotypes." *Why I Burned My Book and Other Essays on Disability*. Philadelphia: Temple University Press, 2003. Print.

Meeuf, Russell. "*Collateral Damage*: Terrorism, Melodrama, and the Action Film on the Eve of 9/11." *Jump Cut: A Review of Contemporary Media* 48 (Winter 2006). Web. 26 July 2012.

Mitchell, David, and Sharon Snyder. *Narrative Prosthesis: Disability and the Dependencies of Discourse*. Ann Arbor: University of Michigan Press, 2000. Print.

Sampson, Fiona. "Globalization and the Inequality of Women with Disabilities." *Journal of Law & Equality* 2:1 (Spring 2003): 16–32. Print.

Shapiro, Joseph P. "Tiny Tims, Supercrips, and the End of Pity." *No Pity: People with Disabilities Forging a New Civil Rights Movement*. New York: Three Rivers, 1994. 12–40. Print.

Snyder, Sharon, and David Mitchell. *Cultural Locations of Disability*. Chicago: University of Chicago Press, 2006. Print.

Suraratdecha, Chutima, Somying Saithanu, and Viroj Tangcharoensathien. "Is Universal Coverage a Solution for Disparities in Health Care? Findings from Three Low-Income Provinces of Thailand." *Health Policy* 73 (2005): 272–84. Print.

"Thailand Wins UN Disability Award." *CNN World*. 5 July 2001. Web. 7 June 2012.

Williams, Linda. "Film Bodies: Gender, Genre, and Excess." *Feminist Film Theory: A Reader*. Ed. Sue Thornham. New York: New York University Press, 1999. 267–81. Print.

Physical Disability and Indian Cinema

Joyojeet Pal

The 2010 film *Lafangey Parindey* centers on a dancer, Pinky Palkar (Deepika Padukone), who becomes blind before a major competition, briefly loses her faith in her abilities, and then is mentored back to excellence on the dance floor by the prizefighter One-Shot Nandu (Neil Nitin Mukesh) who caused her blindness in an accident and who specializes in blind-folded freestyle fighting. The film has an interesting mixed message. On the surface, it emphasizes the point that people with disabilities can achieve and overachieve in what may be considered a mainstream activity for the able-bodied. At the time of its release it was lauded by the popular press for Padukone's attempts at method acting for which she spent several months "[observing] a lot of blind people" to prepare for the role (*Daily*).

But not far beneath the surface of the plot lurks a hodgepodge of stereotypes cloaked by the storyline of a blind protagonist's determination delivered as a fast-paced romance. After the accident, Pinky broods gently over her shattered dreams of being a prize dancer and the guilt-ridden, thuggish Nandu decides to turn Bodhisattva by leading her to redemption. He starts by beating her and nearly drowning her in a vat of water, emphasizing that her desire to overcome her disability needs to be as desperate as the desire to breathe she felt when he was shoving her head underwater. The argument appeals to Pinky, who proceeds to rectify her disability by sharply honing her listening skills with the repentant thug who more or less eliminates any need for sight by giving her an A-grade Shaolin-templesque training on navigating with sound. The film ends on a note that not only suggests that the rectification of disabilities is largely at the will of the individual, but more importantly that the path can be revealed to the weak woman by an enlightened man willing to mete out some tough love.

Disability on Indian screen is not nuanced with mixed messages. From the occasional supercrip portrayal (Hartnett) of Deaf lip-readers and blind people with near sonar ability to sense objects to discourses of dependency around the pathos of disabled life, Indian cinema seemingly encompasses the range of canonical globally prevalent disability stereotypes. Our goal in this article is to examine screen disability in India and propose thematic buckets through which it can be understood. Mass media has a strong impact on how people imagine disability (Cumberland and Negrine; Norden). This makes our study one in which the lines between conceptions of disability derived from traditional social culture and religious texts blur easily with those derived from contemporary screen portrayals. Thus while

109

depictions of sensory superiority, such as blind crime fighters dodging swords, could arguably be attributed to the latter, a number of other portrayals such as disability as punitive or deserving of charity are attributable to a reinforcement of patriarchy that has traditionally come from Indian literature and culture. In this article, we focus mainly on four particular trends on cinema — disability as punitive, disability as dependence, disability as disequilibrium, and disability as maladjustment. We explore the roots of these traditional representations and discuss them as they are portrayed in cinema down the years. In conclusion, we consider some contemporary cinema that has departed from the trends we outline and discuss what this may hold for the future of on-screen depiction of disability.

Disability as Punitive

In the climactic scene of the Malayalam action film *Roudram* (2011), the protagonist (Mammotty) wraps up the film by maiming the chief villain (Saikumar) by nailing his legs under a car. He explains that death would be too easy a resolution by saying: "You deserve a life filthier than death. To repent for the sins you have committed, you must live with this half body, to crawl and feel the hell of life before you die. The scene represents an important punitive theme related to disability across Indian film and literature alike. The villain can pay for his misdemeanors through a simple death, or in the words of the protagonist, be subjected to a fitting ordeal.

Perhaps the most enduring portrayal of dismemberment as punitive is that of the Thakur protagonist from possibly the most-watched film in India, *Sholay* (Sippy 1975). In this film the Thakur police officer (Sanjeev Kumar) has his arms amputated by the bandit Gabbar (Amjad Khan). Unable to avenge himself, he employs two mercenaries to clean out the bandit's gang, but sets up a climactic duel between himself and Gabbar. He begins the duel by noting that even without his arms Gabbar is no match for him and concludes it not by killing Gabbar, but by crushing his arms with spikes. The punishment for evil is not a swift bullet, but an enduring disability similar to the one imposed on the protagonist.

The Thakur in *Sholay* is a critical starting point in the discussion of disability in Indian cinema because its depiction of disability has been parodied in a range of public forums. There have been entire television comedy shows that mock the character without arms, and a popular MTV joke features other characters in the film also losing their hands. Viral videos, often put together by groups of friends and even national advertisements by major corporations, reference the film. For example, Airtel, the country's largest cellular network, has an advertisement that mocks the Thakur's inability to type text messages; Monster.com, the international job search site, features the Thakur as a sports umpire who cannot raise his arms to make signals, followed by the catchline "Caught in the wrong job?"; and Channel [V] India's music television channel spoofs the Thakur's inability to make a "V" sign for a group photo.

One of the earliest films to use the theme of disability as punishment outside of a mythological context was the 1936 Bombay Talkies film, *Jeevan Naiya*. In a drive for social justice through cinema, screenwriter Niranjan Pal (who earlier wrote a blind character as the designer of the Taj Mahal in the 1929 orientalist classic *Shiraz*) used his script as a means of highlighting problems with traditional beliefs, specifically those related to Hindu orthodoxy. In *Jeevan Naiya* the lead character abandons his wife on finding out she is from a family of dancers (thus impure). He is eventually blinded in an accident, left without resources, and nursed back to health and happiness by a woman who, unknown to him, is the same devoted wife he abandoned. Thus, the character's path to enlightenment leads away from his flawed social conceptions and is engineered by means of a "punitive" blindness that sets him at the same level of social exclusion as the woman/wife of ignoble parentage.

One of the most important mainstream films on disability, and perhaps among the first that combined a narrative interspersed with some basic discussion of sign language and independent living for the Deaf was Gulzar's 1972 film *Koshish*. The film has four disabled protagonists, two Deaf, one blind, and a fourth who loses a leg in the course of the film. We examine this film in much greater detail in our discussion of dependence and disability, but one striking aspect of *Koshish* is the troubling turn it takes when the chief antagonist, the female lead's brother (Asrani), pays for his sins towards the Deaf couple by finding himself disabled. The focus on the character's remorse as arising from his own experience of disability is clearly an attempt to calibrate the narrative for popular appeal, but the use of disability as punitive in a supposedly progressive film about disability is telling.

This idea of disability as the ultimate punishment for a range of sins appears across Indian cinema. The philanderer (Rajnikanth) ends up in a wheelchair with impotence that offers a fitting outcome for his lascivious ways (and therein also highlights the de-sexualization of the disabled) in *Netrikkan* (1979). The wicked father-in-law (Pran) is blinded in *Aadmi* (1968); the chieftain of a village of criminals (Pran) is disabled in a police attack in *Kasam* (1988); the drug addict (Kiran Kumar) is blinded in *Jalte Badan* (1973); the evil brother (Asrani) who torments his Deaf sister and brother-in-law is himself crippled in *Koshish*, which he takes as punishment for his acts; the rich, arrogant atheist (Rajesh Khanna) is blinded, unable to buy a new pair of eyes for himself, and eventually finds a benevolent donor only when he repents and turns to god in *Dhanwaan* (1981); and when the protagonist (Pradeep Kumar) comes to kill his nemesis (Iftikhar) in *Mehboob ki Mehendi* (1971), he finds him in a wheelchair and decides that he's not worth stabbing since he is already disabled. Allowing him to live would be worse punishment than death, a conclusion echoing the theme of *Sholay* (1975) that disability trumps death as the worst of fates.

The use of disability in terms of physical disfigurement has receded in cinema, but the theme was common when leprosy was more socially prevalent in India. A landmark Tamil film, *Ratha Kaneer* (1954) pairs western debauchery with consequent traditional punitive reprisal in the form of physical disfigurement. In its narrative, the foreign-returned protagonist Mohanasundaram (M.R. Radha) represents the depravity of western ways — alcoholism, sloth, pride, scorn for traditional values, and sexual promiscuity. His eventual end comes through leprosy, disfigurement, and disablement, which he accepts as a punishment for a life lived poorly and magnanimously hands over his wife (who he can no longer have sexual relations with) to an upright friend. The film ends with the erection of a disfigured statue of Mohanasundaram as reminder to all those who may choose to the path of debauchery. The storyline of *Ratha Kaneer* interestingly mirrors that of Samba, son of Lord Krishna from Hindu mythology, who became a leper in part because he was extremely handsome yet dissolute and was cursed with leprosy by his own father for his sexual debauchery.

The relationship of disability and punishment in Indian cinema is complex as disability can either be seen as punitive or therapeutic, where the tolerance of a disability is a form of self-abnegation that emerges as an act of redemptive righteousness. Both these ideas have strong mythological roots. The idea of self-abnegation most strongly resonates with Gandhari, the queen of Kurukshetra and wife of the blind king Dhritarashtra in the *Mahabharata*. Gandhari's father, King Subala of Kandahar (in present-day Afghanistan) receives an offer of alliance from Bheeshma, the head of the Kuru dynasty, an alliance that cannot be refused. When Gandhari finds out that her soon-to-be husband is blind, she takes a blindfold, ties it around her eyes, and never takes it off except once for the rest of her life (the reasons for which are debated). Gandhari's act of "'disabling herself" raises her in the epic from a mere human to someone with extraordinary powers (*Mahabharata*, Book 1, Chapter 103, Verses 12 & 13)—she is able to grant the boon of near invincibility to her son, she curses Krishna (an avatar of the Lord Vishnu) and eventually causes the annihilation of his entire clan. Her ability to do this is attributed to her status as an exemplar of a *sati* who takes on an ultimate sacrifice for her husband. In perhaps the most Gandhari-esque moment of Hindi cinema, the heroine Usha (Sadhana) in the film *Arzoo* (1965), in an attempt to equate herself with the hero (Rajendra Kumar) who has an amputated foot, places her own foot on a chainsaw.

The standard purely punitive view of disability in Indian cinema has deep roots from multiple sources in mythology and folklore. Among the most important and enduring are the figures of the sage Ashtavakra and the demonesses Surpanakha and Ajamukhi. In all three cases, disability is caused by some infraction, but the distinctions between the stories of each figure are interesting and go to the root of how disability is figured as punitive. Ashtavakra, whose name literally means "eight deformities," is mentioned in the *Chāndogya Upanishad* scripture, and was born disabled. His disability was caused by a curse cast when he was still in his mother's womb. As a young fetus, already very learned because his mother listened in on lectures by scholars during her pregnancy, he made the error of correcting his father, the sage Kahola, when he mis-stated some scriptures. For his act of filial impiety, Kahola cursed Ashtavakra with eight deformities for the eight times that he had committed this transgression. After Ashtavakra is born and grows up, he eventually redeems himself by proving to be a stellar scholar, following which his body is restored to one of perfection. This idea of redemption and the consequent restoring of the able body is a persistent theme in Indian cinema. We discuss this further in the "Disability as Disequilibrium" section below.

In Puranic myth, Ajamukhi, the sister of demon Surapadman, suffers amputation when she attempts to seize Indrani on behalf of her evil brother. Ajamukhi is the reincarnation of Chitralekha, a lovely but debauched Brahmin's wife who is cursed for her lust by a sage, Durvasa, to be reborn with the face of a goat. Thus the lustfulness and demonization of Ajamukhi serves as a setup that strips her of the qualities of ideal womanhood at the point of her amputation. The second character in Hindu mythology with an amputation is Surpanakha, the widowed sister of Ravana and the antagonist of the Hindu epic *Ramayana*. North and South Indian versions of the *Ramayana* differ on the physical description of Surpanakha. The North Indian variants note her as having thinning hair, a dissonant voice, being cross-eyed, and having oversized breasts, whereas the Kamban's south Indian version of the epic notes her as extremely beautiful. Surpanakha's key role in the *Ramayana* arises from her spurning by Rama, the hero of the *Ramayana*, and her subsequent disfigurement by Rama's brother Lakshmana who cuts off her nose in the events that follow her rejection. Surpanakha's fate ultimately leads to the war between her brother and Rama. Surpanakha's disability represents an intersection of both disability, punishment, and gender roles. Her condition is specifically attributed to lust and vanity, a theme that repeats itself in films where women who act against social rules are rewarded through some form of disfigurement. Disability and disfigurement as sexual punishment thus represents its opposite — "the perfect body" — as the trope of desirability. Thus the punishment for departures from the social norm in Indian cinema, especially for female characters, can often be some form of disfigurement.

An early example of a film where disfigurement is pointedly used as punishment is Sohrab Modi's 1958 film *Jailor*. This complex work represents disability in multiple ways. Modi plays a disfigured jail warden whose wife leaves him for a doctor. The wife and doctor are then aptly punished for this debauchery: the doctor loses his eyesight, and the wife suffers facial scarring. She is also jailed in the basement of her own home, kept away from seeing her own child, and eventually dies. The blind doctor, now a roaming mendicant, falls in love with another blind girl, who in turns ends up having her sight restored by the disability-avenged jail warden. Tamil filmmaker K. Balachander used the disability as punishment theme for women a few times in films like *Moondru Mudichu* (1976) where a woman (Vijaya) who lives by her good looks is disfigured in a fire, and in *Arangetram* (1973) in which the protagonist (Pramila), a prostitute, eventually loses her sanity. Likewise, in *Vazhayadi Vazhai* (1972) Pramila (who came to be typecast in "bold" roles) replayed the character of a wife who refuses her husband (and motherhood) to preserve her good looks, engineers a situation for her own sister to marry a disabled man, and both mocks her and causes marital discord. Her comeuppance at the end of the film has her ending up disfigured, separated from her husband, and symbolically lowered in status below her crippled brother-in-law. The specific use of actresses known for playing the roles that went against social convention is an interesting comment on the distancing of the "punished disabled" from the desexualized Polyanna-ish representation of the faultless demure woman, usually the hero's sister (*Saccha Jhootha* 1970, *Vishwanath* 1978, *Naan Vaaza Vaippen* 1979).

Disability as punishment in Hindu mythology is not solely related to individuals' sins in the current birth — a disability can also be "deservedly" acquired in the womb or in previous incarnations. Thus Ashtavakra "deserved" his disability from his scholarly vanity as a fetus and Ajamukhi's fate as a goat-faced woman came from her sins as the lustful beauty Chitralekha in a previous birth. In Surpanakha's case, she is reborn as Kubja, a penitent hunchback. Similarly, the punitive view of disability in cinema is often projected as an outcome of transferred punishment, thus the righteous are disabled for the sins of the evil. The consequent disability then becomes the moral mirror through which the evil are eventually driven to repent upon seeing the plight of the righteous, who bore the punitive consequences of their acts. The classic mythological case of this, of course, was the blind Dhritarashtra himself, who was born blind because his mother Ambika was so repulsed by the looks of the sage Vyasa, Dhritarashtra's father, that she closed her eyes during intercourse.

An early example of a film dealing with disability and its derivative punishment was Manilal Joshi's 1925 mythological/historical *Veer Kunal*, featuring action star Raja Sandow. Kunal, the righteous son of Mauryan emperor Ashoka, is blinded because of court intrigue involving his step-mother, but the film ends with Ashoka realizing that his own sins brought risk to his son's eyesight. Likewise, in the Hindi film *Upkaar* (1967), a wayward brother is eventually moved to regret his actions when his upright brother loses his arms for his sins. In *Kaalia* (1981), the responsible elder brother (Kader Khan) loses his arms, which turns out to be a symbolic punishment for the slacker younger brother Amitabh who gets his act together thereafter. And in *Sone Ka Dil Lohe Ke Haath* (1978), a father's act of murder causes his son to be blinded. In each case, the narrative's resolution occurs through an act of disablement that brings about equilibrium.

The corollary to the idea of disability as punitive is the idea of service for the disabled as a means of repentance for penitent sinners. The redemption of the thug from *Lafangey*

Parindey (2010) follows a long tradition of some of India's top leading men playing roles in successful mainstream films that use this theme. In *Prince* (1969), a bratty alcoholic womanizer Shamsher (Shammi Kapoor) is reformed when he has to pose as the son of a poor blind woman; in *Dushman* (1971), an alcoholic, foul mouthed man (Rajesh Khanna) is turned around by the experience of serving the disabled parents and family of a man he killed; in *Dada* (1979), a murderer (Amjad Khan) is reformed by having to take care of a blind child; in *Mera Dost Mera Dushman* (1984), having to live with a blind woman reforms a dacoit; and in *Satte Pe Satta* (1982), an assassin is unable to bring himself to kill his target — a woman in a wheelchair — which eventually brings him around to being a good man.

At the logical extreme of this trajectory, rectifying the disability of another can provide the ultimate salvation for evil. In *Hawas* (1974) the lustful criminal (Bindu) gets her redemption by donating her eyes to the hero's virtuous blind sister as she lies dying. *Suhaag* (1979) goes a step further as the villain of the piece (Amjad Khan) donates his eyes to the blind hero (Shashi Kapoor) in the last scene and accepts life as a blind man in repentance.

Disability as Dependence

Arguably, the persistent portrayal in popular culture of people with disabilities as unable to live independently has been a very important setback to the independent living movement worldwide. In Indian films, the idea of dependence on charity or on the largesse of heroic characters is quite typical. The following three films are critical examples because they underline the pervasiveness of dependence as a disability theme even when the disabled characters are key figures in a story.

The 2010 *Athmakatha* starring Premlal has two blind protagonists who work at a candle factory. The film has its moments of tragic romanticization around the death of one of the protagonists in a road accident that seems to highlight the dangers of being blind and traveling independently on Indian roads. However, overall the film portrays the protagonists as relatively independent, highlighting one striking fact that most films about vision impairment forgo — the protagonist (Sreenivasan) has no particular desire to be sighted. As the film progresses, we find that his daughter also shares his genetic condition, which will lead to her loss of sight. While her adjustment to this eventuality forms the crux of the film's narrative and the film ends with her losing her sight completely, she is entirely at peace with it. Through a range of strategies, including the use of stock benevolent characters and stereotypical situations (the protagonist is a candlemaker — a job visually impaired people are frequently "channeled" towards in training institutes for the Blind in India), the audience is introduced to a variety of strategies through which the vision impaired may complete their daily activities. Several of these are for effect, but the film still focuses consistently on the idea that someone who is blind may live a full life. That the filmmakers felt the need to say this and thought the story premise would make a good film is a good indicator of just how poorly the idea of independent living has been portrayed in Indian cinema.

The 1964 Rajshri classic *Dosti* features two disabled protagonists, Ramu (Sushil Kumar), who uses crutches to walk and Mohan (Sudhir Kumar), who is blind. At the start of the film, we see Ramu distraught — everything about the state works against him — cars cause him danger on the street, water tanks on the street have no water, people don't respond when he speaks with them, and the only person who does insults him when Ramu requests a job by saying, "What work can be done by someone like you?" Mohan, the blind youth, likewise enters the film asking people to help him cross the street to no response. For most of the remainder of the film, the two youths are shown as being in situations where their disability makes them deeply dependent for their basic existence.

Throughout the film the two youngsters are humiliated for their disabilities; students refuse to accept that a disabled boy is studying in a school, and crowds laugh when the blind Mohan claims his sister is a respectable nurse. To make a living the duo begs on the streets — Mohan sings while Ramu plays the harmonica. The film makes a distinction between the two characters and their respective disabilities when it hits a turning point: Mohan concludes that his friend has a future — since he can see, he can study and potentially have a career of some kind. So Mohan goes forth and ramps up his begging activities, eventually supporting Ramu through his studies and helping him to become successful in life. While Ramu slowly edges ahead in life, the blind Mohan's condition worsens as he is abandoned by his own sister and Ramu alike. The importance of the film *Dosti* cannot be overstated. Not only because of the cultural power of its narrative and its two leading disabled characters, but also because of the timeless appeal of its music. Songs from the film are regularly heard in commuter trains and streets where people perform for spare change. The song Mohan sings as a beggar is particularly common: "*Jaanewalo zara mudhke dekho mujhe, ek insaan hoon, main tumhari tarah*" (Passers-by, turn and see me for a moment, I am also human, like you).

While mental illnesses have frequently been exploited in crude terms in Mumbai and South Indian cinema alike, physical or sensory disabilities, especially of male leads, have seldom been the central theme of mainstream films. Gulzar's *Koshish* is an exception in which the male and female leads (played by Sanjeev Kumar and Jaya Bhaduri, respectively) are deaf-mute, and the third main character (Om Shivpuri) is blind. The film, often seen as a landmark in the portrayal of disability in Indian cinema, opens with sign language alphabet in its credits, and at several points the film takes what may be called an 'educational' stance to its audience by instructing one or another character in the film how a Deaf person may communicate, participate economically, etc. Though the protagonists in the film live independently, at several points their ability to do so is threatened by society and the people around them. An exploitative brother-in-law cheats and steals from them, their own infant child dies because they do not hear him cry, and they are frequently poor and generally depicted as kind-hearted unfortunates. Two sequences in the film are particularly troubling — when the couple watch their infant cautiously to find out if he is deaf. Initially they are much relieved when an aunt tells them that he can hear and speak. Later they run into a panic when they again fear that he may be deaf, only to find out to their delight that he is not.

At the film's climax, we find that Sanjeev Kumar's boss invites him home for dinner and asks him to bring along his son. The scene unravels when the boss offers his daughter's hand in marriage to Sanjeev Kumar's son. Sanjeev Kumar is shocked at first, and signs that there is a huge class schism between the two, at which point the boss confesses with tears that his daughter is Deaf-Mute and he is looking for a patient man for her. As he says this, his face crumples in shame, his body language changes, and the camera focuses on the girl's ears and mouth — ostensibly defective. At this point, Sanjeev Kumar puts aside the class difference and agrees to the marriage, but the son refuses emphatically because he does not want to be with a Deaf person. The ending is particularly disturbing for its combination of class and disability, implying that a disabled girl should expect a class adjustment if she hopes to marry. The boss's search for a patient man reinforces the idea of dependence on a benevolent hearing person for a successful life.

Perhaps the most important disabled character from Hindu mythology is Dhritarashtra, the blind king in the *Mahabharata*, and central character in the war between his sons, the Kauravas, and his nephews, the Pandavas. Dhritarashtra is complex because he has some traits that are atypical for disabled characters in Indian narratives. First, he is incredibly strong — at one point in the *Mahabharata* he crushes a metal statue to powder. He is also not desexualized — he sires 100 sons and one daughter. However, Dhritarashtra remains deeply dependent through the entire epic, on his wife, his sons, and his advisors. For the most part, the critical events in the story emerge from Dhritarahstra's dependence on the judgment of his advisors rather than trusting his own judgment. Arguably the entire conflict in the *Mahabharata* hinges on one key factor — Dhritarashtra's incompetence as a king, his inability to do the righteous thing as he is blinded both physically and metaphorically and only practices statecraft through his advisors. Thus, despite being the regent whose kingdom is fought over in the epic, he is sidelined as a supporting character to the battery of stronger sighted players — his uncle, brother, sons, and nephews.

Besides Dhritarashtra, the other key mythological character representing dependency in disability is Shravan. The slaying of Shravan is a particularly emotive tale in Hindu mythology, typically invoked to underline the importance of filial piety, but more specifically to underline the importance of the family in caring for the disabled. Shravan is not disabled, but his parents Shantanu and Gyanavanti are blind. As a dutiful son, Shravan spends most of his time caring for them, carrying them on his shoulders and tending to their needs. Shravan is eventually killed accidentally by Dasratha, the father of Lord Rama of the *Ramayana*, leading his dismayed father to curse Dasratha for having taken away their only support system. This curse eventually triggers the events that lead to the *Ramayana*.

In Indian cinema, disability is most commonly characterized in terms of dependence, particularly in those films where a disabled character is not the lead player, such as in *Atmakatha*, *Dosti*, or *Koshish*. These characterizations include disabled parents who depend on the goodness of their children or others to survive (*Avtaar* 1983, *Allah Rakkha* 1985, *Jaydaad* 1989, *Laadla* 1994, *Zordaar* 1996), dependent disabled daughters (*Apradhi* 1947, *Patita* 1953, *Aai Phirse Bahaar* 1960, *Dil Tera Diwana* 1962, *Biradri* 1966, *Sharaabi* 1984), dependent disabled siblings (*Payal* 1957, *Apne Dushman* 1975, *Brashtachar* 1989), dependent disabled romantic interests (*Barsaat Ki Ek Raat* 1983) or disabled characters who are purely dependent on the goodness of random do-gooders for their survival (*Deedar* 1951, *Bharosa* 1963, *Marte Dam Tak* 1987). In some films, the disability/dependence relationship is the narrative framework through which the faults of modernity implode. Typically when an older male suffers a disability, such as in *Bharosa*, *Aap ki Parchhaiyan* (1964) and *Avtaar*, their usefulness in the family is immediately perceived as reduced, followed by their dependence, marginalization, humiliation and eventual ejection from their homes, usually by their own children. In such films, part of the extremely popular family melodrama category aimed at mixed-gender audiences, the theme of the disabled parent abandoned by ungrateful children, and reduced to penury and dependence on random benefactors, is not uncommon. These films stress the disintegration of traditional values, using the helpless disabled elder as the tragic indicator of decay resulting from the onslaught of Westernization.

Disabled women are particularly at risk. First, there is the recurrent theme of the difficulty of finding a spouse for a disabled woman and the burden this poses to her male relatives (*Santhi* 1965, *Thokar* 1974, *Saccha Jhutha* 1978, *Naan Vazhavaippen* 1979, *Bhairavi* 1996). Such narratives often feature men taking unusual risks to rectify the situation, like committing crime for a larger dowry, leaving a traditional home to move to urban locations for jobs, and so forth. With the unmarriageable disabled person theme, films often justify some unusually callous action. In the Tamil film *Santhi* (1965)—remade in Hindi as *Gauri* (1968)—a concerned father gets his blind daughter married to a man without telling him she is blind. The daughter is abandoned and considers suicide, though she eventually gets her vision back. Where such a parent does not exist, the alternatives could be worse, such as in *Dhoop Chhaon* (1977) in which Hema Malini plays a woman who loses her eyesight and is thereafter abducted and sold into prostitution or in *Jheel Ke Us Paar* (1973) where a blind woman is sold off as a wife to an evil man. She eventually has her sight restored, at which point it is possible for her to marry the kind protagonist who arranges for her sight to be restored. On the "progressive" end are films such as *Barsaat Ki Ek Raat* (1983) in which a pity marriage happens with a desirable groom, right after the bride's parent delivers a speech on "Who will marry my disabled daughter?"

The importance of a male protector for women with disabilities is commonly reinforced by highlighting the risk of sexual exploitation. Such exploitation of disabled women is frequently dealt with crudely. In films like *Imaan Dharam* (1977), *Insaaf* (1987), *Brashtachar* (1989), *Khuddar* (1994), and *Humko Tumse Pyaar Hai* (2006) blind women are aggressively pursued or sexually assaulted when they don't have a man to look out for them. Perhaps the most egregious plot belongs to the Kannada classic *Katha Sangama* (1975; remade in 1984 in Tamil as *Kai Kodukkum Kai*) in which a blind wife who is the sympathy wife of a rich man is raped by a thug (Rajnikanth in his first Kannada role). The thug then goes on to blackmail the woman, but all ends well when the husband forgives the wife and they live on. The bizarre interpretation of virtue signals two important themes which are remarkably common. First, that the act of being with someone who is disabled is essentially an act of social service. Second, that disability allows for certain anomalous concessions — the pollution of a wife's virtue by another man can be forgiven, but it takes a particularly heroic husband to do that.

Women who are disabled are frequently the object of a man's sympathy or protection, but a disabled man has a much more complex fate in terms of dependence. Disability is typically a proxy for a male character's failure to provide or protect. The underlying theme is the inherently exploitative nature of the social system, which means that men must act to their fullest capacity in order to fulfill their duties to family and society. Disability is figured as an inhibitor that prevents men from doing so. For male characters, the loss of arms has been a very important theme in Indian films, highlighting inability. Examples include the farmer played by Raaj Kumar in *Mother India* (1957), the woodcutter played by Suresh Oberoi in *Lawaris* (1981), the mill worker played by Kader Khan in *Kaalia* (1982), and the cab driver played by Farooque Shaikh in *Toofan* (1989). In each case, characters die after they acquire their disability. The farmer and the mill worker both suffer amputations and are thereafter shown as unable to provide for their respective families, and eventually perish. In *Lawaris* and *Toofan*, the hero's respective sidekicks (Suresh Oberoi and Farooque Shaikh) likewise perish, but for different reasons. In these cases, the amputees are unable to protect women from the lecherous gaze of villains. Both *Lawaris* and *Toofan* feature the often repeated theme of a male star who plays role of social protector and avenger, while his sidekick, lacking the protection of Amitabh (a celestial Buddha), dies. In *Toofan*, specifically, the theme is taken to an extreme — the cab driver's wife is molested and murdered in front of his eyes and his ten-year old son is left the task of protecting him from the attacking villains. The son manages to do this relatively effectively for a few minutes before he is finally overpowered. Thus even the child becomes the "man of the family" replacing the disabled male.

A disabled man dependent on his spouse represents the worst form of dependency in most films, especially in those cases where the disability is acquired. The man is removed from his role as provider and protector, and the consequence is often catastrophic for the family as a whole. Thus in *Mother India*, the disability of the protagonist (Raj Kumar) results in his wife becoming a manual laborer in the fields. The shame and penury of the family is resolved in his mind only when he removes himself as a burden from the family by running away from home. In *Kasauti* (1974) the disability of a husband (Bharat Bhushan) leads his wife to take the role of provider by turning to sex work. In *Pati Patni* (1966), *Zameen Asmaan* (1972), *Vakil Babu* (1983), *Qatl* (1986) and *Vaada* (2005), the protagonist's blindness leads to dependence on a wife who eventually has (or is suspected of having) an affair. The gender complexity of male disability extends to females providing support. Films like *Patita* (1953) *Waqt ka Shahenshah* (1987), and *Sharaabi* (1984) in which supporting a disabled parent forces a daughter to become the provider in a household, come with a whole set of female gender issues in the subtext.

The desexualization of people with disabilities is part of this discourse of dependence as well. This desexualization occurs with both males and females, but is particularly sharp in neutering the disabled male character both sexually and socially. Thus in *Joshila* (1973) the disabled Thakur's wife Rani (Bindu) quite openly flirts with other men and in *Khandaan* (1979) when a disabled older brother is unable to get married, it is suggested that he commit suicide so that the younger brother can marry out of turn without trouble. In light of this desexualization, various films feature a disabled person who tries to engineer a break-up of their own relationship with their non-disabled partner out of apparent consideration (*Deedar* 1951, *Arzoo* 1965, *Kannan en Kadhalan* 1968, *Jal Bin Machli Nritya Bin Bijli* 1971, *Saajan* 1991). On the other hand, while most disabled beggars in Indian films are male, female disabled beggars appear as unprotected sexual objects. In *Sahara* (1958) the protagonist is a beautiful orphan turned blind beggar whose sexual vulnerability is offset by having her sing at temples with objects typically associated with pious mendicancy, such as the *Iktara* instrument typically used by itinerant Hindu and Buddhist monks.

The close association of disability and charity is inherent to all the key religious traditions of India (Miles; Maysaa and Hateb; Gupta 2011) and the appearance of disabled people as recipients of charity in Indian cinema has aimed to underline the idea of a social responsibility. However, one of the most problematic and persistent portrayals in film is the blind beggar. The blind singer/mendicant character derives from a popular folklore figure, Surdas, a 15th century Braj region singer/saint who was a wandering musician for much of his young life. Right from the earliest days of talkie cinema, singer/actor Krishna Chandra Dey (uncle of playback singer Manna Dey and mentor to musician S.D. Burman) sang for films. Since it was typically required that he be given some kind of on-screen role, his default character became a blind beggar, often in films where his only scene would involve singing a song. Dey played Surdas a few times, found much popularity in the industry for his music, and ultimately set the stereotype for the blind singer/beggar that has been replayed consistently over the decades (*Insaan* 1944, *Deedar* 1951, *Parineeta* 1953, *Cha Cha Cha* 1964, *Bahaaron Ke Sapne* 1967, *Pyar Ka Mausam* 1969, *Muqaddar Ka Sikandar* 1975, *Sapnon Ka Mandir* 1991, *Kaasi* 2003).

Historically, actors who played characters with disabilities have frequently been typecast. Blind characters have often been played by a few character actors who had built reputations for tragic roles, a practice that collapses the distance between the persona of the star and the personas of the roles, thereby reinforcing the idea of someone who is disabled as being predictably dependent and pitiable. Thus Nazir Hussain (*Kashmir ki Kali* 1964, *Aap ki Parchhaiyan* 1964, *Prem Pujari* 1970, *Pandit aur Pathan* 1977, *Abdullah* 1980) and A.K. Hangal (*Sholay* 1975, *Sharaabi* 1984, *Ek Chaddar Maili Si* 1986) were repeatedly cast as disabled father figures in tragic roles. Bharat Bhushan several times reprised roles of a blind destitute person (*Pyar ka Mausam* 1969, *Kasauti* 1974, *Shravan Kumar* 1984, *Dariya Dil* 1988). When they were not playing the disabled, all three actors — Hussain, Hangal, and Bhushan — were typecast through much of their later careers as weak or unfortunate characters.

In Tamil cinema, an early example of disability as dependence that has important political implications is the film *Parasakhti* (1951). The film was one of the Dravidian movement's key propaganda productions. Written by politician M. Karunanidhi, it features a number of themes intended to appeal to local masses. When a protagonist loses his leg in the war and finds himself shunned by the system, he starts organizing beggars into a union, implying that the obvious occupation for a disabled man is begging.[1] Perhaps the most problematic portrayal of disability, dependency and pathos appears in Tamil director Bala's film *Naan Kadavul* (2009). Bala, known for a unique brand of violent realism in depicting life in rural and small town Tamil Nadu, centers *Naan Kadavul* around the lives of disabled commuter train performers and mendicants. The film is a particularly grim view of the begging industry and grimly voyeuristic in the vein of the Hollywood 1932 classic *Freaks,* where the body is used as an artifact to underline social incompatibility and ultimately pathos. The film casts disabled individuals, several of them performers in real life, in a narrative of particularly cruel exploitation by the begging mafia. *Naan Kadavul* has been widely cited in popular reviews for its "realistic" depiction of disability, but it does not offer much agency to any of the disabled characters. In its chilling climax, the blind female lead is ritually murdered by the protagonist who offers her *moksha* or release from her disabled life. The portrayal of a disabled life as not being worth living appears in films where a supporting character is disabled (*Mother India* 1957), but more typically in films where a female lead becomes disabled during the narrative, making her attempt suicide or choose banishment over being a burden on the male lead (*Basant* 1960, *Do Badan* 1966, *Kannan en Kadhalan* 1968). In more recent times, *Guzaarish* (2010), which we discuss in detail in the last section, offers a complex view of disability in terms of euthanasia.

The pointed use of pathos in representations of disability has frequently employed the building of tragedy or sentimentality into the narrative. One filmmaker who specialized in this strategy in his "family drama/tragedy" brand of cinema was Tamil filmmaker Bhimsingh who made a series of films with disabled characters in the lead (*Baga Pirivanai* 1959, *Palum Pazhamum* 1961, *Parthal Pasi Theerum* 1962, *Santhi* 1965, *Aadmi* 1968). In Bhimsingh's films disability often functions as a mirror for social duplicities and cruelty wherein disability is shown in terms of extreme sentimentality and helplessness. Disability is ultimately resolved at the end of the film with the protagonist regaining sight, or reversing paralysis or otherwise effecting a cure. Other directors who have repeatedly made films with characters with disabilities include Vinayan (*Vasanthiyum Lakshmiyum Pinne Njaanum* 1999, *Karumadikkuttan* 2001, *Oomappenninu Uriyadappayyan* 2002, *En Mana Vaanil* 2002, *Meerayude Dukhavum Muthuvinte Swapnavum* 2003, *Athbhutha Dweepu* 2005) and Sanjay Bhanshali, whose work we discuss in detail later.

While Bhimsingh's motivations are not clear, the importance of his films as commercial successes is key since most of these films, first made in Tamil, were remade successfully in Hindi. One of the most successful, *Baga Piravanai* (1959) remade as *Khandan* (1965), has a lead character, Ramu, who is paralyzed on one side because of a childhood accident. He is depicted as a pathetic fawning simpleton, intended as an object of the audience's pity and is repeatedly insulted by other characters in the film. His nondisabled brother, with whom he is constantly compared, is sent to school in the city while he is relegated to working the fields. The existence of a single disability — the physical inability to use one arm — is thus extended in eugenic terms to Ramu's other facilities. He is consistently portrayed as stupid, unable to recognize social cues, unattractive, and generally someone in whom to invest only limited resources.

The depiction of disabled characters as fawning unfortunates is common not just when key individual characters are disabled, but even with the broader theme of the disabled as a whole. A remarkably consistent example of this is the portrayal of blind schools in Indian films. These scenes are typically shot by rounding up youths from schools or institutions for the disabled and using them briefly in productions for one or several scenes or songs. In *Parvarish* (1977) a group of blind musicians are gathered by their teacher, played by Vinod Khanna (whose characterization in the film as a blind school teacher is used to emphasize his generosity as a film star), to sing the popular song "*Band Aankh Se Dekh Tamasha Duniya Ka,*" which literally means "see the comic irony of the world through closed eyes."

Anuraag (1972), another film to show a blind school, likewise caricaturizes and openly uses the pity card when a local politician, Amirchand (Madan Puri), gives a speech at the blind school: "Serving these poor young women is a sort of national social service. I ask, what is their fault for being blind? This is God's mistake, which we humans can fix. To remove the darkness from their life, I urge the young men of this country to come forward and make them their life partners." Immediately following this call for rescue marriages, the minister himself refuses to let his own son Rajesh (Vinod Mehra) marry a blind girl. That girl, Shivani (Moushumi Chatterjee), the film's protagonist, is a blind student at the school. The narrative makes it clear that the only way for her to marry Rajesh is if she were no longer disabled, for which she would need a cornea donor. A candidate appears in the terminally ill cherub of a boy Chandan (Master Satyajit), Rajesh's nephew, who ties all the ends together. The tearjerker is resolved when the tragedy of the child's passing is ameliorated by Shivani's restored sight and Chandan's second chance metaphorically. A very similar plot repeats in *Neel Kamal* (1984) where the hero's kid brother, also a dying cancer patient, donates his eyes so that the heroine can see. *Anuraag* was itself remade in Bangla as *Aloy Phera* (2007).

Disability as Disequilibrium

The theme of the "disability cure" — the conceptualization of disability as a state requiring a cure that the narrative achieves however unrealistically — is not unique to Indian cinema, but the frequency with which disability is proposed as a state of disequilibrium is striking. In most Indian films, disability is marginalized, affecting one of the less important characters. When it does impact a protagonist, almost always in relation to a punitive act or stroke of ill luck, it is typically temporary. In no case is this more of a guaranteed formula than when the protagonist is either blinded or paralyzed. The curing of the protagonist reflects his or her return to a state of equilibrium that the "normal" body confirms.

The idea of disability as disequilibrium is tied to the Hindu conception of disability as related to virtuous suffering, which is a central part of the characterization of Gandhari, one of the key characters in the *Mahabharata*. She is the wife of King Dhritarashtra who willingly takes on a blindfold all her life to "virtuously suffer" with her blind husband. Thus disability is her *choice*, one which she chooses consciously never to reverse. This linking of choice, virtue, personal fortitude, and impairment is reflected in the case of mythological Ashtavakra whose disability is understood as a temporary state of disequilibrium, which is eventually rectified when he earns back his perfect body after he excels as a scholar. Similarly, the sinful Samba, son of Krishna, reverses his disability when he works off his leprosy by penitent prayer to the Sun God at the Chandrabhaga River.

In both of the latter two cases, the message is important — repentance and/or hard work can reverse a disability. This seemingly fantastic message has a remarkable number of takers in Indian cinema. In countless films, some act of extreme will or fortuitous and deserved shock will make a person in a wheelchair start walking or even running right away (*Basant* 1960, *Aaj aur Kal* 1963, *Kannan en Kadhalan* 1968, *Naan yen Piranthen* 1972), or a person with a speech impairment start speaking (*Sangeet Samrat Tansen* 1962, *Karma* 1986, *Shor* 1972, *Khol de Meri Zubaan* 1989, *Koyla* 1997). Even more surprising are the cases of a paralysis reversed through an electric shock (*Baga Pirivanai* 1959, *Khandaan* 1965), through a near drowning experience (*Aalayamani* 1962, *Aadmi* 1968), or vision restored through some impact such as an accident (*Nau Bahar* 1952), even hitting one's head on a rock (*Amar Akbar Anthony* 1979) or falling down stairs (*Saajan ka Ghar* 1994) or from a snakebite (*Bairaag* 1976). In addition to all of these, there is an entire Indian genre of mythological or fantasy film featuring vast numbers of examples of the disabled being cured through some form of magic or divine intervention (*Devta* 1956, *Shirdi ke Sai Baba* 1977, *Ajooba* 1991).

The earned reversal of disability trope is particularly striking when the disability is the fault of another. In such cases, the responsibility for restoration often falls to the perpetrator who must engineer a cure through penitence. In *Thulladha Manamum Thullum* (1999), the hero Kutty (Vijay) causes the heroine Rukmini (Simran) to lose her eyesight in an accident. The hero is repentant and eventually reverses the situation by having his dying mother donate her eyes for Rukmini, and thereafter selling his kidney to pay for the transplant. The film ends happily with the emotional reunion of the now successful Rukmini and Kutty, who has transformed himself into the man who has successfully restored what he destroyed: her sight. They live happily ever after with no disabilities, save for the fact that Kutty needs to cut down on his double martinis. This successful film was remade in Telugu as *Nuvvu Vasthavani* (2000).

The plot of a disability caused by an accident and the quest for its reversal through virtuous penitence derives from the popular mythological story of Sukanya from the *Bhagawata Purana*. Sukanya, the beautiful daughter of the Shraddhadeva Manu poked two shining objects she saw in a termite's nest. They turned out to be the eyes of a meditating sage, Chyavana, who was so rapt in his meditation that he was covered in termites. Her poking blinds the sage, so Sukanya's father offers her in marriage to him to compensate for the loss of his eyes. The sage accepts and Sukanya remains a faithful wife who nurses and serves her husband. At a critical juncture, two suitors approach Sukanya, divine twins called the Ashwins (the fathers of Nakul and Sahadeva from the *Mahabharata*), who offer themselves in partnership instead of her blind, old husband Chyavana. Sukanya rejects their overtures and chooses instead to be faithful in service to her husband. The Ashwins, pleased with her chastity, offer her a small test. If she passes, her husband's disability will be reversed. She does and the story ends with Chyavana's sight and youth restored. The story offers the exemplar for the Indian woman: a wife who selflessly serves a disabled husband and through her selfless service gains his able body back. Thus Sukanya is referred to as "Sati Sukanya," a standard-setter for the ideal woman. The Sukanya saga has been filmed multiple times and dubbed in various languages in India (*Sati Sukanya* 1959, *Punyam* 2001).

We see the same plotline in *Paalum Palamum* (1960) and *Saathi* (1968), where the blind protagonist is nursed by a devoted and persevering female partner and eventually regains his sight. While the theme of a dedicated, chaste woman nursing a disabled man to a cure is actually most common in films dealing with mental illness, which we do not discuss much here (see *Khamoshi* 1969 and *Khilona* 1970), it has also been used for paralysis. In a dark twist on the theme, *Anjaam* (1996) features a woman seeking revenge on a disabled man. She decides that it is necessary first to pretend to be his devoted wife/nurse until he is well again before wreaking vengeance.

A woman's devoted service to a disabled man is well in keeping with the ideal of the virtuous woman, but when a man nurses a disabled woman to good health the objective is undeniably to highlight his heroism. In *Aaj aur Kal* (1963) a heroic young doctor/psychiatrist (Sunil Dutt) cures the grieving heroine (Nanda) of her paralysis by using his wit and love. In some films, even though the doctor actually provides the cure, the hero is the man who gets the woman to the operating table, as in *Jheel ke us Paar* (1973), *Sunayna* (1979) and *Humko Tumse Pyaar Hai* (2006).

In no case is the heroism of the "disability curer" in sharper focus than in the 1968 film *Kannan en Kadhalan* where the hero, played by MG Ramachandran (MGR), cures his love interest who is paralyzed from the waist down (Kanchana). She is literally so enthused by his singing that she gets out of the wheelchair and starts walking. The scene (a reprise of an earlier ham scene in which a crooked Jayalalitha gets out of her wheelchair and starts dancing vigorously) came at a time when MGR's popularity was at an unimaginable high. At this point, MGR was already a two-time legislator and his populist films were thoroughly propagandist, pushing the idea of him as a larger-than-life man who looked out for the poor, weak, aged, women and children, and every other group that was excluded economically and socially. Thus playing a hero who cures a disabled person becomes a vehicle to reinforce the heroic persona of the star himself. More dangerously, it emphasizes that disability is only in the mind. All it needs is a good heroic cure.

In a troubling parallel case the upright Dr. Amar (Shatrughan Sinha) cures a young polio-afflicted boy Rahul (Master Tito) in *Aa Gale Lag Jaa* (1974). Dr. Amar's approach is to beat Rahul repeatedly in a closed room until in desperation the young boy gets up and runs towards the door. The weak mind of a child is thus strengthened by Dr. Amar, who understands the right time for tough love. Just as MGR plays the gendered card of taming the child-like mind of a woman who does not understand that the disability is ultimately in the mind of the patient, so Dr. Amar teaches Rahul to toughen up and choose to live an able-bodied life.

Alternatively, the narrative of curable disability may posit the cure as a prize for good behavior, much in the vein of the mythological Ashtavakra or Samba. In this case, righteous people who suffer some form of disability are inevitably relieved of the disability by the end of the film. Typically it is the faultless blind who are cured (*Deedar* 1951, *Nau Bahar* 1952, *Raji en Kanmani* 1954, *Santhi, Gauri* 1968, *Amar Akbar Anthony, Perazhagan*). This cure for the righteous is almost necessary in narratives where the hero is disabled. For the most part, if the lead character in an Indian film — either male or female — is disabled for some reason, this is inevitably reversed. For a hero, often featured as the perfect male, the state of being disabled is inevitably one of disequilibrium that needs to be reversed (*Aalayamani* 1962, *Prem Patra* 1962, *Suhaag* 1994, *Vijaypath* 1994). Usually the only exception to this is when the disability is due to some act of valor, especially war wounds (*Hum Dono* 1961, *Major Chandrakanth* 1966, *Suhaag Raat* 1968, *Prem Pujari* 1970, *Kandukondain Kandukondain* 2000).

In contrast, a female lead character's disability functions to reinforce the male lead's heroism, but an element of disequilibrium remains, necessitating a cure for her regardless. In *Kannan en Kadhalan*, MGR's hero agrees to marry the apparently disabled Jayalalitha out of pity, but she is desexualized as unworthy of a good man. Likewise, in films like *Basant* (1942), *Aaj aur Kal* (1963), *Santhi* (1965), *Jheel ke us Paar* (1973), *Sunayna* (1979), and *Humko Tumse Pyaar Hai* (2006), the consummation of the relationship of the heroine with the hero comes only after the woman has lost her disability. A happily-ever-after ending cannot have one incomplete body.

Disability as Social Maladjustment

The stories of Manthara and Shakuni from the epics *Ramayana* and *Mahabharata* are important sources of the idea of disability as a form of social maladjustment and a pathway to evil. Manthara is the scheming, evil hunchbacked maidservant of King Dashrath's wife Kaikeyi who constantly feeds negativity into the mind of her mistress. She eventually gets Kaikeyi to guilt her husband into banishing her stepson (and Dashrath's heir to the throne) Rama into exile so that her own biological son Bharat can be king. Rama's exile is the turning point in the epic.

Shakuni is a somewhat more nuanced character. Shakuni is the son of Subala, father of Gandhari, the mother of the Kaurava clan and is famously known as the crippled, scheming uncle who cheats in dice and causes the Pandavas and Kauravas to go to war. In one version of the *Mahabharata*'s retelling, Subala and all his sons are imprisoned by the Kauravas and threatened with starvation. Each is given a grain of rice to eat, so Subala decides that they will pool their rice and give it to the youngest son, who will live at the cost of all the others, grow up, and avenge them with the Kaurava clan, using dice with magical powers made from the bones of Subala himself. This youngest son was Shakuni, who grew up both orthopedically impaired and scarred by the experience of his family's decimation. As a result of his disability-marked social maladjustment, he determines to bring about the downfall of his own sister's clan by marriage, which he eventually succeeds in doing by taking them down the path of evil.

Both Manthara and Shakuni are frequently used as models for characters in Indian cinema and have appeared in their own right in media productions of the *Ramayana* and *Mahabharata*. The classic Manthara in the televised version of *Ramayana* was played by Lalita Pawar. The casting of Pawar is particularly significant since she herself had strabismus (a squint eye condition), which led to her being frequently typecast as an evil woman in cinema. Pawar's stereotyping in Hindi cinema was so powerful that the squint in particular, rather than disability in particular, came to be seen as an indicator of evil. The Shakuni stereotype has usually been employed for wicked supporting characters, such as the scheming crippled brother-in-law played by Prem Chopra in *Ram Tera Desh* (1984).

A more common personification of the disgruntled disabled man appears in Rajendra Kumar's superhit film *Gora Aur Kala* (1972) in which the actor played twin sons of a royal family named Gora and Kala who are separated at birth. One grows up good (*gora* meaning white), as a prince, while the other becomes bad (*kala* meaning black), as a bandit. The two terms are indicative of a prevalent dichotomy in Indian narratives: the fair skinned prince is suave, kind, and desirable, whereas the bandit is dark skinned, cruel and, most importantly, has a paralyzed left arm. The grouping of negative characteristics is particularly striking: skin color, looks, and disability come together to make one brother unmistakably evil. The film was extremely successful and was eventually remade in Tamil as *Nerum Neruppum* (1971) starring M.G. Ramachandran. Similarly in the film *Vaali* (1999), Ajith Kumar plays twin brothers, one of whom is deaf. The deaf brother, Deva, is an evil genius of sorts modeled on the "supercrip" personality, with extraordinary lip reading powers. He is however perennially jealous of his speaking twin, Shiva, and constantly schemes against him. Eventually, when the evil twin dies, his soul expresses the sadness of never being able to speak of his feelings towards his brother. The film was remade in Kannada as *Vaali* (1999) and was very successful in both releases.

Both the Kala and Deva characters are fundamentally maladjusted. This theme of maladjustment is remarkably common with the characterization of maladjustment ranging from disgruntled evil to caricaturized comic with a full spectrum of poignant or pitiable in the middle. The key to this representation of maladjustment is the mismatch between disability and the required embodiment of a standard hero. Because of the cultural perception of this mismatch, there are at this writing only a handful of films in all of Indian cinema in which the lead protagonist is permanently disabled and stays that way through a film. Even in these unique narratives, the sense of maladjustment remains central to the characterization, reflecting the disconnect in cinema between the figure of the hero and the presence of disability.

Filmmaker Sanjay Bhansali's three films—*Khamoshi: The Musical* (1996), in which the protagonists are deaf-mute, *Black* (2005), in which one protagonist has Alzheimer's and another is deaf-blind and mute, and *Guzaarish* (2010), in which the protagonist has quadriplegia—are particularly salient and complex examples of this dynamic. Not commenting on Bhansali's own personal perceptions of disability or reasons for picking scripts that feature it repeatedly, the consistently alternating narrative of pith and fortitude in his films strongly reinforces an othering view of disability in India.

Khamoshi features Nana Patekar and Seema Biswas as a deaf-mute couple who bravely face a number of difficulties in raising their children (one of whom dies). The film uses some rudimentary Indian Sign Language (ISL), but even though it uses more sign per se than *Koshish* (1972), the portrayal of deafness as deficit is often disquieting. The central theme of the film is the importance of music in the lives of two of the four characters: the hearing mother (Himani Shivpuri) and the hearing daughter (Manisha Koirala) of Nana Patekar. Through most of the film, Patekar and Biswas claim to "hate music" which itself is disappointing to their daughter who wants to be a musician. The film frequently turns to the value of rhythm and notes in the lives of Helen and Koirala who love dancing and singing, yet both are required to sacrifice their love of music for the deaf couple through a series of situations. This comes to a climax when Koirala starts screaming inside their home to make a point about this family dynamic to her suitor who wants to encourage her to have a career in music. She says in frustration, "Scream and shout, there is nobody who can hear you here."

Perhaps the most unsettling facet of the film is its emphasis on exaggerated situations in which the characters are insulted for their disability. At the start of the film Patekar is told "You have no option but to beg. I pitied you because you were deaf, but you cannot handle any job." When he does have a job as a salesman, he is dehumanized by its logistics. He takes his daughter along door-to-door as an interlocutor in scenes that reverse the role between adult and child, thus placing more agency in the child who rattles off the sales-pitch and reducing the father to the menial carrier of goods. Later in the film, Patekar burns a hand and a doctor tells his employer, "Why do you keep such disabled people at work. Because of his not being able to hear, any mishap can take place," following which he is promptly fired. While exclusion from the workplace is central to the lived experience of disability in India, the use of melodramatic cruelty in films caricaturizes its economic reality and turns the individual into a recipient of charity by focusing pointedly on an inability to perform one kind of task or another and highlighting the economic burden disabled parents (assumedly) are on their children.

The choice of Nana Patekar in the lead role in *Khamoshi* is interesting because he had already come to be stereotyped as an actor who played maladjusted, usually unhinged characters. In the film, Patekar is frequently volatile and histrionic in difficult situations, reinforcing the idea that deafness is not compatible with social living. Besides the repeated references to his incompetence at work, the deaf couple are generally awkward whenever they are around hearing people, complicating situations such as their daughter's marriage planning by behaving oddly in front of the in-laws. When Patekar dismisses a suitor for his daughter, the man eventually protests, "Okay go ahead, keep your daughter in 'your world.'" Patekar then proceeds to violently throw his daughter out of their home when she finally desires marriage, to which she responds, "I was never a child, only a voice for you [...] I have supported you all your life, given you support and help, now it is your turn." Through most of the film, the relation of dependence flows from the daughter to her parents, a striking inversion of social norms.

The film climaxes with Patekar making a poignant speech in which he apologizes for how difficult his daughter's life has been because of having deaf-mute parents and acknowledges how helpful she has been in their own lives, finally ending his speech with how grateful he is to his son-in-law for giving his daughter a much better life than he himself could have given her. The film ends with Koirala lying in a coma while her father dances in the hospital room hoping this will revive her.

The portrayal of a character with a disability either voluntarily or through association behaving in a manner appropriate for a child helps not just confirm their maladjustment, but their pitiful dependence on the socially mainstream figures in the film. This pattern appears in several different variations. One of the most common ways it is achieved is by having a disabled character (especially a blind one) fooled by another (sighted) character into believing some alternate state of affairs. Such "misleading" can be caricaturist, such as in *Kakakuyil* (2001), remade as *London* (2005) in Tamil and *Golmaal* (2006) in Hindi, in which a crew of crooked protagonists trying to fool a blind old couple through fake identities. Or else it appears in films featuring the "for the best of the already burdened blind person" theme, such as *Zakhmon ka Hisaab* (1993) in which a blind mother is made to believe that her husband is alive and well though he is dead. Likewise, there is the "disabled deserve a break" theme of *Imaan Dharam* (1977) in which the two protagonists (Amitabh Bachchan and Shashi Kapoor) want their blind neighbor (Aparna Sen) to be happy. So they pretend that her application to sing at a large contest has been approved and take her to an empty rented auditorium where they pretend there is a massive audience in attendance to whom she tearfully sings, "I wish I could see all my audience members." She is portrayed as a particularly pathetic character, frequently telling her suitor to go chase after the light elsewhere instead of the darkness in her life.

Physical disability as a source of social maladjustment is fairly common in supporting character roles where the exploitation of the disabled character adds some spice to the film without having any real bearing on the plot. These include the occasional sidekick, such as the cynical disabled farmer Malang (Pran) from *Upkaar* (1967) who sings songs about the evil in the world around; the dancing army veteran with an amputated foot Balbir Singh (Utpal Dutt) from *Imaan Dharam* (1977); the crippled gymnast Jasjit (Pran) from *Don* (1978) who ends the film performing a tightrope escape between two buildings holding two children and a walking stick; and the singing, skateboard-riding street beggar/informant Abdul (Mazhar Khan) from *Shaan* (1982). In most of these films the disabled character acts as a minor and vulnerable player, and often ends up as an extension of the hero's patriarchy by being situated among the broad range of people who share a patron-client relationship with the hero, including the children, women, and the sick. A great example of this pattern is the film *Kalicharan* (1978) in which the hero (Shatrughan Sinha) has to face a socially maladjusted street fighter (Danny Denzongpa) in hand-to-hand combat. Only when the duelists are face to face does the hero realize that the fighter has only one leg. In line with his heroic image, he ties one foot to offer his opponent a "fair fight" and the two men engage in a stick-fight on one leg each. Through much of the remaining film the fighter turns over to the good side, moved by the generosity of his opponent who adopted a disability to fight him.

Perhaps the strangest use of disability as maladjustment in Indian cinema is that of the disability fake. In *Punjabi House* (1998), remade in Hindi as *Chup Chup Ke* (2006), the hero pretends to be mute for financial benefit. In the Tamil film *Sollamale* (1998), remade in Hindi as *Pyaar Diwana Hota Hai* (2002), the hero pretends to be mute to win over a woman, but on being discovered as not being disabled, cuts off his tongue to stay true to his disability. Pretending to be blind for some form of benefit has historically been frequently employed. Perhaps one of the earliest films to do this was Mohan Bhavnani's *Prem Nagar* (1940) in which the hero goes blind but upon regaining his sight continues to pretend to be blind in order to perceive people's true attitudes towards him. Similarly, the combination of charity with disability fraud has been a convenient means of depicting disability, as with the street beggar who feigns blindness in *Baat Ek Raat Ki* (1962), or films in which feigning blindness is a means for the hero to appear harmless while plotting some form of revenge, as in *Parvarish* (1977), *Vaada* (2005) or *Chess* (2006). There are also a host of films in which pretending to be blind is a ploy used by men to appeal to the sympathy and thereafter love of women. These include *Johar Mehmood in Hong Kong* (1971), *Poikkal Kuthirai* (1983), *Dil* (1990), *Badshah* (1999), *Kandaen* (2010), and *Rascals* (2011).

Finally, there is the disturbing trend of films where disability as social maladjustment is integral to the comedy. The success of this theme is evidenced by its repeated use across languages, perhaps among the most common of which is the use of multiple disabilities as part of a comedy-of-errors. Examples include the Hindi film *Hum Hai Kamaal Ke* (1993) a remake of *See no Evil Hear no Evil* (1989) featuring Kader Khan as deaf and Anupam Kher as blind, which was again remade in Tamil as *Andipatti Arasampatti* (2002) with Mansur Ali Khan and Pandiyarajan, and yet again in Hindi as *Pyare Mohan* (2006). Similar themes are used in the Tamil films *Ennavale* (2000), *123* (2002), and *Tom, Dick, and Harry* (2006), in which the interactions between blind, deaf and mute characters are used for comic intent. In *Mujhse Shaadi Karoge* (2004) the entire gamut of disability is rolled into a single character, Duggal (Kader Khan), who has a disease that gives him a new disability each day of the week. He has a sign outside the door of his home that indicates the disability of the day. In the film he is blind, mute, deaf, and cognitively impaired.

The underlying premise of disability as maladjustment across all of these films is that the disabled character cannot be viewed with the same lens as the rest of the characters; thus whether it is the villainy of the Shakuni type figure, the melodramatic pathos of the deaf couple and their longsuffering hearing relatives in *Khamoshi,* or the celebrated side-kickery of the Jasjits or Abduls, the central idea is that the maladjusted are fundamentally not reasonable, regular folks. In each of these cases that we discuss as maladjustment, the condition of being disabled is caricaturized to be more than the sensory or functional impact of the impairment itself. Disability results in the character being relegated to an object of righteous scorn, derision, pity, or comedy. In short, the state of disability necessitates a reaction of some kind from the other 'normal' characters, and in turn from the audience itself.

The New Disabled

> *I suggested to the director that my role be turned into that of a blind man just [...] I wanted to challenge myself as an actor. I felt that the man has a lot to say but I did not want it to look preachy [...] We are not showing him as a fakir, he is a modern man, so beyond a certain point it would have been very boring with this man continuously talking about life and how it should be. The thought of him being blind turned the film upside down but it made the film's message deeper [...] Playing him as a blind man was very exciting for me.*
>
> —Anupam Kher on his role in the 2012 film
> *Chhodo Kal Ki Baatein* (*Express*)

> *I interacted with a lot of paraplegic patients before taking up the film. Before that I used to be irritable and edgy, but they taught me to live. My character of a paraplegic touched my heart.*
>
> —Hrithik Roshan on his 2010 role in
> *Guzaarish* (Dabholkar)

> *This is a good beginning, in time as we evolve as a society, it will become easier to see reason in the concept of [passive] euthanasia as a boon for those who are suffering to a degree, which you and I cannot even imagine.*
>
> —Hrithik Roshan on the 2011 Indian Supreme Court
> verdict on passive euthanasia (*Times*)

Anupam Kher's comments on his role in the 2012 film *Chhodo Kal* reflect an unusual period of transition in the portrayal of disability in Indian cinema. On one hand, he seems to fetishize playing a character with vision impairment as a test of his abilities as an actor and to endorse the assumption that disability produces or legitimizes wisdom in the vein of the blind seer character of Western culture. On the other hand, by at least publicly reflecting on the experience of playing a disabled character, Kher opens the door for discussion. Similarly, Hrithik Roshan's interview in the *Times of India* on his experience of portraying a paraplegic's legal case for euthanasia in Sanjay Bhansali's *Guzaarish* (2010), based loosely on *Mar Adentro* (*The Sea Inside,* 2004), reinforces assumptions by extolling disability for the life lessons it offers the nondisabled. Yet it also marks a moment of public discussion about disability with Roshan's subsequent comments on the Indian Supreme Court decision in favor of passive euthanasia for those in a persistent vegetative state (PVS). Kher's and Roshan's statements are examples of the increasingly common phenomena of prominent Indian leading actors reflecting on disability and its portrayal in the media, but they also betray the extent to which the idea of a disabled person as a standard participant in social or economic circles is still so alien in India, and how deeply ingrained is the need to view disability through a lens of pity or heroism as part of our national discourse.

While the portrayal of disability in film in the period leading up to the early 2000s was offensively caricaturist, a new wave of cinema is changing the portrayal of disability on screen. There are two aspects to this new movement. First, a small subsection of popular films have narratives that reduce blatant denigration, although the sentimentalizing of disability is still deeply prevalent and very effectively sold to the market. A second related factor is that disability itself has become a fairly valuable avenue for actors to emphasize their talent, similar to the way in which playing a disabled character became a fairly strong indicator of Academy Award success in the late 1980s and early 1990s. The sheer list of awards that have gone to the actors playing a disabled character since the 2000s in the Filmfare and Filmfare South best actor and actress awards speaks to this: Amitabh Bachchan for *Black* (2006) and *Paa* (2009), including the National Award, Vikram for *Kasi* (2001) and *Pithamagan* (2003), including the National Award, Surya for *Perazhagan* (2004), Mohanlal for *Thanmatra* (2005), and Shah Rukh Khan for *My Name is Khan* (2010). Actresses included Rani Mukherji for *Black*, Kajol for *Fanaa* (2007), and Pooja for *Naan Kadavul* (2009).

Casting lead actors as disabled characters has precedent in a few films that, despite falling to stereotypes, nonetheless set the stage for portraying people with disabilities as regular protagonists, in relationships with mainstream partners. Sai Paranjpe's *Sparsh* (1980) for the most part remains unparalleled in this regard. In the film Nasseruddin Shah plays a blind school principal who has a relationship with one of the volunteers at the school. The film does not sentimentalize the relationship. Instead, it highlights social expectations and assumptions about pity and dependence, and the role these play in coloring relationships between disabled and nondisabled people. The following year Singeetham Srinivasa Rao made *Raaja Paarvai* (1981), which featured Kamal Haasan as a blind violinist living independently. While the film is not sternly unsentimental, it nonetheless emphasizes a perfectly reasonable romantic relationship between disabled and nondisabled mainstream characters. More importantly, the use of Kamal Haasan in the lead role brought to cinema a disabled character who appears to be a "regular" person. The film ends on a bright note with a *Graduate*-like escape where the heroine, played by Madhavi, dumps the groom selected by her family and, in her wedding dress, bolts with Kamal Haasan.

The recent re-emergence of disability in cinema with a hint of an empowered bent has not only brought a range of disabilities to the screen, but has also brought actors with disabilities. Deafness and deaf-blindness are characterized in *Pattiyal* (2006) in which the hero is a deaf assassin; in *Black* the two protagonists are deaf-blind-mute and an Alzheimer's patient respectively; and in *Mozhi* (2007) the lead actress is deaf. In the biggest hit of 2009, *Nadodigal*, Deaf actress Abhinaya appears opposite the lead actor who is hearing. She was instantly popular and went on to score supporting roles in a number of major productions. The same year, blind actor Nasser Khan played a sighted person in the film *Shadow*. The actor Ajay Kumar, who has a growth deficiency and is also known as Guinness Pakru (for being the shortest actor in the world), has typically played comical supporting characters or fantasy characters such as the prince of dwarves in *Adbhuta Dweepam* (2005). He landed a starring role as the father of Jayaram, a major Malayalam star, in the 2010 hit *My Big*

Father. The same year, Bala, who earlier dealt with subjects of disability in *Kasi* (2001) and *Pithamagan*, released *Naan Kadavul*, which featured an entire star cast of disabled performers.

However, if we read into the narratives of these films, we find a lot that is unsettling. *My Big Father* has a number of derogatory references to Ajay Kumar's size, repeated poking fun at his character. In a comic scene his own son chases the running father (Kumar) and traps him in a rubbish bin. A hero treating a parent in such a manner would never be shot in any popular film featuring nondisabled actors and characters. *Naan Kadavul* (2009), a disconcertingly provocative film, deals with itinerant performers and beggars, and creates an intentionally freakish visual ethic where the disabled body is an object of voyeurism. In the name of realism, the disabled characters are exploited and sometimes abused on screen, and the chief female protagonist — a blind commuter train singer — is eventually murdered in the name of sympathy by the hero who offers her *moksha* (deliverance). The film was both critically acclaimed and well received in popular circles for its apparent foray into the underbelly of the begging underground. The disturbing nature of its narrative on disability, however, has not found much discussion.

A number of other mainstream films have been released in recent years about a range of conditions, although they rarely get serious discussion in the public sphere. These include Progeria (*Paa* 2009), Alzheimer's (*Thanmatra* 2005; *U Me aur Hum* 2008), dyslexia (*Taare Zameen Par* 2007), autism (*My Name is Khan* 2010), and cerebral palsy (*Angel* 2011; *Vinmeegal* 2012). While some of these films indeed move closer to an inclusive view of disability as part and parcel of society, and several are significant on multiple levels because they discuss concepts that have never been featured before, there are still far too many films at the other end of the spectrum that continue the strong foundations of othering that years of Indian cinema have facilitated. In a country where studies show that even a vast number of the disabled themselves consider the role of a past birth as playing a part in one's disability, things like the public discourse of disability in popular culture are of critical importance.

Notes

1. In an interesting piece of political trivia, the amputee protagonist sets up an Unamutror Maruvazhvu Nilyam (Disabled Rehabilitation Center). Years later when Karunanidhi, the writer of the film, became chief minister of the state, he set up the likewise named Pichaikarar Maruvazhvu Nilyam (Beggar Rehabilitation Center) in much the same vein as in the film.

Works Cited

Cumberland, Guy, and Ralph Negrine. *Images of Disability on Television*. New York: Routledge, 1992. Print.

Dabholkar, Reshma Kelkar. "I was in Depression: Hrithik." *Times of India*. 24 Oct. 2010. Web. 27 July 2012.

Daily Bhaskar. "I am Like *Lafangey Parindey* Heroine: Deepika Padukone." *Daily Bhaskar*. 27 Aug. 2010. Web. 27 July 2012.

Express India. "Playing Blind Man in *Chhodo Kal* was Challenging: Anuparn." *Express India*. 4 Apr. 2012. Web. 27 July 2012.

Gupta, Vijay Bhushan. "How Hindus Cope with Disability." *Journal of Religion, Disability & Health* 15:1 (2001): 72–78. Print.

Harnett, Alison. "Escaping the 'Evil Avenger' and the 'Supercrip': Images of Disability in Popular Television." *The Irish Communications Review* 8 (2000): 21–29. Web. 27 July 2012.

Maysaa, S. Bazna, and Tarek A. Hateb. "Disability in the Qur'an: The Islamic Alternative to Defining, Viewing, and Relating to Disability." *Journal of Religion, Disability & Health* 9:1 (2008): 5–27. Print.

Miles, M. "Disability in an Eastern Religious Context: Historical Perspectives." *Disability & Society* 10:1 (1995): 49–70. Print.

Norden, Martin F. *Cinema of Isolation: A History of Physical Disability in the Movies.* New Brunswick: Rutgers University Press, 1994.

Times of India. "Hrithik Hails Nod for Passive Euthanasia." *Times of India.* 11 Mar. 2011. Web. 27 July 2012.

Extra-Textual Reveals

Disability, (Sort of) Queer Sexuality and a Military Coup in *Battlestar Galactica*

ALYSON PATSAVAS

It takes a certain perversity to critically engage with disabled, queer images on screen. When they do appear these images simultaneously hold the promise of something more, something beyond the heterosexual and able-bodied norm plaguing most television and film narratives, and yet the inevitably tokenistic and flat representations prove always disappointing. The few available examples of disabled queer characters either use disability as a mere extension of and metaphor for queer sexual difference (see Davidson) or use the queer disabled character to shore up able-bodied heterosexuality (see McRuer). Still, I relish the perverse practice of anticipation and frustration with these disabled queer images always looking for ways to, as Carrie Sandahl suggests, queer the crip and crip the queer. She states, "Queering describes the practice of putting a spin on mainstream representations to reveal latent queer subtexts" while "[c]ripping spins mainstream representations or practices to reveal able-bodied assumptions" (37). Together, queering the crip and/or cripping the queer is the (arguably hopeful) practice of looking for points of rupture embedded in the often politically whitewashed characterizations of plucky crips and corporately endorsed queers: a practice of reading against the network television and mainstream film versions of flexible heterosexism and ableism that *tolerate* disability and/or queerness on screen as long as they serve a function for the straight, able-bodied characters and narratives (McRuer 16–28). It is with this perversity that I turn to the hit SciFi network television show *Battlestar Galactica's* portrayal of Lt. Felix Gaeta (Alessandro Juliani).

Battlestar Galactica (2004–2009), a remake of the markedly less successful 1978–79 television show with the same name, aired a total of 73 episodes.[1] It garnered, and continues to garner, scholarly, critical and fan acclaim for its gritty realism, sharp writing and dedication to creating complex characters, the use of disability as characterization notwithstanding.[2] In the series' dystopic, post-apocalyptic future humans face near annihilation at the hands of Cylons, the show's version of cyborgs, which look human but are actually machines. The Cylons wage a surprise nuclear attack on the humans and force the few survivors to flee their planetary homes and seek refuge in space. These survivors form a makeshift fleet, which is protected by the only remaining military ship, the Battlestar Galactica. The series tells the story of their journey through space as they hide from the pursing Cylons and search for a mythical planet called Earth to make a new home. There are twelve different Cylon models (and multiple copies of each model) and part of the show's drama comes from the suspense of uncovering the identity of the Cylons, some of whom reside undetected in the human fleet. Adding to the suspense, some of the Cylons are programmed to think that they are human. The narrative tension derived from this plot structure provides the background to its mutiny narrative arc.

Gaeta is a communications officer in the show's military fleet, who, in the fourth and final season, gets his leg shot and eventually amputated, setting him on a narrative trajectory not unfamiliar to disability scholars. He dons a prosthetic leg and goes from being a loyal military man to an embittered and mutinous officer who leads a military coup and eventually dies for his disloyalty. *BSG* uses disability as a form of characterization to mark Gaeta as a symbol of fleet-wide discontent.[3] Meanwhile, situated safely within the confines of a tangential web series called *Battlestar Galactica: Face of the Enemy,* featured on the SciFi network's website, two queer love stories involving Gaeta unfold. The webisodes reveal that Gaeta is involved with another male officer, Lt. Louis Hoshi (Brad Dryborough), and a (female) Cylon. Despite his name (pronounced Gay-ta), the main narrative of *BSG* makes no reference to Gaeta's sexuality, either in the three and a half seasons leading up to the military coup or in the episodes composing the mutiny arc. The webisodes aired in the middle of the fourth season between the time that Gaeta sustains his injury and the development of the mutiny arc.

In what follows I explore the way that both *BSG* and *Face of the Enemy* utilize Gaeta's disability and queer sexuality, respectively, to accomplish the same narrative function. Each explains Gaeta's role as the leader of a military coup, ostensibly offering a reason or justification for his disloyal actions. Reading these two narratives together, however, undermines the use of disability and sexuality as narrative explanation. Combined, they present a tangentially queer, disabled character that arguably exceeds the stock characterization offered in each individual narrative. Examining each narrative on its own, I "crip" *BSG*'s use of disability, uncovering how the show deploys disability to construct Lt. Felix Gaeta as the embodiment of broader social tensions over a proposed alliance between humans and their enemy *and* conversely personalizes Gaeta's motives for starting a military coup in response to this alliance. I argue that for disability to function in this dual way — as both embodiment of the whole and individually embodied personal motivation — the series must first invest Gaeta with the tensions of the fleet and then divest him of this broader significance through a process of individualization. I then "queer" *Face of the Enemy*'s use of what I will call a (sort of) queer sexuality to justify Gaeta's mutinous actions to argue that the show introduces these relationships to personalize his motives. Finally, I examine the two narratives together to argue that the addition of *Face of the Enemy* to the *BSG*-verse signals a place where stock characterizations of disability begin to break down.

Lt. Felix Gaeta and the Materiality of Metaphor

David Mitchell and Sharon Snyder argue that narratives use disability because "[p]hysical and cognitive anomalies promise to lend a "tangible" body to textual abstractions; we term this metaphorical use of disability the *materiality of metaphor*" (47–8). At its simplest, *BSG* uses Gaeta's disability as a material metaphor for the tensions the fleet feels over the proposed alliance. Gaeta's injury and the subsequent prosthetic leg he uses depict the painful coming together of humans and machines. Gaeta's injury gives form to a textually abstract anxiety that a proposed alliance between the humans and a group of Rebel Cylons (who separate from the other Cylons after a civil war) induces in the human fleet. The proposed alliance comes after three seasons of attacks, an apocalypse and a brutal military occupation, all at the hand of the Cylons. As such, it proves hard for the characters, and the audience, to accept. However, Galactica's military and civilian leaders believe that the alliance offers the best chance of human survival. Gaeta becomes the figurehead of those that believe otherwise.

Gaeta sustains the injury that causes his disability in the episode in which the alliance is first proposed, setting up the correlation between his disability and the alliance. A crew of military officers separates from the rest of the fleet to search for an alternative route to Earth. Tensions run high among this frustrated crew who are eager to return to the fleet. A Cylon boards their ship and proposes an alliance, promising the humans help finding Earth in exchange for their help fixing a broken ship. The ship's captain, Capt. Kara "Starbuck" Thrace (Katee Sackhoff), agrees, but the rest of the crew demands that they return to Galactica. A fight ensues, and as tensions boil over, the crew attempts to relieve Starbuck of command. Gaeta, supporting the rest of the crew, tries to direct their ship back to the Galactica, but a crewmember loyal to Starbuck shoots him in the leg to stop him ("Faith" 4.6).

BSG draws out this shooting scene in order to visually embody the damage the conflict causes. When the gun goes off, the camera cuts to show the gaping hole in Gaeta's leg, the protruding bone, the oozing blood and the frantic attempt to patch him up. Emily Russell argues narratives often frame the body (specifically relying on blood and pain) as a conduit toward the real (70). The visceral/visual representation of Gaeta's injury conveys the seriousness of his wounds and thereby the seriousness of the conflict, conferring a reality or heightened sense of realism on the conflict. Moreover, lingering on Gaeta's wounds allows the camera to redirect the viewer's gaze onto Gaeta's body. While the preceding sequence of camera shots cut from Starbuck to the dissenting crew members in quick succession, allowing the tension to build between them, the camera shots focusing on the wound cut between various focal points on Gaeta's body. The site of the tension becomes Gaeta's body rather than the less tangible tensions between Starbuck and the rest of the crew.

As the crew stabilizes Gaeta's leg, the tension dissipates. Several crewmembers move Gaeta (off-screen) to a bed. Starbuck then admits her mistake and compromises in a way that allows her to pursue the truce without putting the rest of the crew in danger. She separates herself from the crew by taking a smaller ship to the Cylons, which allows her to accept the alliance but not risk the crew. Her decision temporarily tables the conflict that the alliance poses. Much like Gaeta's removal from the visual field of the screen, the immediate impact of the proposed alliance gets removed as Starbuck sequesters the "threat" of the alliance to a single ship: a threat that now resides firmly within Gaeta's body.

After Starbuck, the separated crew and the Rebel Cylons return to the fleet, *BSG* solidifies the link between Gaeta's injury and the alliance with a series of cuts between Gaeta in the hospital area of the ship and negotiations between the Cylons and humans. The first sequence back aboard the Galactica shows medics rolling Gaeta into the hospital area of the ship. The camera then cuts directly to the Rebel Cylon leader, Number Six (Tricia Helfer), sitting before Admiral William Adama (Edward James Olmos), the ranking military officer and President Laura Roslin (Mary McDonnell), the civilian leader. She tells them of the Cylon civil war that fractured their fleet and officially proposes the alliance. The show cuts between the dramatic tensions of the hospital room as viewers wait to see whether

Gaeta will "lose" his leg and the less visible tension of the conversation discussing the alliance. By paralleling these two scenes, the show gives the viewer a visual marker through which to read the unfolding drama between the Cylons and the human leaders.

BSG positions Gaeta's amputated leg as a metaphoric amputation of the human fleet, which loses an essential part of its humanness (its distinctiveness from the machines) by integrating with the Cylons. Much like the integration of the Cylons into the human fleet, the integration of Gaeta's prosthetic into his leg causes significant pain at the point of connection and the series uses that pain as a way of giving materiality to the struggles that follow the alliance. Schleifer suggests that "pain [is] the most corporeal sensation, precisely because with it ... there is nothing but body" (Schleifer 150).[4] The series relies on this notion that pain reflects the ultimate corporeal experience in order to work through the less tangible pain of the alliance by transferring it into corporeal pain within Gaeta's amputated leg. However, this transfer is not as simple as setting Gaeta up as a material metaphor and then letting that metaphor run its course. Rather, the series deploys specific cultural assumptions about pain — that it is a deeply individual and personal experience (see Scarry) — in order to both set up Gaeta as the embodiment of less tangible sociopolitical pain and to facilitate a necessary process of separating Gaeta from the rest of the fleet. The series uses corporeal pain as a tool to individualize Gaeta's motivations for the mutiny arc because the narrative can only resolve the conflict that the alliance proposes by individualizing Gaeta from the fleet.

A Military Coup: Corporeal Pain/Corporal Punishment

Gaeta's job as a communications officer makes him the literal voice of the fleet. He tells the Admiral (and the viewers) when Cylons approach and if there's a problem aboard Galactica or other ships in the fleet. His position makes him a natural representative of the fleet's temperament. Nicole Markotić and Sally Chivers argue that "the disabled body often exists primarily as a metaphor for a body that is unable to [move forward]" (2). Gaeta's disabled body represents not just the inability of *a body* to move forward, but also the inability of *bodies* to move forward. However, as Rosemarie Garland-Thomson tells us, the disabled body stands in opposition to other, normative bodies. She writes "the very act of representing corporeal otherness places [the disabled character] in a frame that highlights their difference from ostensibly normate characters" (Garland-Thomson 10). Garland-Thomson suggests that this marked difference from the normate or able-bodied (i.e., normal) characters makes iconic disabled characters like Captain Ahab and Tiny Tim easily identifiable and memorable. In order to construct the mutiny as widespread and Gaeta the representative of widespread feelings, the series has to work against prevailing notions that disability signifies a very personal and private tragedy.[5] For as much as *BSG* links the tensions of the alliance to Gaeta's body, as the mutiny plot begins to unfold the show deemphasizes his disability in order to deliberately link his feelings with others in the fleet.

We see this played out most fully in a confrontation between Starbuck and Gaeta. The two sit in a mess hall with a crowd of people around and almost instantly begin to fight. Starbuck admonishes Gaeta for his "bad attitude" which she blames on his disability. She says, "Fifty billion people are dead and I'm supposed to give a frak about your leg?" ("A Disquiet Follows My Soul" 4.12). Gaeta responds by just smiling and glossing over the comment. He tells Starbuck that soon there will be a reckoning for those that collude with the Cylons. This response aligns Gaeta's disability with the coming reckoning/mutiny but does so in a way that minimizes Gaeta's personal anger. He barely reacts to her repeated references to his disability throughout the exchange, and simply keeps returning back to the topic of the alliance. Starbuck verbally identifies Gaeta's anger with this leg in order for Gaeta to disavow this reading with his continued focus on the fleet's anger over the alliance.

Moreover, Gaeta remains seated throughout the exchange. The only visual sign of his disability in the entire scene is when he sits down at the table. Even then, the camera shows his crutches only briefly. We never see his prosthetic or his leg and as soon as he sits he discards the crutches under his chair. For the most part all corporeal traces of disability from this scene vanish. As Starbuck walks out of the room (followed by only two people), the rest of the crew remains and looks to Gaeta. He tells one of them to shut the door and the scene ends with the camera looking in on the group as the door closes. Ronald D. Moore indicates that the director carefully constructs this scene in order to convey just how widespread the frustration that Gaeta represents is (Podcast Commentary on "A Disquiet Follows My Soul"). I would add that the director accomplishes this by deliberately framing Gaeta in such a way as to minimize his disability.

Similarly, in a scene where Gaeta sits in a meeting with the leading military officers discussing the integration of Cylon technology into the human fleet (a meeting that Gaeta arguably would not otherwise be part of), *BSG* downplays Gaeta's physical presence and instead highlights his voice in the scene, constructing him as the voice of the people. The Admiral, his son, two Cylons and a man married to a Cylon discuss a deal that the Cylons propose. They offer to give the humans their technology in exchange for citizenship status within the fleet.[6] The camera looks in on the meeting, focusing on the Admiral and the other military officers who discuss the request and the resistance that they will surely face within the fleet. Gaeta sits in the background of the scene. He interjects into the conversation only to express his disbelief that the Admiral even considers the proposal. Like the scene in the mess hall, the camera features Gaeta primarily from the waist up, disembodying him in a way that almost removes his disability from the frame.

Thematically, *BSG* complicates rigid lines between humans and Cylons. Characters we recognize as human for three seasons suddenly turn out to be Cylons, and Cylons in the series often act more "human" than some of the human characters. The mutiny arc develops in a way that reiterates this overall thematic message. Gaeta stands for an antiquated view of human/Cylon difference that the series wants to move beyond. Therefore, for as much as the series invests in constructing Gaeta as the voice of the fleet, it equally divests him of that symbolic meaning in order to advance the narrative. The series accomplishes this by refocusing on Gaeta's corporeal body, using disability to do so. As the mutiny takes shape, the camera frames Gaeta's prosthetics with a low angle and close-up shots to draw our attention to Gaeta's disability and create a visual correlation between it and the mutiny plot. We see this most clearly in a scene where Gaeta officially acts on his (and the fleet's) angst. He meets with a man named Tom Zarek (Richard Hatch), a malcontent criminal/revolutionary turned vice-president whom the show constructs as the embodiment of bad politics, power-hungry behavior and morally ambiguous ethics.[7] The meeting between the men opens with a shot of Zarek washing his hands. The camera faces him as he talks about the costs and consequences of a revolution. Zarek steps away from the sink to reveal Gaeta, who sits on a chair in the center of a prison cell (where Zarek is currently being held for his own efforts to resist the alliance). At first the viewer sees Gaeta in profile and Zarek stands blocking Gaeta's prosthetic from view. As Gaeta replies to Zarek, saying, "I've thought about the consequences," Zarek steps away to reveal Gaeta's prosthetic ("A Disquiet Follows My Soul").

BSG visually reveals Gaeta's disability in this moment, establishing Gaeta's leg as both a consequence of the alliance that has already occurred and as a tool of characterization that marks Gaeta as the figurehead of the mutiny who will carry out the consequences yet to come of aligning with the Cylons. Furthermore, Gaeta's prosthetic limb angles toward the camera while his other leg angles away. This makes his prosthetic loom disproportionately large and draws the viewer's eye to it. The menacing portrayal of Gaeta's prosthesis here works to enhance the menacing nature of Zarek and Gaeta's meeting. It also serves to reintegrate Gaeta's body into the mutiny narrative. His disability becomes the foremost important visual marker of the scene.

As the mutiny sequence unfolds the *BSG* increasingly highlights Gaeta's corporeality by highlighting his pain. In a series of scenes interspersed throughout the Galactica mutiny arc, Gaeta reaches down into the leather attachment of his prosthetic (which unrealistically fits so loosely that he can reach his hand inside) to scratch the flaking and irritated skin. The series uses these moments of expressed pain to signal Gaeta's increasing isolation from the fleet. For instance, before the mutiny develops Gaeta sits in the ship's hospital waiting for the doctor. The camera closes in on Gaeta's leg at the amputation site. He scratches and winces at what we visually see as the cracked and red stump. The camera, however, does not linger on the leg. Rather, it moves up to frame Gaeta above the waist in order to draw focus on his verbal complaint that the leather attachment for his prosthetic chafes and hurts. When the doctor's assistant, Layne Ishay (Kerry Norton), tells him that he will have to wait because the doctor is busy treating two Cylons, Gaeta expresses his frustration with the doctor's priorities, which by extension represent the Galactica command's failure to alleviate human pain in favor of treating (read: accept, help and comfort) the Cylons. In response to Ishay, Gaeta lists the problems of the fleet, saying sarcastically, "The fleet's a mess ... but hey, gotta make sure the Cylons are taken care of" ("A Disquiet Follows My Soul"). He chides the doctor for ignoring his pain, while the episode plays up this ignored pain to illustrate Gaeta's growing discontent. Meanwhile, Ishay empathizes with him and apologizes for both his suffering and the inattention of the doctor, effectively witnessing Gaeta's pain and frustration, validating it, and thereby reaffirming Gaeta's position as spokesperson for the fleet. Sara Ahmed contends that the act of witnessing pain grants it "the status of an event, a happening in the world, rather than just the 'something'" that the body feels (29–30). Visually representing this act of witnessing, the show transforms Gaeta's pain into an event that Gaeta and Ishay share. Gaeta's pain happens not just within his body but also through empathy within the experience of other characters. However, as the mutiny develops the series decreases the empathy reflected back at him, increasingly containing Gaeta's pain within his body.

Early in the mutiny Gaeta and Zarek walk down the hall with a group of armed officers. As Gaeta reaches down to rub his leg the viewer sees Zarek in the background watching with concern, while the other officers pause at Gaeta's wince. The men take visual notice of Gaeta's pain but do not verbally acknowledge it as Ishay did. Still, the other mutineers reflect Gaeta's discomfort back to him, witnessing it in both the personal and political sense, calling his pain forth (if slightly less prominently) into the world of Galactica and into the moment of the mutiny. However, the camera subsequently pulls back from this scene to focus on Gaeta's entire body as he lumbers down the hall, wincing with each step. By the end of the mutiny, the camera entirely isolates Gaeta's expressions of pain from the rest of the crew. Alone in the Admiral's quarters (which for this brief period belongs to Gaeta), he sits down, unbuckles the attachment for his prosthetic, and cringes as he removes it. Cultural understandings of pain configure it as an intensely personal experience and the show capitalizes on these assumptions within this scene.[8] The viewer takes in Gaeta's isolation through seeing him alone with his pain as the camera pulls back to show the empty room around him, accentuating Gaeta's isolation, which will increase according to narrative needs as the season unfolds.

The fleet will not be able to move forward more united than ever if Gaeta ends the mutiny serving the same metaphoric purpose as he did when it began. When Admiral Adama — held prison and awaiting execution — regains control of his Rebel human captors, he gives them the option of joining him in retaking command, which they do (with the exception of one character who symbolically refuses). The quick shift in allegiance represents the reunification of the fleet. Individualizing Gaeta's disability makes this shift both possible and plausible. The more attention that the episodes call to Gaeta's leg pain, the more the audience perceives this pain as the source of his actions rather than recognizing him as the symbolic representation of the human losses fleetwide.

Admiral Adama and the supportive mob now marching behind him storm the command center and re-take control of the Galactica. The Admiral orders Gaeta and Zarek taken away and executed.[9] As Gaeta awaits execution, he smiles and talks easily about his life before joining Galactica and before the Cylon attack. He expresses resignation, saying to another character, "I'm fine with how things turned out" ("Blood on the Scales").[10] Gaeta retains his calm even as the scene cuts to him and Zarek tied to two chairs facing a firing squad. In Gaeta's final moment before death he looks down at his leg as the camera cuts to reveal his cracked and flaking stump. The director features Gaeta without his metal prosthesis here in a moment of entirely "human" corporeality signifying his anti–Cylon position. After lingering on his leg, the camera pans back up to Gaeta who says, "It stopped." The gunshots go off as the screen cuts to black.

We can read the significance of Gaeta's final utterance on several levels. One might suggest "It stopped" simply marks that resolution of the conflict: the pain stops because the anxiety that it signifies has been exercised. Gaeta's leg, free of the painful prosthesis, literally and physiologically stops hurting while the fleet metaphorically and politically stops hurting, having now fully embraced the alliance. The show acknowledges the weight of the decision to align with the enemy through Gaeta's death.[11] Gaeta's loss of limb and the loss of Gaeta satisfy the need to acknowledge the "cost" of the alliance in a way that creates narrative closure. Granted, the series works hard to divest Gaeta from this symbolism so that his final utterance solidifies the process of disability individualization by suggesting that, for Gaeta, death is the only relief from his physical anguish. But this individuation, in turn, facilitates his larger narrative function. By ultimately constructing Gaeta's motivations as personally situated within his disability, the viewer feels good about a death that brings him relief. Disability (and the inevitable death that follows) allows the story to neatly wrap up. This construction of Gaeta's leg as a metaphor dovetails with Gaeta's death, which sit solidly within a broader narrative tradition of disabled characters either being cured or killed at the end of stories.[12] All in all, *BSG* provides an illustrative example of *how* the narrative use of disability works through the representational bind that emerges when a disabled character individually embodies broader social conflicts. Gaeta's disability ultimately appears on screen as just another narrative device and/or example of stock characterization.

(Sort of) Queer Love

The Emmy-nominated webisode series *Battlestar Galactica: Face of the Enemy* aired on the Sci-Fi website between December 12, 2008, and January 12, 2009, after Gaeta's injury but before the mutiny arc. Much like episodes from a television show, the webisodes aired serially during this time. *Face of the Enemy* features Gaeta and several other characters from *BSG* and serves as an extra-textual narrative connected to the *BSG universe*. Most simplistically, *Face of the Enemy* presents two love stories that complicate Gaeta's disability as motivation for the coup by presenting an alternative narrative explanation for his actions. Notably, while the webisodes aired between the first half of season four (marked 4.0 on the DVD) and the second half (4.5), *Face of the Enemy* was written and filmed after the entire fourth season had been filmed (Podcast Commentary on "A Disquiet Follows My Soul"). The writers and producers of the series fail to comment on the reason for the addition, but the content of the webisodes suggests that it fills a narrative gap left by *BSG*. *Face of the Enemy* evidences the inadequacy of disability to account for a major character shift in which Gaeta transitions from a dutiful colonial officer and generally likable supporting character to a mutineer whose death the viewers easily accept. Although *BSG* makes no direct reference to the webisodes, these love stories infuse Gaeta's actions in *BSG*'s narrative with the ghost of an alternative explanation for his mutinous actions that undermines the function disability plays.[13] However, like all ghosts, *Face of the Enemy* is haunted with its own stereotypical conventions, as it constructs Gaeta's queer sexuality as little more than an opportunistic narrative device (similar to its use of disability) to further individualize Gaeta's action.

    Face of the Enemy opens with Col. Saul Tigh (Michael Hogan), the ship's second in command, ordering Gaeta on a mandatory rest leave to better recover from his injuries. Gaeta reluctantly departs on a small transport ship that, due to a system's malfunction, leaves him, three other humans and two Number Eight Cylons, both called Sharon (Grace Park) lost in space.[14] With limited oxygen and no promise of rescue, one of the Sharons begins secretly killing crewmembers. Through a series of flashbacks we learn that this particular Sharon (each copy has their own unique experiences) had a relationship with Gaeta.[15] During that relationship Gaeta unknowingly gave Sharon sensitive information that lead to the deaths of untold humans. Gaeta learns of her betrayal during the course of *Face of the Enemy* and subsequently attacks and kills her. Eventually Gaeta returns to the fleet, changed by the revelation of this betrayal and motivated to start the mutiny that follows. Again, I reiterate that *BSG* makes no mention of this sequence because, practically, it wasn't conceived of or written until after the *BSG* narrative was completed.

    In *Face of the Enemy* "Episode 1" the viewer learns that Gaeta and Hoshi are lovers. *BSG* makes no direct reference to Gaeta's sexuality in any of its 73 episodes. Yet *Face of the Enemy* reveals two relationships in its ten-webisode run. The show codes both relationships as (sort of) queer and uses them to frame Gaeta's motivations for starting the coup.[16] First, Sharon seduces and tricks Gaeta into helping the Cylons and this revelation constructs Gaeta's distrust of the alliance and his mutinous actions as resulting from her betrayal. Sharon is played by the rather feminine Grace Park and unambiguously gendered female on screen; however she is a machine and therefore technically an "it" from the majority perspective of the humans. Shira Chess contends that *BSG* depicts all Cylon/human relationships as queer because the fleet ostracizes humans who have sex with Cylons through labels like "toaster lover" (Chess 88).[17] Gaeta's relationship with Sharon carries the same transgressive valence. Similarly, I also cautiously call Gaeta's relationship with Hoshi queer because it is only one of two acknowledged gay or lesbian relationships within the world of *BSG*.[18] Notably, both of these relationships appear outside the main narrative of the series (both were revealed in extraneous storylines). This alone could make Gaeta and Hoshi's relationship queer in the broader sense (as in non-normative).

However, I qualify my use of queer marker because the show deliberately normalizes both relationships in a way that attempts to make them less queer. Moreover, I do not want to simply label a non-normative relationship queer because doing so elides the politics that undergirds queer.[19] Judith Butler suggests that "queer" is a site of collective contestation (228). Queer connotes affiliations across identity categories made in order to, as Butler suggests, contest norms. In other words, just because something defies normative heterosexual representations does not mean that those representations inherently challenge that norm (McRuer 29–30). As such, labeling either of Gaeta's relationships as queer without qualification fails to recognize the political undertone of the term. More importantly, *Face of the Enemy* deliberately depoliticizes both of these relationships, making them only "sort of" queer.

Face of the Enemy uses a narrative of romantic love and care between Gaeta and Hoshi in order to normalize their relationship. When Gaeta's ship goes missing, Hoshi convinces one of the commanders to give him a ship to search for Gaeta. Having no idea where to look, Hoshi and his pilot search randomly. Hoshi believes that the universe will guide him to Gaeta, and the narrative plays this belief out to suggest that Hoshi's love literally saves Gaeta. The show combines this overly romanticized rescue with little physical affection between the two men to present what we might call an acceptable gay relationship, i.e., one overly monogamously attached yet passionless. Benshoff and Griffin argue that films often present overtly gay characters, when they appear on screen at all, as "desexualized, depoliticized, and removed from any sociocultural context" (262). *Face of the Enemy* attempts to similarly naturalize Gaeta and Hoshi's relationship by presenting an already established romance nearly devoid of on-screen physicality. While this presentation resists the traditional (often tiresome, tedious and trite) "coming out" narratives found in mainstream LGBT representations, *Face of the Enemy's* integration of their relationship obscures any political position or challenge to heteronormativity. The men share only one kiss on screen, and the actions that buttress the kiss (the looks that they exchange, a hand on Gaeta's cheek, a smile) do more to establish their intimacy than the actual kiss, but even this intimacy bespeaks care more than it does passion ("Episode 1").

By downplaying the kiss, the scene effectively whitewashes the couple of any sexual intimacy. This contrasts with the markedly more passionate kiss that Sharon and Gaeta share in a flashback scene where candles line the frame, the lighting is dim, and they slowly approach one another with drawn out sexual tension. Similarly, Gaeta and Sharon's second kiss aboard the lost ship takes place in equally dim lighting; as they lean in Sharon pauses while Gaeta tells her that he has someone else in his life and then moves in for an intense and passionate kiss. In some ways, their passion helps to neutralize the relationship between Gaeta and Hoshi by eclipsing it with Gaeta's sexual desire for a woman (though the show eventually undermines this reading).

In perhaps the most striking confirmation of Gaeta's queer function in the narrative, if we read *Face of the Enemy* alongside *BSG*, we see that Gaeta's homosexuality shores up the able-bodied heterosexuality of the entire fleet. As mentioned, *BSG* depicts the fleet in disarray before the mutiny. The figurative mother of the fleet, President Roslin, has effectively abandoned her duties, leaving the fleet's figurative father, Admiral Adama, to hold the fleet together. He proves inadequate to the task without her. The mutiny threatens the family unit (the fleet) and the parents (both leaders) rally to defend it. In an overly dramatic and romantic scene Roslin flees Galactica for the safety of a Cylon ship where she can regroup to challenge the mutiny while Adama stays to defend their floating home base ("The Oath"). Gaeta's death at the close of the mutiny allows the heterogeneity of the fleet to be retained as exemplified by the reunification of Adama and Roslin at the end of "Blood on the Scales." Roslin returns from the Cylon ship to Adama, who stands ready to embrace her (the two are in fact figured as a mature romantic couple, although their romance is consistently sublimated and kept subordinate to their public roles).

Culpably Gay: Betrayal as Justification

Much like the presence of disability on screen, queer sexuality requires a narrative explanation and both of these relationships are no exception. Gaeta and Hoshi's relationship presents a backdrop to Gaeta and Sharon's relationship. Despite the passionate kiss that Gaeta and Sharon share, *Face of the Enemy* quickly concedes that Gaeta is unequivocally gay. Gaeta's transgression with Sharon — giving her the names of human "resistance fighters" during a several-months-long Cylon occupation on a planet the humans deemed New Caprica — is cast as a mistake of bad judgment. As *Face of the Enemy* develops, Sharon intimates to Gaeta that she tricked him into helping the Cylons by playing into his fallibility as a human male. She chides him, saying, "I'm a woman. And a Cylon. I didn't seduce you. Hope did" ("Episode 9"). Her censure suggests that Gaeta should have known better than to fall for her because she is a Cylon *and* because she is a woman. Not only does the series foreclose any chance of fluid sexuality, it suggests that Gaeta should never have been tempted by Sharon's seduction in the first place because of his sexuality. Sharon's reproach (and Gaeta's sexuality) constructs Gaeta as naïve, but naïve in a way that makes him culpable. If he were a heterosexual male then the (presumably heterosexual male) audience could sympathize with and understand this seduction. *Face of the Enemy* introduces Gaeta's gay sexuality in order to derail this identification and thereby implicate him in the deaths on New Caprica, which ultimately facilitates the ease with which *BSG* literally discards Gaeta (and his body) after the Galactica mutiny.

While *BSG* constructs Gaeta's disability as the "reason" or "justification" for his mutinous actions (as Ronald Moore explicitly states in the podcast commentary of "Blood on the Scales"), *Face of the Enemy* presents Sharon's betrayal as his "real" justification. The webisode draws a distinct difference between Gaeta's feelings about Cylons before Sharon reveals her betrayal and afterward. Before the transport ship leaves the Galactica, Gaeta displays annoyance at another human crewmember who bemoans the presence of Cylons on the ship. Gaeta looks disapprovingly as the man calls the Sharons boarding the ship "toasters" ("Episode 1"). Yet, at the end of *Face of the Enemy*, Gaeta expresses outright anti–Cylon sentiment. Colonel Tigh tells Gaeta that the Admiral will not investigate the deaths aboard the lost ship because he does not want to risk the alliance. Gaeta responds by emphatically telling Tigh that there should not be an alliance. Then Gaeta demands to speak with the Admiral directly. Tigh questions why, and Gaeta responds by telling him, "Because you're a Cylon, Sir" ("Episode 10"). His blatant refusal to speak to Tigh (the same commanding officer whose orders he obeyed just days earlier) marks the beginning of his shift toward the leader that he becomes in the Galactica mutiny arc and locates that shift firmly in response to Sharon's betrayal.

Crip/Queer Futurity

In splitting my analysis between *BSG* and *Face of the Enemy*, I do not mean to suggest that the webisodes do not address (i.e., use) disability. Gaeta's disability facilitates *Face of the Enemy's* narrative by providing the propulsion for the storyline: Gaeta must take a leave from work to recover from his injury, which puts him aboard the lost ship. The webisodes establish the care and intimacy between Gaeta and Hoshi by having Hoshi give Gaeta morpha (the show's version of morphine) and describe the lengths he went to in order to get the morpha for Gaeta. Each time Gaeta injects himself with morpha *Face of the Enemy* transitions into a flashback. Here the pain of Gaeta's disability, quantified through the frequency with which he uses the morpha, serves a similar function as pain does in the main *BSG* narrative: it marks a process of individualizing Gaeta's motives. The painkillers cause Gaeta to slip into a dreamlike state that facilitates the flashbacks through which Gaeta (and the viewer) learn of his relationship with Sharon, the relationship that leads Gaeta to start the coup.

In discussing disability in theater, Victoria Ann Lewis (1998) suggests that parallel constructions of disability and race, class and/or sexuality provide an emergent dramaturgical strategy for combating stereotypical and stigmatizing representations of disability by presenting complex and multilayered characters (527). While I share the belief in the *possibility* of parallel constructions, *BSG* and *Face of the Enemy's* presentation of a tangentially gay, disabled character falls short of fulfilling this potential. *Face of the Enemy* arguably complicates Gaeta's character by conferring sexuality onto a disability character, a rarity in itself. However, my initial reading suggests that the extra-textual nature of this narrative undermines the effect of this addition. Moreover, the addition of two (sort of) queer narratives does not destabilize the stereotypical use of disability to propel narratives forward and give materiality to nonmaterial tensions. The addition of Gaeta's sexuality merely reiterates the individualized narrative that *BSG's* use of disability creates.

That said, disability studies scholars will arguably have to wait a long time before mainstream film and/or television offer representations that in no way fall into the prevailing disability stereotypes. Similarly, queer studies and queer theory may face a dreary future of critiquing the appearance of gay, lesbian and bisexual characters that function to reestablish heteronormativity. Where does that leave us, then? Are we locked into continually interrogating the failures of Hollywood to move beyond disability stereotypes or continually tracing the ways that network television uses queer characters in the service of a politics of tolerance?

Jose Munoz suggests that "we gain a greater conceptual and theoretical leverage if we see queerness as something that is not yet here" (22). Munoz argues for a queer relationality grounding in a future collectivity and advocates squinting — straining our vision beyond the here and now to locate glimpses of this queer futurity (22).[20] Reading Gaeta's (sort of) queerness from this position challenges us to squint through the deployment of sexuality as a narrative device to locate a complexity in Gaeta's sexual desires. It challenges us to "queer" Gaeta in a way that sees sexual desire both within Gaeta's kiss with Sharon *and* within the care shared by Gaeta and Hoshi. Moreover, it fosters a crip/queer collectivity to do so, relying on crip theory and crip perspectives that recover sensuality and sexuality within acts of care like those between Hoshi and Gaeta. This crip/queer futurity invites us to read the passion that Gaeta shows for Sharon as casting doubt not on Gaeta's sexual desire for Hoshi but on the possibility of containing sexuality within rigid identity categories. It excavates the potential for a crip/queer collectivity where a disabled character can have fluid sexual desires, even if that potential (for now) remains sequestered within the extra-textual webisode narrative.

An orientation toward a queer/crip futurity would see the *possibilities* that Gaeta's character in *BSG* and *Face of the Enemy* signals and work toward developing those possibilities. For instance, the webisodes themselves (much like fan fiction, comic books and video games based on television or film narratives) open up an increasingly expanding space for characters to exist beyond the confines of the network television show. These additional narratives sanction viewers to imagine rich lives for characters beyond those offered within the text. Similarly, *Face of the Enemy* invites viewers to imagine a life for Gaeta beyond the episodes of *BSG* and beyond the sexually neutered portrayal of disabled characters. The webisodes suggest that Gaeta's character exceeds, or can exceed, the (sort of) queer, disabled narrative offered. It provides us with just a hint of a queer crip character from which we might locate a way beyond the redundant, and often oppressive, use of disability and sexuality as narrative devices.

I end, then, with an indulgently campy allusion to Admiral Adama's opening speech in *Battlestar Galactica: The Miniseries: The road to this crip/queer futurity will not be easy. It will be long and arduous, but we will get past the stereotypical representations of disability and sexuality on screen.* Of course, like Admiral Adama, I would be lying if I said I knew how to get there. But as Munoz suggests, this futurity is not so much a place as it is a process of contestation.

Notes

1. This number does not include *Battlestar Galactica: The Miniseries* (2003). IMDB lists the miniseries as separate from the other 73 episodes and for consistency's sake I adopt this demarcation as well.

2. For critical essays on *BSG* see Potter and Marshall as well as Steiff and Tamplin. To convey the extent of its popular acclaim: the series was nominated for three Primetime Emmys, named the top television series of 2005 by *Time* magazine, took home the prestigious Peabody Award in 2006 and received an additional 22 awards. All in all the show was nominated for a total of 46 awards.

3. Emily Russell details the pervasive use of the disabled body as a signifier of problems within the social body or the body politic. See her introductory chapter for more information, and for a historical look at the construction of the social body see also Mary Poovey's *Making a Social Body: British Cultural Formation, 1830–1864.*

4. See also Elaine Scarry's *The Body in Pain: The Making and Unmaking of the World* and Jean Jackson's *"Camp Pain": Talking with Chronic Pain Patients.*

5. For more on the social perception of disability as an individual problem and personal tragedy see Longmore ("Screening Stereotypes" 34), Norden (*Cinema of Isolation* 4) or Rosemarie Garland-Thomson (*Extraordinary Bodies* 22).

6. Though clearly not part of this paper, this citizenship narrative offers an interesting and complex critique of U.S. discourses and debates about citizenship within the context of 'illegal' and 'alien' immigration.

7. Simply pairing Gaeta with Zarek signifies to the viewer the danger that Gaeta and the fleet are in.

8. See Tobin Siebers ("In the Name of Pain") for a more specific discussion of the ways that cultural discourses configure pain as an individual problem.

9. I have refrained from discussing Zarek's role in the mutiny for brevity's sake. However, it's worth noting that the show carefully separates Gaeta and Zarek, at times showing Gaeta adamantly opposed to Zarek's methods (especially when Zarek orders the entire Quorum executed). This separation allows Gaeta to remain a sympathetic character even as the viewer may disagree with his actions.

10. Gaeta utters these words to Dr. Gaius Baltar (James Callis). Baltar's significance in this scene should not go without mention, as he plays a morally suspect character throughout the show. Gaeta almost kills Baltar (twice) because of Baltar's morally questionable actions. Yet, in the end Baltar sits with Gaeta and shows him empathy, marking Gaeta's fall from grace (so to speak), but also softening this scene with an air of intimacy between the men.

11. While Zarek dies along with Gaeta, the show asks us to see his death as justifiable because Zarek murdered the Quorum (the show's version of the Senate) in an effort to consolidate his power. Viewers accept his death as punishment for this act whereas we are meant to read Gaeta's death as tragic but necessary.

12. See Longmore for a discussion of the "Better dead than disabled" sentiment in film (137).

13. There is no way to know how many BSG viewers saw the webisodes or when they viewed them. However, this number ultimately proves secondary to what the webisodes' addition signals: a narrative gap left by disability's use as metaphor.

14. There are many copies of each of the 12 Cylon models so there are hundreds of Sharons in the Cylon fleet.

15. Gaeta and Sharon were together during the New Caprica Cylon occupation. Gaeta gave Sharon the names of human resistance fighters that the Cylons captured because she told him that she wanted to help set them free. Instead, she used the list to determine whom the Cylons would kill, assuming that the names Gaeta gave her were high value operatives.

16. I add the qualifying "some way" to acknowledge both the contested definition of queer and to draw attention to the ways that the show attempts to normalize the queerness it presents.

17. Chess' analysis only focuses on human men who have sex with Cylon women rather than human women who have sex with Cylon men. This is hardly due to an oversight by Chess. Rather, *BSG* features only two sexual relationships between Cylon men and human women. Notably, both relationships were established before the two men were revealed to be Cylons. Sam and Kara's relationship was essentially over when the series revealed Sam to be a Cylon and Chief Tyrol's marriage to a human woman deteriorated once he learned of his Cylon status. While outside the scope of this paper, there's a rich reading available in the show's depiction of sexy, forbidden and transgressively heterosexual human male and Cylon female relationships, which speaks to the assumed male viewer in a titillating way.

18. The other relationship is between Admiral Caine (commander of the Pegasus) and a Six, which is also revealed outside of the main narrative of *BSG* in a two-hour *BSG* special entitled *Razor*. Their relationship ends when Admiral Caine discovers that the Six is a Cylon and subsequently orders her tortured.

19. For a discussion on the depoliticization of gay politics see McRuer, *The Queer Renaissance*.

20. Notably, Munoz does not see this queer futurity as a distinct site as much as a continual process of working toward a "better" future through on-going critically queer engagement with oppressive forces.

Works Cited

Ahmed, Sara. *The Cultural Politics of Emotion*. New York: Routledge, 2004. Print.

Battlestar Galactica. Perf. Edward James Olmos, Mary McDonnell, Jamie Bamber, Trisha Helfer and Katee Sackoff. Universal Studios, 2004–2009. DVD.

"Battlestar Galactica." *IMDB.com*. IMDB.com, INC. 2011. Web. 7 Aug. 2011.

Battlestar Galactica: Face of the Enemy. Perf. Alessandro Juliani, Grace Park and Jessica Harmon. SyFy.com, 2008–2009. Web.

"Battlestar Galactica: Face of the Enemy." *IMDB.com*. IMDB.com INC, 2011. Web. 7 Aug. 2011.

Battlestar Galactica: The Miniseries. Perf. Edward James Olmos, Mary McDonnell, Jamie Bamber, Trisha Helfer and Katee Sackoff. Universal Studios, 2003. DVD.

Benshoff, Harry M. and Sean Griffin. *Queer Images: A History of Gay and Lesbian Film in America*. Oxford: Rowman & Littlefield, 2006. Print.

"Blood on the Scales." Dir. Wayne Rose. *Battlestar Galactica*. Perf. Edward James Olmos, Mary McDonnell, Jamie Bamber, Trisha Helfer and Katee Sackoff. Universal Studios, 2009. DVD.

Born on the Fourth of July. Dir. Oliver Stone. Perf. Tom Cruise, Raymond J. Barry and Caroline Kava. Universal Pictures, 1989. DVD.

Butler, Judith. *Bodies That Matter: On the Discursive Limits of "Sex."* New York: Routledge, 1993. Print.

Chess, Shira. "The C-Word: Queering the Cylons." *Battlestar Galactica and Philosophy: Mission Accomplished or Mission Frakked Up?* Eds. Joseph Steiff and Tristan D. Tamplin. Chicago: Open Court, 2008. Print.

Chivers, Sally and Nicole Markotić. *The Problem Body: Projecting Disability on Film*. Columbus: Ohio State University Press, 2010. Print.

Davidson, Michael. *Concerto for the Left Hand: Disability and the Defamiliar Body*. Ann Arbor: University of Michigan Press, 2008. Print.

"A Disquiet Follows My Soul." Dir. Ronald D. Moore. *Battlestar Galactica*. Perf. Edward James Olmos, Mary McDonnell, Jamie Bamber, Trisha Helfer and Katee Sackoff. Universal Studios, 2009. DVD.

"Faith." Dir. Michael Nankin. *Battlestar Galactica*. Perf. Edward James Olmos, Mary McDonnell, Jamie Bamber, Trisha Helfer and Katee Sackoff. Universal Studios, 2009. DVD.

Garland-Thomson, Rosemarie. *Extraordinary Bodies: Figuring Physical Disability in American Culture and Literature*. New York: Columbia University Press, 1997. Print.

Jackson, Jean E. *"Camp Pain": Talking with Chronic Pain Patients*. Philadelphia: University of Pennsylvania Press, 2000. Print.

Lewis, Victoria Ann. "The Dramaturgy of Disability." *Michigan Quarterly Review* 37.3 (1998): n. pag. Web. 8 Feb. 2013.

Longmore, Paul. "Screening Stereotypes: Images of Disabled People in Television and Motion Pictures." *Why I Burned My Book and Other Essays on Disability*. Philadelphia: Temple University Press, 2006. 131–146. Print.

McRuer, Robert. *Crip Theory: Cultural Signs of Queerness and Disability*. New York: New York University Press, 2006. Print.

Mitchell, David T. and Sharon L. Snyder. *Narrative Prosthesis: Disability and the Dependencies of Discourse*. Ann Arbor: University of Michigan Press, 2000.

Munoz, Jose Esteban. *Cruising Utopia: The Then and There of Queer Futurity*. New York: New York University Press, 2009. Print.

Norden, Martin. *The Cinema of Isolation: A History of Physical Disability in the Movies*. New Brunswick: Rutgers University Press, 1994. Print.

"The Oath." Dir. John Dahl. *Battlestar Galactica*. Perf. Edward James Olmos, Mary McDonnell, Jamie Bamber, Trisha Helfer and Katee Sackoff. Universal Studios, 2009. DVD.

Potter, Tiffany, and C.W. Marshall, eds. *Cylons in America: Critical Studies in Battlestar Galactica*. New York: Continuum, 2008. Print.

Poovey, Mary. *Making a Social Body: British Cultural Formation, 1830–1864*. Chicago: University of Chicago Press, 1995. Print.

Russell, Emily. *Reading Embodied Citizenship: Disability, Narrative, and the Body Politic*. New Brunswick: Rutgers University Press, 2011. Print.

Sandahl, Carrie. "Queering the Crip or Cripping the Queer? Intersections of Queer and Crip Identities in Solo Autobiographical Performance." *GLQ* 9: 1–2 (2003): 25–56. Web.

Scarry, Elaine. *The body in Pain: The Making and Unmaking of the World*. New York: Oxford University Press, 1985. Print.

Schleifer, Ronald. *Intangible Materialism: The Body, Scientific Knowledge and the Power of Language*. Minneapolis: University of Minnesota Press, 2009. Print.

Siebers, Tobin. "In the Name of Pain." *Against Health: How Health Became the New Morality*. New York: New York University Press, 2010. Print.

Steiff, Josef, and Tristan D. Tamplin. *Battlestar Galactica and Philosophy: Mission Accomplished or Mission Frakked Up?* Chicago: Open Court, 2008. Print.

Healer? Assassin?

Ben Hawkins, "Cure," "Disability" and Missions in HBO's *Carnivàle*

JOHNSON CHEU

HBO's *Carnivàle* is fraught with religious symbolism — the symbolic battle between good and evil, an allegory for today's political climate — and a look anew at freak shows and normality. Set in the Dust Bowl Depression years of the mid–1930s, the show focuses on intersecting lives of the performers and producers of a carnival traveling west, the locals who encounter them, and a demagogic preacher based in California and his flock. Ben Hawkins (Nick Stahl), who joins the carnival in Oklahoma, is arguably the series' primary protagonist. He turns out to have an "ability" to "heal" those who are diseased, disabled, sick or even dying, which is central to the multi-layered, complex, intersecting storyline. For Ben's character, the relationship between disability and curing is complicated by the fact that his healing powers are apparently a zero-sum game. Whenever he heals or gives life, he must take it as well, as if there is only so much able-bodiedness or life force to go around. For Ben, "healing" and disability are thereby linked by an economy of redistribution that is also deeply enmeshed with an idea of "mission." In an interview on HBO's website, *Carnivàle*'s creator Daniel Knauf has this to say about the second season:

> You know the Ben Hawkins character is going to become more and more activated. He knows what he's supposed to do now. The man that goes into Management's trailer at the end of episode 12, he's been set off on a task. Now it's not necessarily gonna be something that he wants to do. And it's not something that he feels good about doing all the time. But he has to do it. He's compelled to do it ["HBO *Carnivàle*"].

As Knauf asks, "Is he a healer? Is he an assassin or both?" How are viewers supposed to read Ben's curing of a little girl's (Lilli Babb) legs against or alongside his strangling of Professor Lodz (Patrick Bauchau)?

The question of whether Ben Hawkins is a murderer or a healer or perhaps both, his position in relation to disability, and the question of cure are issues with which this essay wrestles. *Carnivàle,* with the freak show as its ever-present backdrop and with disabled characters who may have a healer in their midst, offers, I believe, a new way of understanding cure and disability beyond the age-old image of the disabled person as freak. I should note here that though there are distinctions to be made between a disabled person and a freak—

145

for instance, a person of small stature who likely would have been called a "dwarf" or "midget" during the days of the commercial freak show versus a freak show performer who swallows swords—for the purposes of discussion of *Carnivàle* I am collapsing both kinds under what Rosemarie Garland-Thomson terms enfreakment. Enfreakment "emerges from cultural rituals that stylize, silence, differentiate, and distance the persons whose bodies the freak-hunters or showmen colonize and commercialize. Paradoxically, however, at the same time that enfreakment elaborately foregrounds specific bodily eccentricities, it also collapses all those differences into a 'freakery' a single amorphous category of corporeal otherness" (10). Because *Carnivàle* collapses all its characters under the banner of the freak show, it is appropriate to do so in this examination.

A forerunner to *Carnivàle* and the freak show it presents is Tod Browning's 1932 cult classic *Freaks. Freaks* is a film in which disabled people are shown doing everyday activities such as eating, drinking, joking and so forth. *Freaks* as Robin Larson and Beth Haller note, moved disabled persons from a "celebrated exotic attraction" to a "pathological, scientific specimen" (Larson 164). This distinction is important if for no other reason than what engendered public protest of *Freaks* as Larson and Haller note, has become a non-issue in Knauf's *Carnivàle*—the freaks of *Carnivàle* live their lives with little protest or revulsion on the part of others. Knauf's series would likely not exist without the fore-runner *Freaks,* something that Knauf himself acknowledges in an interview with theage.com.au:

> Knauf says so-called "freaks," people born with striking physical anomalies, have always inter-ested him, and it is a fascination that probably grew from having a father confined to a wheel-chair by childhood polio.
> "People defined him by that disability, it all had to do with the wheelchair," says Knauf. "One of the beautiful things about Tod Browning's work in *Freaks* is, five seconds after being shocked or even repulsed by their appearance, you stop seeing it and just start taking them as a person. That's what I wanted to play with, and hope I was successful with it" [Tuhoy].

Given *Carnivàle's* mix of futuristic or apparently supernatural elements, such as Sofie Apol-lonia's (Diane Salinger) telekinesis, within a dramatic context of the early twentieth century American freak show, the progression of American society's acceptance of disabled people at-large is key to twenty-first century domestic viewers' acceptance of Knauf's *Carnivàle* universe. Before turning to *Carnivàle* and Ben Hawkins, in particular, I turn to constructions of disability and of the Freak Show as background for the ideas explored in this essay.

A Place to Belong: Disability, the Freak Show, Cure and the Body

Scholarship in Disability Studies has both reflected and helped spur on this "new" understanding of the disabled body and disability experience as something more than just a "defective" body. While "disability" is a term largely imbued with medicalized notions of an impaired body, scholars such as Carol Thomas and Jenny Morris have articulated a dis-tinction between the terms "impairment" and "disability." In this new configuration, "impairment" generally refers to physiological and psychological conditions of the body, while "disability" encompasses a larger cultural understanding of disability experience, including teasing, stigma, the history of institutionalization, literary and media represen-tations of disability, and so forth.[1] In this way, the configuration of "impairment" refers to the body as a corporeal entity, while "disability" refers to a societal and cultural phenomenon, an identity. James I. Charlton sums up the social construction of disability this way:

> People with disabilities are significantly affected by the way in which culture(s) explain the cause of their disabilities (God's will, reincarnation, witchcraft); the images disability evokes (the sick/deformed body); and how they are described (cripple, invalid, retard). These interact to produce the way society at large is socialized to think about disability. Socialization works on simple symbols, simple repetition. Over and over the myth as message is repeated: disability = sickness/deformation; sickness = helplessness and deformation = abomination; helplessness = protection and abomination = asexuality; asexuality = childlike; childlike = helpless/protection; helpless/protection = pity; pity = disability [Charlton 68].

This distinction between impairment and disability is important for it posits a difference between physical bodily state (impairment), and socio-political-cultural status (disability).[2] As such, the freak show characters in *Carnivàle* can and certainly do have impairments (the bearded lady, the telepathic Apollonia, and so on), but how society ostracizes them and how they function as/in their own world with their own set of rules is largely a product of how the nondisabled or able-bodied world view and respond to those folks who produce and perform in the freak show. How, too, the freak show or revival attendees (representing main-stream society) view their own impairments and Ben Hawkins's ability to cure them, often as part of either the freak show or of a religious gathering, is also important and will be explored later.

In his chapter entitled "Freaks and the Literary Imagination," from *Freaks: Myths and Images of the Secret Self,* Leslie Fiedler writes:

> The real world of show Freaks [... has] turned human prodigies into metaphors for something else: the plight of the artist, the oppression of the poor, the terror of sexuality, or the illusory nature of social life. They provide us, therefore, with no satisfactory clue to what it is like to be a performer of one's own anomalous and inescapable fate [273].

The freak show or freak oddity has often been thought of as the physical embodiment of those in society called "grotesque." Freak shows, as Fiedler and others note, were at once repositories for the disabled, those considered abnormal, unsightly, grotesque, but also, in ways, an empowering mechanism for the disabled. At a time when job opportunities for the disabled were limited, the freak show served as a means for disabled persons to sustain a livelihood, albeit using their disabilities as commodities to do just that.[3] The freak show then, was both a literal place where the disabled and different can exist, but also a place where the *idea* of the freak was presented to and consumed by the larger populace. While the freak show itself has since receded into the annals of twentieth-century carnival history, the pervasive idea of the freak as someone outside the boundaries of societal normalcy remains. As Robert Bogdan claims in *Freak Show: Presenting Human Oddities for Amusement and Profit,* "Freak is a frame of mind, a set of practices, a way of thinking about and pre-senting people" (3).

The idea of freak as oddity and as a measure of social boundaries can be traced back to a time before the twentieth-century. As Chris Baldick tells us in his work, *In Frankenstein's Shadow: Myth, Monstrosity, and Nineteenth-Century Writing,* the monster is a being or cultural embodiment that has a specific societal purpose "to reveal the results of vice, folly, and unreason as a warning to erring humanity [...] The monster is one who has so transgressed the bounds of nature as to become a moral advertisement" (10–12). To be monstrous, then, is to teach others proper behavior by illustrating the results of breaking socially accepted codes of conduct, disobeying parents, laws, or norms, or altering nature.[4] The characters in *Carnivàle* are not, of course, monsters in the traditional sense of Frankenstein, but they exist in *Carnivàle* as a band of travelers; their presence in a town is always temporary, and they are nearly always separated from the townies. They are needed only to run a carnival or host a prayer meeting, so they always exist on the boundaries of the rest of society. In addition, in the episode of Clayton "Jonesy" Jones' (Tim DeKay) tarring and feathering that I discuss later, it is quite evident that the carnies have their own social and moral code. In this way, though they are not monstrous per se, they do experience a certain degree of social isolation and possess abilities that mark them as different. The position of the freak show characters of *Carnivàle* as outsiders generates critical dramatic potential in relation to the regular townies, but it is the presentation of "freaks" as both oddities and as a means of profit, and the idea of illusion, that is important in understanding how the construction of cure operates in the text. (In terms of illusion, as Fielder, Bogdan, and Baldick all point out, there is some question as to whether Ben's abilities as a healer are indeed "real" throughout much of the series.)

In this section, I began with outlining the difference between impairment and disability (one as material, the other as constructed) and the idea of freaks as both real and as socially imagined as grotesque or odd. Before turning to Ben Hawkins, it is necessary to explore one more theoretical idea, the idea of medical cure, at least briefly.

Horacio Fábrega, Jr., notes in *The Evolution of Sickness and Healing,* "Members of all societies encounter disease and injury and develop social practices to cope with their effects" (1). Fábrega contends that the epistemology of medicine consists of a sickness side which "announces, communicates, and expresses the sufferings of conditions of disease and injury, and of the healing side which is but the response aimed at comforting, undoing, relieving, fixing, minimizing and, if necessary, drawing to a close that suffering" (290). While I do not want to dwell on the idea of suffering here, what is of importance is a supposed duality that exists between the body as sick or the body as well, or to put it *Carnivàle's* terms, the body as deformed or the body as healed, the body sick or the body as cured.

While not about film and media per se, Lois Keith's book *Take Up Thy Bed and Walk: Death, Disability and Cure in Classic Children's Fiction* explores the idea of cure quite directly, tying it to the way that disabled characters operate and are represented in fiction. She writes, "From the 1850s, up until very recently (and even now writers kill or cure their disabled characters with worrying ease), there were only two possible ways for writers to resolve the problem of their character's inability to walk: cure or death" (5). Of course, Jonesy doesn't die after being tarred and feathered late in the series, though he comes close, but for the intervention of Ben Hawkins, an example of why Ben's position as a supposed healer is so important. Moreover, if one goes back to the idea that sickness/wellness are bodily states, both medically and socially defined, then cure of the sickness or of the impairment is understood to be a finite end to suffering, and/or in the case of Jonesy, a restoration to a whole bodily state (he is no longer crippled). In other words, buying into the duality between sickness/wellness, disease or disability/cure, as the mainstream audience who attend the freak shows and religious gatherings of Brother Justin Crowe (Clancy Brown) obviously do, then the power of cure enacted in Ben's abilities are understood to be a positive. In this way, cure, whether through faith healing, divine intervention, or medicine, must be understood to be a positive gain. One's life and body are indeed made better via cure. Thus, the familiar equation is: disability/freak = negative, cure/nondisabled bodies = positive.

My goal, in pointing out the constructedness of disability, cure, sickness, etc., is not to negate the presence of actual medical cures for diseases, nor is it to invalidate pain or the actual lived experience of people who may desire such medical cure. Rather, outlining these terms and ideas and exploring them through the character of Ben Hawkins and the series *Carnivàle* may help to understand how they shape the ways in which the disabled and nondisabled view each other in the world.

Ben Hawkins, Healer: Murder, Power, and Control

At the end of Season 1, viewers get their first glimpse of Ben Hawkins as a murderer. (I am discounting Ben's mother Flora Hawkins's [Lucinda Jenney] death, which Samson [Michael J. Anderson] later charges Ben with allowing because at that point neither Ben nor viewers understand his abilities). In this finale, Ben strangles Lodz with his bare hands so that Ruthie (Adrienne Barbeau) may live. The closing shot of episode 12 shows a close-up of Ruthie gasping awake. This murder is personal for Ben Hawkins, who upon strangling Lodz says with full vengeance, "Take a good look, you son of a bitch." In contrast, once Ben understands from Management (Linda Hunt) that his ability to cure or change a life means another has to die, he does not want to hurt someone he knows. In fact, he does not want to hurt anyone if he can help it. He attempts to strangle a stranger in a bar in exchange for Ruthie's life, and also he slices his own throat — his life for Ruthie's. Both of these actions are thwarted. Upon slicing his throat, Ben sees a flurry of visions and Management's voice is heard, "It doesn't work that way. You are meant for greater things. This is who you are." Henry "Hack" Scudder (John Savage) then appears and says, "You must make a choice. I'm sorry." Touching his hand to Ben's throat, Scudder heals him. Later, confronting Management, Ben still shows he's conflicted about his power, telling Management, "I ain't like you. God takes what's his, man don't take it back." But management tells Ben that God is not responsible for Ruthie's fate, Lodz is. And the killing of Lodz at the hands of Ben ensues.

Earlier in the series, viewers are led to see Ben's ability to cure as fake. At a gathering of townsfolk, viewers see a shot of a cloaked Sofie[5] (Clea DuVall) as the "planted" sick person for Ben to cure. One could read the idea of cure as being socially constructed as a scam in this scene, which is important both in understanding Ben Hawkins's gradual evolution and acceptance of his mission. For if Ben does not fully understand or believe in his power, then of what use is it beyond lucrative carnivalesque entertainment? Depicting Ben's ability to cure as socially constructed is the viewers' first glimpse of the idea that perhaps cure is not all it's cracked up to be. Again, this is not to say that pain/impairment/disease does not exist; rather questioning the power of cure, whether it's real or possible, is, in effect, saying that perhaps one ought not to be so dependent on the idea of cure — that one ought not to view it as a magical elixir or panacea without consequences. When Ben Hawkins saves Ruthie's life, cure/healing becomes real, but there is a cost: the life of Lodz. In this moment Ben Hawkins is indeed both a healer and a murderer.

In Elizabeth Grosz's *Volatile Bodies* she writes:

> Within the Christian tradition, the separation of mind and body was correlated with a distinction between what is immortal and what is mortal. As long as the subject is alive, the mind and body form an indissoluble unity [...] Within Christian doctrine, it is as an experiencing, passionate, suffering being that generic man exists. This is why moral characteristics were given to various physiological disorders and why punishments and rewards for one's soul are administered through corporal pleasures and punishments [5–6].

If one reads Ben's actions in the above instances in light of Grosz's assertions, then viewers are meant to read bodies (and souls) as intertwined and connected along a system of punishments and rewards. In this way, we can argue that on the plane of rewards and punishments, Lodz and Ruthie do not exist separately — that reviving the body and soul of Ruthie necessitates the killing of the body and soul of Lodz; that Ben's actions result in a zero-sum gain.[6]

Another transformative moment for Ben Hawkins in his relationship to his ability is his healing of Jonesy from near-death and the healing of Jonesy's lame leg. In this extended sequence, Ben comes upon Libby Dreifuss (Carla Gallo) and Jonesy after Jonesy has been tarred and feathered by a gang who blame him for the accident of the Ferris wheel that causes the death of one of the men's wives. Ben sends Libby to his truck on the roadside ("So you don't get hurt") and proceeds to bring life to the nearly-dead Jonesy, who awakens confused and peeling bits of tar from his body, and who eventually discovers that his lame leg is healed as well. "I fixed that too," Ben Hawkins simply says.

Before Ben heals Jonesy, he looks up at vultures circling overhead; Jonesy subsequently awakens encircled by a bunch of dead vultures. In these two actions — Ben's sending Libby away to protect her and in accepting that vultures will die for Jonesy — viewers encounter a different Ben Hawkins from the vengeance-filled one who murders Lodz. With the healing of Jonesy, Ben accepts his power and attempts to control the life that is sacrificed. To be sure, in doing so, he is making a judgment about which lives or kinds of lives are more valuable and which are less. But, in doing so, he is also attempting to ensure that the hurt he causes through healing is as minimal as possible for the humans he encounters. There will be other vultures and water lilies, but there is only one Libby. Some may still see him as a murderer, but at least he is aware of the consequences of his actions and takes action to mitigate them. He's a murderer and a healer both, with a conscience.

Moving Life: Cure, Gains, and Quality of Life

One of Ben Hawkin's final acts as a "healer" is the most telling. After the "accident" on the Ferris wheel in which the carnies try to kill Brother Justin, a barely-alive mother lies next to her dead boy and mumbles repeatedly, "Take me not my son, take me not my son." In a wide-angle shot, viewers see Ben kneeling down towards the mother, as the camera zooms in on a close-up of his face so that no one milling about the wreckage may see what he is doing. "Are you sure this is what you want?" he questions the mother. Unlike his killing of Lodz, which was filled with vengeance and where he was still wrestling with the idea of God v. Man, and unlike the healing of Jonesy, where he understands what the price is and he tries to control who or what loses life, in this scene he cedes the decision of a healing's cost to the person who will pay it. She affirms her desire, and within moments she's dead and her lifeless son is alive and asking for her. Samson has witnessed this whole exchange from a distance, and suggests to Ben that he can win away Brother Justin's flock by healing the sick, but Ben replies:

> BEN HAWKINS: I can't just conjure up a healing from scratch.... It doesn't work that way. All I do is move life.
> SAMSON: So you heal someone...
> BEN HAWKINS: ...I gotta hurt someone else ["New Caanan," episode 24].

For me, the phrase "All I do is move life" is of key importance, both in Ben's understanding of his ability, and for the construction of disability more generally. Often, disability is constructed as a loss, and cure or healing is a gain. However, with this phrase, Ben reminds viewers that his ability has a profound cost. The idea of cost, I believe, is central to a different understanding of disability from that of impairment, of simply bodily functional loss. By reminding viewers that his ability has a cost, the series asks viewers to question, in effect, whether "cure" is simply and always a gain, as it has so often been portrayed to be. If, in point of fact, Ben simply "moves life" from one being (human or animal) to another, then is it even necessary to think in terms of "gains" and "losses" when it comes to the disabled or ill, both within the series and outside of it in our own lived realities, our own world? Jonesy, after all, was able to have a full life with his crippled leg. Though the series certainly presents Jonesy's "normal" leg, which he is joyous about, as positive, the healed leg is incidental to the fact that Ben Hawkins has saved his life. In fact, Jonesy has to hide it and pretend he is still crippled thereafter in order to protect Ben.

What is at work I would argue is an idea of the body that is not wholly Cartesian, that neither functions wholly on a mind/body dualism, nor on dual planes of the well and sick.[7] Rather, a body is in and of itself a body, regardless of the presence or absence of a mind, for it is we (society, readers and viewers) who assign value to that body. It is we who see crippled bodies as "less than." Rather than negating the social constructedness of disability by thinking about bodies as just bodies, *Carnivàle* instead highlights the distinction between disability and impairment by reminding us that it is we who have constructed experiences upon that body, and who bear responsibilities therein.

As I have said earlier, it is not my intention to negate the presence of actual medical cures for diseases, nor is it to invalidate pain or the actual lived experience of people who may desire such medical cure. I don't think that *Carnivàle* is trying to do that either, for it is quite apparent that disease and pain do exist. The power to cure and heal is still, though, within the world of *Carnivàle*, presented to viewers as something beyond the reach of "ordinary" humans. It is relegated to Ben, to Brother Justin, and ultimately to Sofie. In other words, the power of cure lies not within ourselves but within those who have "abilities" that ordinary humans do not. This is not shocking in and of itself, perhaps, for there are indeed many diseases and disabilities in the real world for which humans have not yet found a cure. Making Ben Hawkins question such powers and ultimately perceive their cost and limitations — for he simply "moves life" — in turn asks viewers to question the idea of cure as a magical elixir. Perceiving and seeking cures for pain and suffering presumes that the townspeople see their lives as better after curing than before — that one kind of life is ostensibly more valuable than another. But Ben simply "moving life," as he sees it, without assigning value calls into question valuation itself, particularly of those who are "different." Ultimately, the series is an examination of the question: is one life more valuable than another? And if it is, what or who makes it so? Moreover, if cure is re-imagined in *Carnivàle* as something that carries with it gains and losses, then what, besides pain or ailment, does a person lose in the face of cure? If disability is more than just a bodily impairment, what might society and/or a Disabled person lose by curing it?

Series creator Knauf asks viewers to question whether Ben Hawkins is a healer, an assassin or both. If viewers are to understand him and his power to heal/cure as limited, as coming with a cost, then he is most certainly both, for as he heals/cures, he must assassinate something or someone else, though that may not be how the nondisabled see the idea of cure. Much more intriguing, for me at least, is the idea that Ben Hawkins may, indeed, be neither. If Ben Hawkins "moves life" without, in the instance of healing/cure of the mother/son, assigning a value to the life he moves, then the idea of determining someone's quality of life lies not in someone else's hands but in one's own. Ben Hawkins may have the power to "move life" but it is for the bearer of that life to determine what that life ultimately *means*. The series ends rather quickly after this episode with the Ferris wheel and turns its attention away from Ben largely to deal with Sofie and Brother Justin, an arc that pertains more to thematic ideas of good and evil than to actual cure (e.g., Sofie's decision about power at the end of the series). This is, of course, not to negate Ben's role in the narrative, but simply to say that once he appears comfortable in his own skin, so to speak, the power that he possesses and its importance to others ceases to be central to the storyline, at least in the way of actual cures. By the series' close, Ben Hawkin's supposed powers appear to have receded into the realm of acceptance, like the acceptance of many other characters in the series and their "enfreakment" status — a normalization that Knauf appears to intend. Ultimately, *Carnivàle's* point when read through the dynamics of cure may be that the determiner of one's quality of life ought to depend not on another's ability to alter one's body, but, clichéd as it may sound, on one's ability to fashion for oneself a life worth living. Perhaps Ben Hawkins's mission is not to offer someone the magic of cure; rather his mission may be to get one to see the magic already possible in one's own life, and the potential cost of altering that life.

In the first anthology of its kind to integrate the humanistic field of Disability Studies with Biblical Studies *This Abled Body: Rethinking Disabilities in Biblical Studies,* editors Hector Avalos, Sarah J. Melcher and Jeremy Schipper collect a number of essays that explore disability as a social construction applied to Biblical stories. In their essay, "Jesus Throws Everything Off Balance: Disability and Redemption in Biblical Literature," David Mitchell and Sharon Snyder contend, "Jesus as a prophet engaged in faith healing treats disability as any other socially made obstacle in that bodies may be revised into less cumbersome experiences. Whereas the removal of social barriers delimits the environment as the target of social intervention in cure/resurrection/redemption narratives, bodies are fixed to fit an unaccommodating environment" (179). At the end of *Carnivàle*, Ben embodies such a position. Neither he nor anyone else denies that he possesses a power that others do not. Rather, it is how he understands bodies and the limits of his powers that is critical and that has changed. Bodies are merely vessels, into which life can be "moved," that are of equal value in Ben's way of thinking to the obstacles or impairments (e.g., Jonesy's lame leg) placed upon them. Disability becomes a socially made obstacle like any other. What is at issue in *Carnivàle* is not just a re-thinking of disability as a "less than" social or bodily state, but also a re-thinking of the power of someone to cure or alter that state. Noted feminist and Disability Studies essayist Nancy Mairs ponders such ideas in her book, *A Dynamic God: Living an Unconventional Catholic Faith*. She writes:

> I can't count the number of times I've been told, often by strangers as they observe my crippled form, "God never sends us more than we can handle." I know they mean to comfort me for what they assume, quite wrongly, to be a wretched fate, so I grit my teeth and smile — but weakly. I despise pious clichés not merely because they falsify experience (most of us face, from time to time, more than we can handle) but because they distance and distort the "Holy."
> "God" doesn't "send" the events of our lives for good or ill. What happens, happens ... we recognize that God, though infinitely mysterious, is no magician, is indeed not an entity at all but rather an eternal unfolding in which all creation — even Winchester [her cat], even I — have our parts and bear our responsibilities [53–54].

What happens, happens. Earlier in this chapter I asked the question, "If disability is more than a bodily impairment, what might society or a Disabled person gain or lose by curing it?" Perhaps we would lose an idea of the body that is not wholly Cartesian, that does not function wholly on a mind/body dualism, or perhaps as stated earlier, an idea of the body that exists on dual planes of the well and sick.[8] A body is in and of itself a body, regardless of the presence or absence of a mind, for it is we — society, readers and viewers — who assign value to that body. It is we who see crippled bodies as "less than." Rather than negating the social constructedness of disability by thinking about bodies as just bodies, doing so instead highlights the distinction between disability and impairment by reminding us that it is we who have constructed experiences upon that body, and who bear responsibilities to find and/or create joy (and sorrow) therein.

Carnivàle offers viewers not only a different way of thinking about particular "enfreaked" bodies and lives beyond just a socially constructed "less than" state but also the need to think about the power that one has over one's own life and the ability of someone to make meaning in their lives. The carnies lived their lives regardless of Ben Hawkins's power, which even he views as limited by the end of the series. He is not a magician, an arbitrator of joy and sorrow, of good and evil in people's lives. People must look, ultimately to themselves, not to a healer and the idea of a "healed" or "cured" body to make meaning in their lives.

Notes

1. For more on the impairment/disability distinction see such texts as Mairian Corker and Sally French's "Reclaiming Discourse in Disability Studies" in *Disability Discourse*; Jenny Morris's *Pride Against Prejudice: Transforming Attitudes To Disability;* and Carol Thomas's "Theorizing disability and impairment" in *Female Forms: Experiencing and Understanding Disability*. Though not the only writers to invoke the distinction, U.K. scholars commonly use the term "disabled people" as opposed to the more common United States usage of "persons with disabilities" (PWD). This signifies a different understanding of personhood in relation to disability. The term disabled person is akin to "African American person," "gay person" and so on. It denotes identity, whereas PWD, intentionally or not, denotes disability as an add-on descriptor, a non-essential unrelated to core identity categories like race, ethnicity or sexual orientation. Therefore, my citing of U.K. theorists is intentional in exploring identity issues of disabled persons.

2. The terms "disabled" and "able-bodied people" historically allude to the idea of impairment. The combination of "disabled" and "nondisabled people" is gaining parlance in Disability Studies to signify cultural identity. Utilizing the term "the able-bodied," serves a dual purpose of referencing the historical use of the "disabled/abled" paradigm, which is grounded in impairment, while simultaneously recognizing the reclamation of naming as part of the process of claiming a disability identity.

3. See Rosemarie Garland-Thomson's edited collection *Freakery: Cultural Spectacles of the Extraordinary Body*.

4. Semantic differences exist between the terms "freak" and "monster" (freak is a term applied to freak shows; monster is generally associated with horror movies). Both are terms that imply the grotesque as I use it in this chapter, so I use both terms "freak" and "monster" somewhat interchangeably here.

5. *Carnivàle*'s site and DVDs sometimes spell Sofie as Sophie. This essay uses Sofie for consistency.

6. The idea that dual qualities of good and evil exist in the same body can be traced to the Albigenses sect of Catholicism. In thinking about the value, gains, and losses of bodies, the idea that every body encompasses the same qualities points toward a more uniform way of thinking about bodies, hence the importance of the Albigenses' thought. I am indebted to my colleague Professor Roger Brenahan for information and clarification of this point. An overview of the principle can be found here: http://www.newadvent.org/cathen/01267e.htm.

7. See Grosz's Introduction in *Volatile Bodies* for a concise overview.

8. See Grosz's Introduction in *Volatile Bodies* for a concise overview.

Works Cited

"Albigenses." *New Advent*. New Advent.Org. 2009. Web. 26 Feb. 2009.

Avelos, Hector, Sarah J. Melcher, and Jeremy Shipper, eds. *This Abled Body: Rethinking Disabilities in Biblical Studies*. Atlanta: Society of Biblical Literature, 2007. Print.

Baldick, Chris. *In Frankenstein's Shadow: Myth, Monstrosity, and Nineteenth-Century Writing.* New York: Oxford University Press, 1987. Print.

Bogdan, Robert. *Freak Show: Presenting Human Oddities for Amusement and Profit.* Chicago: University of Chicago Press, 1988. Print.

Carnivàle: The Complete Series. HBO Home Video. 2006. Television.

Charlton, James I. *Nothing About Us Without Us: Disability, Oppression, and Empowerment.* Berkeley: University of California Press, 1998. Print.

Fábrega, Horacio, Jr. *Evolution of Sickness and Healing.* Berkeley: University of California Press, 1997. Print.

Fiedler, Leslie. *Freaks: Myths and Images of the Secret Self.* New York: Simon & Schuster, 1978. Print.

Garland-Thomson, Rosemarie, ed. *Freakery: Cultural Spectacles of the Extraordinary Body.* New York: New York University Press, 1996. Print.

HBO Carnivàle. Home Box Office. 2009. Web. 9 Nov. 2009.

Keith, Lois. *Take Up Thy Bed and Walk: Death, Disability and Cure in Classic Fiction for Girls.* New York: Routledge, 1991. Print.

Larsen, Robin, and Haller, Beth. A. "The Case of Freaks: Public Reception of Real Disability." *Journal of Popular Film & Television* 29.4 (Winter 2002): 164–172. Print.

Mairs, Nancy. *A Dynamic God: Living an Unconventional Catholic Faith.* Boston: Beacon Press, 2007. Print.

Mitchell, David, and Sharon Snyder. "Jesus Throws Everything Off Balance: Disability and Redemption in Biblical Literature." *This Abled Body: Rethinking Disabilities in Biblical Studies.* Eds. Hector Avelos, Sarah J. Melcher, and Jeremy Shipper. Atlanta: Society of Biblical Literature, 2007: 173–184. Print.

Morris, Jenny. *Pride Against Prejudice: Transforming Attitudes to Disability.* London: The Woman's Press, 1991. Print.

Thomas, Carol. *Female Forms: Experiencing and Understanding Disability.* Buckingham: Open University Press, 1999. Print.

Toto, Christian. "Canceled (for Now): Die-hards Fight to Save TV Faves." *Save Carnivàle.* July 2005. Web. 24 Feb. 2011.

Tuhoy, Wendy. "Freaking Hell." *theage.com.au.* 16. Dec. 2004. Web. 15 Feb. 2011.

"Are they laughing at us or with us?"

Disability in Fox's Animated Series *Family Guy*

SIMON MCKEOWN AND PAUL A. DARKE

If the writers of a particularly pathetic cartoon show thought they were being clever in mocking my brother and my family yesterday, they failed. All they proved is that they're heartless jerks.
— Bristol Palin, referring to depictions of Down Syndrome on *Family Guy*

Almost all media research on disability (e.g., from Barnes to Norden to Davis) has clearly shown that disabled people are one of the few social groups where all rules of intelligent and civilized engagement in the cultural (and increasingly political) sphere do not apply. Disability is usually "open season" for the media where disabled subjects can be objectified, pitied, or exploited in equal measure. It is a bleak picture: Western culture traditionally perceives disability and disabled people as different, separate, and something entirely disconnected from ordinary life. Social behaviors and cultural institutions, compounded by non-disabled ignorance and lack of exposure, perpetuate disabled people's exclusion and negation. A 2010 U.K. survey reported that 90 percent of Britons had never had a disabled person in their home and 53 percent believed that most people in British society see disabled people as inferior (Dugan). The media follows suit.

When disability is depicted in mainstream media it is usually scripted as either heroic, pitiable, or freakish. Some of the most respected broadcasters in the world regularly produce material that if it were applied to race or gender or sexual preference would be universally condemned or even banned. The BBC, for example, regularly features programs that cast disabled people as heroic victims, such as *Beyond Boundaries* (2005, 2006 and 2008), a "reality" show where disabled contestants are arbitrarily lumped together and given an extensive endurance test with the goal of achieving the seemingly impossible: crossing a jungle. If, let's imagine, broadcasters or television producers challenged a group of Afro-Caribbeans or Afro-Americans to, for example, ascend Mount Everest so that viewing audiences could marvel at their success or be enthralled by their failure *because — wow — they're black*, the audience and critical feedback would be crushing.

Another U.K. broadcaster, Channel Four, a supposedly progressive broadcaster with a legally required remit to engage with marginalized social groups, quite happily showcases journalists whose only purpose is to travel the breadth of the world to find the world's tallest, smallest, or in their eyes weirdest person to humiliate, gawk at and generally annoy. Witness Mark Dolan in *The World's ... and Me,* a travel documentary-cum-modern-freak-show featuring twelve episodes airing from 2008 to 2010. In each episode, as the program's site advertises, "Mark Dolan comes face-to-face with human extremes" (*The World's*). In the first episode, "The World's Smallest Man and Me," Dolan travels to a remote region of Inner Mongolia to meet and, it seems, hold, view and treat like a doll, the smallest man in the world: He Pingping. In order to do this Dolan disturbs Pingping's family's New Year celebration and pays the family a year's worth of income to spend a short time with an extremely annoyed Pingping. The program thankfully translates Pingping's irritation and his flat admission that he does not like Dolan. This is truly disturbing television openly based on sensationalized exploitation. What is there to like in this type of relationship between disability and television? It does little more than reinforce the view of disability as unfamiliar or alien otherness that should be treated differently from supposedly standard embodiment.

In the few occasions broadcasters do try to produce inclusive and intelligent television, it usually just ends up being both odd and usually of little quality (in any sense of the word). The U.K. broadcaster Channel Four's six-episode comedy mockumentary *Cast Offs* (November – December 2009) is a fine example of good intentions creating the worst kind of disability representation. *Cast Offs* features a group of disabled people who are "abandoned" on an island in a faked reality TV setting. Despite quality performances by the cast — occasionally touching on pure comic genius — episodes leave the audience feeling that they are intended to be watching little more than exotics in a zoo.

The bias of any individual program, though, is not the whole story. Beyond the representation of disability in *Cast Offs* or any other show lies the larger issue of resource distribution. The real essence of effective cultural representation is not just what we see on screen but the behind-the-scenes engagement with the ethics of production. When disabled actors do get a chance to play on mainstream screens they are often compromised before the program begins by limited or stereotyped roles, reduced bargaining power, lower pay, even lower investments in their career promotion by industry insiders, and pervasive discrimination in casting regardless of acting talent or experience. One could argue that if the door is closed on an individual level, why should we expect it to open at the cultural institutional level? But it could be argued that the same was (and is still) true in relation to issues of race, gender and sexuality, yet mainstream broadcasters have actively worked to change attitudes. Such active cultural progressiveness does not extend to disability with perhaps few, very few, exceptions.

One exception is Fox's animated series *Family Guy* (1999–2001 and 2004-present), which features a dysfunctional family living in the fictional Rhode Island town of Quahog. *Family Guy* is known for its pointed gags about current events, political figures, and public icons, which places it squarely within a long-established tradition in English-language cartoon satire reaching back at least to the nineteenth century. In the U.K. one of the most startling satirical magazines, *Punch, or the London Charivari* (1841–1992 and 1996–2002), established the idea of combining insightful, perceptive drawings of real people with often searing satire. Throughout its long history *Punch* lambasted British politicians often exposing them as fools (Allingham). Cartoons have gone on in many media to become political and personal bazookas launched at those most needing derision. Cartoons and animations have become an essential part of our democracy aimed at undermining the crass, the hypocritical and the foolish. *Punch* proved its ability to shock and amuse the Victorian world. Modern day animations shock and amuse us now in a similar way. It is no coincidence that Fox's irreverent and culturally critical *The Simpsons* (December 1989 — present) is one of the most loved and well-known cartoons of all time.

But cartoons are strange: they offer a world where the suspension of disbelief is not only essential but quite often warped. Where else would we accept the torturing of a cat as entertainment except in MGM's *Tom and Jerry* (1940–1958) or in *Tom and Jerry's* modern incarnation *Itchy and Scratchy*, which appears as a television show within the cartoon world of *The Simpsons*? Cartoons and animations can extract maximum effect from expression, movement, action and dialogue. They combine the fantastic skills of the caricaturist, the wit of the street comedian, and the sophistication of a cultural critic. Badly written, directed or produced animations can exhibit all the same components of substandard television fare: animations can be vicious, crass, simplistic, stupid, bullying, and ultimately destructive. During the Second World War the German Nazi propaganda machine made cartoons that stereotyped and denigrated Jews, both in dialogue and visual depictions. The United States has the Censored 11, a group of *Looney Tunes* and *Merrie Melodies* animations made in the 1930s and 1940s that were withdrawn from distribution by United Artists (UA) in 1968 after heavy criticism for their racist portrayal of African Americans (Lehman). Apologists argue that the work represents a reflection of society at the time and that criticism is therefore inappropriate. Whatever your opinion, history shows the cultural power of the apparently simple medium of the cartoon. It is a unique medium, which can be used very effectively to exploit any vulnerability, weakness or characteristic for progressive or reactionary purposes.

Family Guy is the brainchild of its producer, Seth MacFarlane, who also performs a number of the voices for the show's characters. An excellent full history of the series, including its broadcast highs and lows and summaries of every episode, can be found on Wikipedia (which is itself a sign of the show's establishment as a staple of popular culture). *Family Guy's* huge success is also evident in its audience figures, global syndication, DVD sales, spin-offs, cross-marketed action figures, and in the rise of the careers of its voice artists, producers and creators. The show's popularity, along with that of *South Park* (Comedy Central, 1997–2011), *Beavis and Butt-Head* (MTV, 1992–2011) and *King of the Hill* (Fox, 1997–2010), has led to a proliferation of adult animated comedy series as a mainstay of television schedules: *Archer* (FX Network, 2009–2012), *Ugly Americans* (Comedy Central, 2011–2012), *The Life and Times of Tim* (HBO, 2008–10) and *Bob's Burgers* (Fox, 2011) to name but a few.

Family Guy's reputation rests on the show being, as its creator Seth MacFarlane has repeatedly stated, "an equal opportunities offender." It aims to use, abuse and exploit every stereotype there is about people whether they are gay, black and disabled, or straight, white and nondisabled — or any other possible combination of human type. Many of the other adult animated series share this quality of shocking, wildly irreverent, politically "incorrect" humor. The element that makes *Family Guy* different is that it is also seemingly obsessed with disability. Almost all scripted shows on television, animated or not, inevitably feature disability in some way through a character, issue, situation or storyline. *Family Guy* does all this plus much more throughout the 165 episodes of its first nine seasons (1999–2011).

The show has made fans of many disabled viewers, especially for one of its main characters, the neighbor and drinking buddy Joe Swanson. Joe is a policeman who happens to use a wheelchair and who often gives and receives jokes based on his impairment as a paraplegic. He is one of the most popular and significant mainstream characters on television to use a wheelchair since Ironside in the 1960s and 1970s. Apart from *Family Guy*'s depiction of Joe Swanson, the show also features a remarkable array of disabled characters, including the father figure, Peter Griffin, who is technically "mentally retarded" and a number of recurring characters: Jake Tucker, a little boy who has a deformed face he is ashamed of (in at least 15 episodes); Seamus, an old seaman with no legs or arms with wooden replacements (20 episodes); the "Greased-up Deaf Guy" (6 episodes); Opie, Peter's fellow worker who is "mentally challenged" yet is promoted over Peter (10 episodes); and Herbert, an elderly Roman Catholic pedophile who uses a Zimmer Frame who also has a "crippled" dog called Jesse who is paralyzed from the midriff down and drags his body around (more than 45 episodes).

Family Guy also features numerous "cut-away" gag sequences — small, seemingly irrelevant asides or sketches — within the narrative to add humor to the plotline. The creators are equally fond of using disability in these cut-away sections. For example, in one sequence Peter plays footsy with Heather Mills under a table while on a date, kicking off her false leg, and Marlee Matlin appears as a "farter" who does not know she farts because she's deaf. Beyond Mills and Matlin, the following have appeared in animated form: Margot Kidder, Kristy McNichol and Van Gogh (with jokes about mental illness); Magic Johnson (AIDS); Beethoven (deafness); Ray Charles (blindness); Helen Keller (deafness and blindness); Lou Gehrig (degenerative disease); Michael J. Fox (Parkinson's disease); Liza Minnelli (obesity and dysfunctional family matters); Kenny Baker and Gary Coleman (short stature); and Joseph Merrick, the Elephant Man, who is seen on a date with a petty blond complaining about her looks. Even fictional disabled characters are utilized for disability jokes, such as Mr. Magoo; Rocky Dennis (Eric Stoltz's character in the contemporary Elephant Man film *Mask*, 1985); Cyrano De Bergerac; Lucky the Leprechaun; Freddy Kruger; Elmer Fudd; Andre the Giant; Fat Albert; FDR's "Midget" Press Secretary (who is called "adorable" as he announces the bombing of Pearl Harbor); and Winnie the Pooh's depressed donkey friend Eeyore (whose depression is due to the nail in his anus).

Clearly disability is a key component of *Family Guy*. This essay will look at a single episode that has courted more controversy than usual, "Extra Large Medium" (Season 8, episode 12), which focuses on a young woman, Ellen, with Down syndrome. It was directed by John Holmquist, a former director of the children's animated series *Rugrats* (Nickelodeon, 1991–2004) and written by Steve Callaghan with lyrics and music by Seth MacFarlane and Walter Murphy, respectively. This episode originally aired on Fox in the USA on February 14, 2010 (released on DVD in late 2011). It features a reference to Ellen as the daughter of former Presidential candidate Sarah Palin, which inspired the Palin family to attack the show for its exploitation of learning disability. It also features the "Down Syndrome Girl" song, which went viral on YouTube.com and led to the show's nomination for a Primetime Emmy Award for Outstanding Music and Lyrics at the 62nd Primetime Emmy Awards in 2010. (Ironically, *Family Guy* lost to *Monk*, a series about someone with Obsessive-Compulsive disorder [USA Network, 2002–09].)

Family Guy: *"Extra Large Medium"*

"Extra Large Medium" focuses on the teenaged Chris and his one-year-old brother Stewie. In *Family Guy* fashion, Chris is obese, lacks confidence and is a very low achiever at school, while Stewie is an effeminate prodigy, probably gay, who sports an English accent and a giant oblong head. Stewie is also the series' sharp-tongued, mother-hating egomaniac whose articulate speech is understood only by the family's talking dog. At the beginning of the episode, the two of them get lost in a forest. Fearing they will never be found, they confess to each other the one thing they will definitely do if they are rescued. Chris states that he will ask a particular girl at school, Ellen, out on a date. Stewie vows to run for public office *again*. Three subsequent sequences follow the narrative arc of Chris's effort to follow through on his promise. In the first, Chris takes Stewie to his school to introduce him to Ellen and ask her out. Second, Chris prepares for his date with Stewie's help and the two brothers sing "Down Syndrome Girl" together. Finally, we see the date at the restaurant followed by Chris and Ellen going back to Ellen's home. *Family Guy*'s episodes often feature multiple subplots, which in this case includes an unrelated riff on popular beliefs about psychics through the boys' mother who is a believer and their father who temporarily becomes a psychic. Thus, as you can see, this is not an ordinary family.

The jokes start early in the episode with a very simple, yet ingenious, disability adaptation gag. Lost in the woods at night, Stewie starts to dig a hole, so Chris asks him what he is doing. Stewie tells Chris he likes to sleep on his side and promptly places part of his unusually shaped head in the hole. The joke functions on more than one level, as does much of the episode, demonstrating an awareness of disability and a depth of social analysis beyond what it might superficially appear to be in one quick viewing. Stewie's on-the-fly adaptation works as physical comedy highlighting his head size, a joke everyone can get, but it also works as disability comedy about a disability reality: that the environment often calls for spontaneous adaptations that require thinking outside the box. Instead of a pillow, use a hole. The ingeniousness and ridiculousness of Stewie's solution is as much an inside joke about the practical challenges of living with disability as it is about Stewie's head itself. This same sophistication is consistent throughout the episode.

Once rescued, Chris takes Stewie to school with him (again, in *Family Guy* fashion, there is no logic to this) and points out Ellen. This would be the moment in which many narratives would make the show "about" Down syndrome and the inspiration or lessons the nondisabled characters can gain from Ellen's "misfortune." Instead, *Family Guy* gives us a classic rite-of-passage story, remaining focused on Chris' genuine interest in Ellen and his anxiety about dating. At the same time, the episode doesn't dodge Ellen's Down's either. It is represented in the brothers' dialogue as a reality, but no more than that—as if Ellen simply had one of many forms of human difference found in high-school populations, which of course she does. Chris tells Stewie that Ellen has Down's and that he thinks she's sweet and has adorable eyes, and Stewie accepts this, replying. "The spacing seems a tad off but [...] All right, I'm on board." "Yeah," Chris says, "isn't she special?" meaning it in the way boys mean it when they are falling in love. "That's the way the State of Rhode Island would put it," Stewie cracks in reference to educational labeling practices that Chris doesn't perceive. Stewie's initial skepticism about Chris' romance is in keeping with his character as he finds everything a bit alien and functions as the show's meta-cultural commentator. His Rhode Island crack is in keeping with this persona: it isn't simple labeling. It points acerbically to the fact that various government entities actively define otherness and that nomenclature can be used to create otherness irrespective of the diverse individuality of any population. The fact that Stewie himself has a disability—or at least a prominent physical difference that requires environmental adaptation in the same episode—reinforces the critique: either Stewie is the pot calling the kettle black, or he's the pot observing that we're all potentially subject to getting called something.

In this same scene, Ellen picks up Stewie and squeezes him, prompting Stewie to deadpan that she probably once "owned a bunny, but not anymore." This joke, along with the consistent reference to Ellen's very strong arms and hands in every scene in which she appears, constitutes a clear reference that few have picked up on given *Family Guy*'s fame for cultural and literary in-jokes: the learning disabled character Lenny in John Steinbeck's *Of Mice and Men* (1937), which has been adapted to film three times and performed on stage for more than seventy years (even by Learning Disability theatre groups). The novel is a longstanding core text in U.S. and U.K. literature courses and one of the top ten most read books in U.S. high schools ("John Steinbeck"). The reference is clear: Lenny kills both a rabbit and the girl of his dreams with his strength, which constitutes both his greatest asset and his disability-related tragic flaw. Lenny is the most striking example of the stereotypical characterization in cultural depictions of figures with learning disability as having poorly modulated strength, but he's not an uncommon type. Although Lenny does not have Down syndrome, the episode reinforces the link over the next two scenes as Ellen uses her strength to vigorously embrace people and animals. This extended joke functions just as Stewie's Rhode Island crack does — as a spoof on stereotyping itself — in a brilliant reproduction of it that undermines its seriousness.

With its invocation of labels such as "special" and the cultural specter of Lenny, the scene suggests that physiological differences are real but their meanings are socially constructed. It effectively teases apart Ellen herself — in the full vividness of her appearance as a person with Down's — from common stereotypes of Down's and learning disability, and as we shall see — from the narrative arcs that would typically be the core function of a character with Down's in a story script. The bottom line, *Family Guy* suggests, is that characters (and by extension people) just are who they are. Ellen has Down's. Stewie has a head like a Subway sandwich. Chris lacks confidence. So what? The point is actually about *how* they relate to each other, not "*what*" they "are." The rest of the dialogue in this scene features Chris admitting to Ellen that he likes her and the two of them arranging a date with the focus on Chris' courage in actually following through with that painful first approach to his teenage crush.

Neither this scene nor the rest of the episode contains a "meaningful" discussion of any "problems" associated with dating someone with Down Syndrome: there is no hesitation, no criticism, no derision, no pity, no appeasement, and no external social questioning of this plotline. The date is just matter of fact. Chris' anxiety remains squarely focused on his own appearance and attractiveness, not on Ellen's Down's. Yes, it's a spoof because Chris doesn't apparently comprehend that Ellen's Down's automatically places her lower on the socially determined potential-mate attractiveness scale. But it's a tremendously subversive spoof because laughing at the episode at that level alone requires us to adopt the labeling Stewie sarcastically throws out rather than responding to Ellen the way Chris does: as an individual. *Family Guy*'s brilliance is that its comedy consistently undermines the crass stereotypes, social presumptions, and cheap jokes that it so blatantly parades, not the least because it doesn't actually take them seriously. That makes it harder for us to take them seriously either.

In the second sequence, Stewie offers to help Chris prepare for his date and in doing so starts to dance and sing "Down Syndrome Girl." This mock musical scene has Stewie pulling down a bathroom blind that has Ellen's face on it while Chris gazes and swoons. As they continue singing, Stewie dresses up as Ellen with a wig and stilts and romantically dances with Chris. On the mention of the excessively strong hugs, the image of Ellen on the blinds changes to Ellen squeezing a bear whose head pops off. The song speeds up to its finale with Stewie sending Chris off to his date with Ellen by sliding down the banister and pushing him out the door while his final high-pitched note shatters the windows. The Emmy-nominated lyrics with their wildly irreverent lines in which Stewie urges Chris that he "must impress that effervescing/Self-possessing, no BS-ing/Down syndrome girl" are widely available online.

Is Ellen a stereotype? Of course she is. But stereotypes are not automatically regressive representations, perhaps especially in animated comedies that satirize stereotypes themselves as the sacred categories of contemporary culture. Richard Dyer writes in *The Matter of Images: Essays on Representations* that "the role of the stereotype is to make visible the invisible, so that there is no danger of it creeping up on us unawares; and to make fast, firm and separate what is in reality fluid and much closer to the norm than the dominant values system cares to admit" (16). All of the characters in *Family Guy* are stereotypes of one kind or another — in this Ellen is not alone. But the stereotypes of *Family Guy* spoof the illusions and elusions upon which the mythologies of the American Family and the American Dream depend. The lyrics of "Down Syndrome Girl," for example, pair prototypical suburban "normality" — a middle-class teenager getting ready for a first date while his brother supports him — with surprising "abnormality" — the date has Down's, a fact the characters celebrate with no apparent irony. The juxtaposition reveals the stereotypes that appear naturalized in earnest narratives. Seen through the romps of *Family Guy*, even the stereotypes of Downs lose their steam. They no longer have the monolithic power that comes from being taken at face value.

Patricia W. Linville et al. note that "stereotyping is a matter of degrees" (198). Unlike archetypes, which allow very little deviance from their intended meaning, stereotypes are polymorphous even within the same context or text. *Family Guy* implicitly recognizes this dynamic by anticipating the audiences' expectation of the veracity of stereotypes of Down syndrome. These stereotypes are so common and so dominant in cultural representations of developmental disability and Down's that we expect them to hold true even in satirical animations. Rather than playing it straight, *Family Guy* gives us an Ellen that embodies both our expectations and their reversal. In doing so, the show demonstrates its awareness of how stereotyping functions socially and in narratives, how to undermine its stability, and how to use animation to transcend audiences' expectation in order to create a more nuanced understanding of an issue and to explore the progressive potential of animation.

Simply put, by pulling stereotypes out and parading them, *Family Guy* pulls *us* out of stereotyping. This dynamic is articulated as fundamental to the show in another episode, "FOX-y Lady" (Season 10, episode 7). Peter, the father figure, writes his own animation about disabled ducks called "Handi-Quacks" in a typical *Family Guy* lexicon gag, which he submits to Fox (*Family Guy*'s own broadcasting company). Meg, the daughter, remarks of the script that "none of this stuff makes sense." Yet Peter argues that people will relate to it because they will see themselves in it. He pitches the aim of "Handi-Quacks" to a fictional Fox producer with the same description that could be used to pitch *Family Guy* itself:

We fire the jokes at you like an automatic weapon of comedy. We throw a curveball joke at you — hits you on the head! You go: WOW — what happened! We take you on a little trolley ride down story lane: you're having a good time and enjoying our little tale — thinking you know what's coming — Boom — left turn. You don't know how it happened; you don't know where you are but you like it. You're watching the show. The ducks are saying stuff. You're yukking it up — you're laughing, your sides are hurting. All of a sudden you realize you're feeling something too: when did that happen? When did the Handi-Quacks become people I care about? When did they become like welcome guests in your home whose weekly visits the whole family eagerly awaits?

Significantly, the wheelchair using duck in the "Handi-Quacks" pilot is voiced by Peter's wheelchair-using neighbor Joe Swanson. Clearly, *Family Guy*—its creators and writers—demonstrate they know the issues surrounding disability, they know models of disability, and they know the nature and paradigms of comedy representation.

In "Extra Large Medium's" third sequence in the Chris and Ellen storyline, the two finally go out on their date. It begins in an apparently high-class restaurant where Ellen reveals that her mom is the former governor of Alaska. Then she gets dictatorial. "Now, get up and come over here and give me a shoulder massage," she demands. "Boy," Chris replies, not a little intimidated, "you're tougher than a Doggie Dominatrix." When the couple return to Ellen's house she continues in the same vein, demanding that Chris get his "fucking arse" inside the kitchen and make her an ice cream sundae. When he does, she berates him for making it the wrong way: "Do you hear me say put chocolate sauce on there?" When he tries to apologize, she mocks him, making his subservient status clear: "You thought what? You know, if you want access to this temple [Ellen points at her own body], you'd better pay me proper tribute." Chris finally cracks, throwing the sundae to the ground:

> I don't care how hot you are! I don't much like being treated this way. You know, I used to hear that people with Down syndrome were different than the rest of us. But you're not. You're not different at all. You're just a bunch of arseholes like everyone else.

Chris leaves Ellen's house and meets up with Stewie, who congratulates him for having the courage to go out on the date. "I'm just sorry I never got to make out with her," Chris replies. "That's okay," Stewie responds "She would've crushed your scrota into a diamond with her robot-strength hand." What's ultimately going on in this scene is a conflict between equal partners without pity or glamorization. Chris remains physically attracted to Ellen. He leaves her not because she has Down's, but because she's mean to him — she's turned out to be "not different" from everyone else. Ellen has turned out not to be a cute poster child of "special abilities" with a stereotypical sweet and cheerful "Down syndrome personality." She is idiosyncratically opinionated, vividly individualistic, and has the same potential capacity for disappointing boys as other three-dimensional girls, both animated and real.

Dyer writes that the effect of the call to positive imagery depends upon "prior assumptions: whether what is positive about [disability] is the degree to which it is like [normal] life or the degree to which it differs from it." In other words, the call to use "disability correct" imagery *per se* can be retrograde if it reinforces the very basis of our oppression by insisting upon imagery that is simply an image of pseudo-normality. Pseudo-normality can be appealing and reassuring for those of us who are willing and capable of passing as "normal." But it is ultimately exclusive and counter-productive. *Family Guy* simply turns "normal" and "abnormal" upside down, reversing their expected positions. In "Extra Large Medium" Chris, a son in the series' "ordinary" American family, requires the most enabling from his younger brother to make it through the storyline, while his classmate Ellen, the Down Syndrome student, remains independent throughout and requires no such hand-holding.

The episode has Chris saying "arsehole" and Ellen saying "fuck," uncharacteristic words for the series. By trading expletives, *Family Guy* gives their interaction verisimilitude as a dramatic incident typical of everyday teen relations. Rather than "normalize" Ellen by providing some sort of representation of her ability to appear and function as nondisabled, the episode keeps Ellen's appearance and qualities true to both her Down's and her individual personality, and places "normal" elsewhere — in the language of both kids. Significantly, the word "retard" — an obvious go-to for American humor in relation to learning disability — never appears. Its pointed absence constitutes a critique of its frequent cultural use, pointing to the corrosive association the term reinforces between incompetence and learning disability.

Family Guy's "Extra Large Medium" is not without its critics. Sarah Palin interpreted the show's reference to herself as Ellen's mother as mocking the existence of her own son Trig, who was born with Down syndrome in 2008, calling it "another kick in the gut" on Facebook. With the support of the cable network Fox News (a separate entity from Fox) where she works as a paid commentator, Palin created a small media firestorm about the use of Down syndrome on *Family Guy*. In an interview with media pundit and popular show host Bill O'Reilly, Palin observed that "the world is full of cruel, cold hearted people who would do such a thing" and that "those in the special needs community are some of the most loving and compassionate people in the world. So why pile it on them and make their lives that much more challenging?" O'Reilly replied, "I agree with you. Look, this guy MacFarlane is a hater" ("Sarah"). On the other hand, Andrea Fay Friedman, who voices Ellen for *Family Guy* and is a professional actress with Down syndrome, supports the show and has offered her own critique of Palin's response:

> I guess former Governor Palin does not have a sense of humor. I thought the line "I am the daughter of the former governor of Alaska" was very funny [...] In my family we think laughing is good. My parents raised me to have a sense of humor and to live a normal life. My mother did not carry me around under her arm like a loaf of French bread the way former Governor Palin carries her son Trig around looking for sympathy and votes [Linkins].

For confirmation that the creators of *Family Guy* are not simply exploiting disability for regressive and divisive comedy, we need look no further than an earlier episode, "No Meals on Wheels" (Season 5, episode 14) in which Peter opens a restaurant that becomes a popular eatery for disabled people, much to his disappointment. His distress is exacerbated when a local newscaster describes the restaurant as a place where "the elite without feet meet to eat." Arguing that he wants to run a "cool establishment" and "cripples are not cool," Peter bans his disabled customers with a sign that reads: "No Shirt / No Shoes / No Legs / No Service." His neighbor, the wheelchair-using Joe Swanson, is the primary recipient of Peter's discrimination. Peter continues his campaign to rebrand his restaurant as disability-free by obtaining a photograph of the attractive actor Mark Harmon (who stars as Special Agent Gibbs in the CBS show *NCIS*), who epitomizes the "normal" model able-bodied American male as an illustration of how cool by definition means "not in a wheel."

Peter, however, winds up in a wheelchair. Once there, he cannot cope physically or accessibility-wise, even for a short time. Attitudes towards him become negative and he is obviously excluded in a number of ways. A brief montage sequence occurs to the soundtrack of Elton John's 1983 hit "I Guess That's Why They Call It the Blues" in which Peter experiences a lack of physical aids, an inaccessible home, lots of steps, people throwing stones, and being patronized and excluded as a goalie in a soccer match. With his new awareness of the tyranny of "cool" and his own ableist ignorance, Peter goes to Joe Swanson and apologizes for discriminating against both him and his friends (the disabled). While the representation of Ellen in "Extra Large Medium" is more subtle in its comic dissection of contemporary social perceptions of disability than "Meals on Wheels," it is nonetheless just as pointed. It offers a striking critique of learning disability imagery, a commentary on the acceptability of relationships between the learning disabled and the non–learning disabled, and pushes the boundaries of representing disability in ways that have barely been touched upon by other mainstream television or cinema media. For this we should welcome *Family Guy*'s "Extra Large Medium" into the canon of disability works as a bold step forward. To adapt Bristol Palin's phrase: all they proved is that they know what they're doing.

Works Cited

Allingham, Phillip V., ed. "Punch, or the London Charivari (1841–1992)—A British Institution." *The Victorian Web*. Faculty of Education, Lakehead University, Thunder Bay, Ontario. 21 Feb. 2011. Web. 15 Dec. 2011.

Barnes, Colin. "Media Guidelines." *Framed: Interrogating Disability in the Media*. Eds. Ann Pointon and Chris Davies. London: British Film Industry, 1992. 228–233. Print.

Davis, Leonard J., ed. *The Disability Studies Reader*. New York: Routledge, 1997. Print.

Dugan, Emily. "*IoS* Investigation: Our Patronising Approach to 10 Million Disabled Britons." *The Independent*. 5 Sept. 2010. Web. 15 Dec. 2011.

Dyer, Richard. *Heavenly Bodies: Film Stars and Society*. New York: St. Martin's Press, 1986. Print.

_____. *The Matter of Images: Essays on Representations*. London: Routledge, 1993. Print.

_____. *Now You See It: Study on Lesbian and Gay Film*. New York: Routledge, 1990. Print.

_____. *Only Entertainment*. New York: Routledge, 1992. Print.

_____. *Stars*. London: British Film Institute, 1990. Print.

"John Steinbeck." *Wikipedia*. 9 Aug. 2010. Web. 20 Aug. 2010.

Lehman, Christopher P. *The Colored Cartoon: Black Presentation in American Animated Short Films 1907–1954*. Amherst: University of Massachusetts Press, 2007. 113–114. Print.

Linkins, Jason. "*Family Guy* Actress Responds to Sarah Palin's Criticism." *The Huffington Post*. 20 Apr 2010. Web. 20 Aug. 12.

Linville, Patricia W., Peter Salovey, and Gregory W. Fischer. "Stereotyping and Perceived Distributions of Social Characteristics: An Application to Ingroup-Outgroup Perception." *Prejudice, Discrimination and Racism*. Eds. John F. Dovidio and Samuel L. Gaertner. Orlando: Academic Press, 1986. 165–20. Print.

Norden, Martin F. *The Cinema of Isolation: A History of Physical Disability in the Movies*. New Brunswick: Rutgers University Press, 1994. Print.

"Sarah Palin on Tea Party Extremism, *Family Guy* Down Syndrome Joke." *Fox News*. 17 Feb. 2010. Web. 20 Aug. 2012.

Steinbeck, John. *Of Mice and Men*. New York: Penguin, 1993. Print.

"The World's Smallest Man and Me." *The World's ... and Me*. BBC Channel 4. 20 May 2008. Television.

Choreographing Disability

Stigma, Handicapability and
Dancing with the Stars

HEATH A. DIEHL

Dancing with the Stars (hereafter *DWTS*) represents one of a handful of reality television offerings that celebrates the medium of dance. Over the duration of its first twelve seasons, the program has served as a platform for a diverse range of celebrities, with respect to age, body type and skill level, to explore the worlds of competitive ballroom and Latin dance in front of millions of avid fans around the world. Two of the all-star cast contestants have been explicitly identified on the show as physically disabled: Heather Mills,[1] a charity campaigner, former model and Beatle ex-wife with a prosthetic leg, and Marlee Matlin, an Oscar-winning actress who is deaf. The juxtapositioning of mobility and sensory impairment with competitive dance poses a set of logistical and interpretive challenges and choices to all parties involved in making and viewing the "reality" of this reality show: the show producers, hosts and judges, celebrities engaged in the competition, and members of the audience.[2] This essay examines the complexity of the intersecting dynamics of perception and narrative that the appearance of disabled contestants on *DWTS* involves. It offers an extended analysis of Marlee Matlin's performance and the ways in which the show casts her as a brave underdog, propagating conventional narratives and constructions of "disability."

DWTS borrows heavily from the classic American game show format by staging a competition between contestants vying for a much-coveted prize. Rather than a bedroom set or a trip to Hawaii, *DWTS'* prize is the Mirrorball Trophy, a gaudy metallic trophy atop of which is affixed a shiny disco ball. Celebrities who make it into the finals can also expect to earn a sizable paycheck that has been estimated at up to $350,000. But whether celebrities compete for ten weeks or just one, they will not go home empty-handed. As at least one source confirms, "every star receives $150,000 for the first six weeks of rehearsals and the first two live shows. Then as each week goes by, they make an extra $10,000 then $20,000, then $30,000 for surviving each elimination" (Donovan). Unlike the classic game show format, however, the fates of *DWTS* contestants do not turn on the flip of a playing card (*Card Sharks*), the spin of an oversized slot machine (*Joker's Wild*), or the well-timed press of a plunger (*Press Your Luck*). Rather, *DWTS* contestants must demonstrate some degree of athleticism and artistry. In this respect, *DWTS* shares some similarities with televised professional sporting events. Prior to the first live televised performances, celebrities and their professional dance partners must endure six weeks of grueling rehearsals, sometimes as many as six hours a day, six days a week. As the season wears on and the contestants hone their dance skills, rehearsals often extend to as many as eight hours a day.[3] Celebrities who do not fulfill their rehearsal obligations not only perform poorly, but also earn less money (Shuter; EBRADY).

DWTS also borrows from the conventions of reality television, which functions not by revealing the mundane, but by constructing the bizarre from whatever elements it can exploit to create "reality" at its most dramatic. As Pam Meister, a blogger for *Big Hollywood*, notes: "Would you want to watch a show about the true reality of everyday lives? Watching someone mop the floors, go to the grocery store, pick up the kids from school, realize at dinnertime that there's no spaghetti sauce in the cupboard and having to run out to the store for the third time that day? Watching paint dry might be more exciting." Christopher C. Cianci echoes Meister, noting that "the success of a reality show is heavily dependent upon the creativity or innovativeness of the show's concept" (364). *DWTS* has often sought to attract the type of media buzz that such innovativeness generates through the selection of its contestants. As Noah Davis writes:

> The inclusion of Heather Mills signals that *Dancing*'s producers are struggling for publicity [...] Mills' leg is amputated below the knee, a fact [host Tom] Bergeron alludes to in the first segment [...] Her appearance generated considerable media hype for *Dancing*, much of it revolving around the possibility that she could lose her leg during a dance. Tasteless, yes, but effective [...] her participation brings the circus freak show element of *Dancing* to an all-time high.[4]

The media frenzy surrounding the casting of Mills ultimately turned on two common cultural narratives about disability: (1) the violability of the amputee's body (in comparison to the intact nondisabled body) and (2) the potential fallibility of the prosthetic device. The online gambling site Bodog.com "opened bets on whether [Mills'] prosthetic leg would fly off during a dance routine" as soon as the cast was announced (De Leon). The possibility that Mills' leg might come flying off during a passionate Rumba or a lively Quickstep — a possibility heightened by the unpredictability of the live show format — added enough "difference" to the by-then predictable format of *DWTS* not only to generate revenue for Bodog but also to rejuvenate viewer interest in the show itself. The commercial exploitation of Mills' disability demonstrated most strikingly in the betting on her impairment becoming disruptively visible reiterates a familiar ideological link between physical disability and social stigma, underscoring a common generic feature of reality television programming: its ideological conservatism.

The conservative bent of much reality television programming should not be surprising given the form's indebtedness to literary realism. As Catherine Belsey observes in an oft-quoted passage:

> Classic realist narrative ... turns on the creation of enigma through the precipitation of disorder which throws into disarray the conventional cultural and signifying systems.... But the story moves inevitably towards *closure* which is also disclosure, the dissolution of enigma through the reestablishment of order, recognizable as a reinstatement or a development of the order which is understood to have preceded the events of the story itself [70].

Classic realist narratives, in other words, often initially seem more transgressive and progressive than they actually are. Whether we are talking about realist drama (e.g., Ibsen's treatment of venereal disease in *Ghosts*), realist fiction (e.g., Chopin's treatment of sexual experience in *The Awakening*), or reality television (e.g., *The Real World*'s treatment of race relations among youth), "realism" as a genre tends to begin with "controversial" subject matter drawn from the everyday lived realities of its readers that is posited as inherently problematic for conventional perception (Belsey's enigma). The enigma, however, cannot survive within the realist narrative; rather, it must first be exposed as an enigma and then be expunged from the narrative in order for resolution to occur, and narrative and ideological order to be reestablished. With respect to reality television, readers need only consider how frequently disruptive forces (e.g., the promiscuous and mouthy vixens on *The Bachelor,* the argumentative and ill-trained sous chefs on *Hell's Kitchen,* or the cocky but tone-deaf singers on *American Idol*) are eliminated from shows. Through the elimination — or in Belsey's terms "dissolution" — of these disruptive forces, narrative order is restored, but that narrative order comes at a cost. For disabled persons on reality television programs, the expurgation of enigma often translates to the recapitulation of traditional and traditionally limiting narratives about physical ability. In what follows, I will examine the kinds of ideological narratives about disability that are constructed around the appearance of Marlee Matlin on *DWTS*.

In at least one noteworthy respect, *DWTS* shares some commonalities with other "call-in-and-vote" reality programs. From the granddaddy of the genre, *American Idol*, to its many progeny — including *So You Think You Can Dance, America's Got Talent,* and even *Idol* alum Paula Abdul's short-lived *Live to Dance* —such glorified popularity contests[5] are characterized by the element of unpredictability that often forces viewers to consider questions like "How does an Adam Lambert lose to a Kris Allen?" or "How does Chris Daughtry not make it into the finale?" *DWTS* executive producer Conrad Green has suggested that "call-in-and-vote" reality program results at times run counter to what viewers expect because when non-experts (i.e., the viewing public) are given the power of the vote, they sometimes judge the performance by non-relevant (to the performance genre) criteria (like star persona, popularity/likability, etc.), making the likelihood of unexpected results inordinately high (Rizzo).

Over the course of its now twelve-season run, *DWTS* has produced at least two memorably unpredictable moments linked directly to the "call-in-and-vote" format. During the fifth season of the program, Cheetah Girl Sabrina Bryan and her professional dance partner, Mark Ballas, were heralded by *DWTS* judges and fellow contestants as the frontrunners, yet during week six, Bryan and Ballas surprisingly were eliminated from the competition — an elimination that later was voted "2007's most shocking TV moment" ("Sabrina Bryan"). The second example occurred during season 11 of *DWTS* when contestant Bristol Palin unexpectedly earned a spot in the finale, prompting a firestorm of conspiracy theories that speculated everything from the probable (e.g., "Sarah Palin has the entire Tea Party movement and everyone on her PAC email list dialing and robo-texting like madmen after every episode") to the outrageous (e.g., "Christine O'Donnell cast a spell on *DWTS* phone lines") (Guthrie, Free Britney).

The unpredictability of America's vote is matched only by the unpredictability of the "live" moment of performance. In *Presence and Desire: Essays on Gender, Sexuality, Performance*, Jill Dolan writes, "There's something in theater's presentation of the live, palpable, endangered body onstage, viewed by live, palpable, equally endangered audiences, that retains a certain power" (152). The "certain power" to which Dolan refers is the sense that "anything can happen." And over the years *DWTS* has enjoyed more than its fair share of "anything can happen" moments. During its inaugural season, soap opera actress Kelly

Monaco barely avoided a Janet Jackson-like wardrobe malfunction when the straps of her costume broke during a performance of the Samba ("DWTS Most Memorable"). Season five competitor Jennie Garth took an embarrassing tumble at the end of a Quickstep routine when her professional dance partner, Derek Hough, stepped on her dress (Blackmon). During season seven, Lance Bass lost his shoes during a performance of the Jitterbug and Cloris Leachman lost her wig during a performance of the Jive ("DWTS Most Memorable"). Perhaps the most unpredictable moment of *DWTS* history, though, occurred during season five when Marie Osmond dramatically fainted on the dance floor following a performance of the Samba ("DWTS [U.S. TV Series]"). In each of these moments, the immediacy and the urgency of the live broadcast heightened the suspense of the performance while the unexpected nature of each blunder underscored its "certain, [palpable] power."

This element of "unpredictability" appears closely linked to producers' decisions to include contestants with disabilities in the cast. The value of such casting for the networks is derived from the framing of disability as a physiological wildcard — a deficit or abnormality that constitutes a form of Belsey's enigma — and that introduces the possibility of unanticipated outcomes through the drama of individual striving. This construction is consistent with the medical model of disability.[6] From the first week of competition, Matlin's participation on *DWTS* was framed by this discourse. In his lead-in to Matlin's inaugural Cha Cha Cha, host Tom Bergeron announces, "Throughout our past five seasons we've had some stars with various physical challenges. Heather Mills had one artificial leg [...] Up next a woman who will dance even though she can't hear the music" (Season 6, Episode 2). A clip package — that is, a montage of shots and scenes chronicling the events of the previous week leading up to the live partner dance, including dance rehearsals, camera confessionals, and the like — follows Bergeron's opening remarks. These clip packages (along with the judges' commentary) typically figure quite prominently in the development of contestant personas and the portrayal of their capacities on *DWTS*. In Matlin's first clip package of the season, her dance partner, Sanchez, recalls: "When I first met Marlee I was so excited, I was like 'Oh my God, that's Marlee Matlin, she's got an Oscar!' Then I was like [screams] 'She can't hear.' I didn't know what I was gonna do with that" ("Episode 2"). Like Bergeron, Sanchez focuses on the fact of Matlin's deafness as an unpredictable conundrum. When Sanchez exasperatedly says, "I didn't know what I was gonna do with *that*," he not only reinforces a medical model understanding of Matlin's deafness as an individual deficit, but also uses medical model discourse to heighten the drama and suspense associated with Matlin's impending live performance.

To view Matlin's participation on *DWTS* in medical model terms is necessarily to view Matlin as an underdog, a stock character of reality programs dramatically valuable for the capacity to inspire. This point was repeatedly underlined by the judges' critiques. Following the week one Cha Cha Cha, judge Bruno Tonioli calls the performance "unbelievable and life-affirming" ("Episode 2"). During week three, judge Len Goodman compliments Matlin on her Jive, noting, "Marlee, you never cease to amaze me. The Jive is such a fast, difficult dance when you've got good hearing and to dance it as sharply as that without hearing I think you did a great job" ("Episode 5"). Following her performance of the Samba, Tonioli comments, "I cannot believe the things you can actually achieve" ("Episode 9"). The next week following a disappointing Mambo, Tonioli maintains, "Well, it's always life-affirming watching you. What you do, it *is* unbelievable" ("Episode 11").

Matlin's underdog status reached a dramatic climax during the sixth week of competition when Matlin and Sanchez were slated to dance the Samba, a Latin dance that, according to Sanchez, "is all about the rhythm of the music. You can't skip a beat." During a one-on-one confessional in the clip package that week, Matlin admits, "Sometimes I feel like my deafness holds me back and Fabian gets frustrated with me." The couple's live performance that week was riddled with problems. Although the judges critiqued the dancing, they also reflexively referenced Matlin's disability and offered the sympathy its casting and construction within the show was designed to elicit. Judge Carrie Ann Inaba acknowledged that Matlin was "out of sorts," but followed up by praising her for being quite "a trooper." Goodman uncharacteristically side-stepped the problematic technique, noting: "when I think of you and look at you and realize you can't hear any of that music I think you do a great job" ("Episode 9"). On only a handful of occasions during Matlin's tenure on *DWTS* did the judges focus on the actual choreography that she performed as a dance competitor. Instead they focused on the framing of her performance as that of a deaf woman: excellent dancing was "amazing" *or* "unbelievable" *given that* she can't hear the music; substandard dancing was nevertheless "a great job" *given that* she can't hear the music. Matlin was never a dance contestant. She was always a *deaf* dance contestant whose performance must always necessarily have been seen in relation to disability.

The underdog narrative enables a contestant story arc that, in the case of disability, casts the individual as afflicted victim in order to construct a narrative of individual tragedy and triumph over the odds that engages nondisabled audiences. James Valentine describes these story arcs as follows:

> Narratives of tragic loss can be used to emphasize the vulnerability of a principal character. This is especially the case in disabled dramas, where vulnerability arouses sympathy for the character [...] Yet such characters are also constructed with the virtues that attract our admiration: they must be heroic in the face of adversity. Heroism combines with narratives of loss and deficiency to turn the tragic story around. This effectively individualizes the problem and places the responsibility on the disabled person, not on the society that is disabling [711].

One particular moment on *DWTS* provides a striking example of how nondisabled viewers were quite overtly invited to sympathize with Matlin as a victim-hero by virtue of disability. During the clip package that preceded Matlin and Sanchez's Quickstep, Sanchez praises Matlin's performance of the Cha Cha Cha from week one, exclaiming, "Girl, you were awesome last night. It was fantastic. Could you hear? Could you hear the band?" ("Episode 3"). Although Matlin had in the previous week's clip package described herself as "profoundly deaf" ("Episode 2"), Sanchez here seems unable to reconcile Matlin's solid performance of the Cha Cha Cha with her inability to hear the music. In response, Matlin asks Sanchez to "imagine if you are in the shower and the door's closed and there's music playing in the other room and you're trying to listen to it." The camera then cuts to a clip of the previous week's Cha Cha Cha with the music and soundtrack altered to "simulate" Matlin's disability in a manner calculated to elicit sympathy by dramatizing the gap between the way in which hearing audience members experience sound and the way in which Matlin does. In some significant ways, the simulation represents a co-optation of the deaf person's hearing impairment in much the same way that Johnson Cheu discusses the co-optation of the blind person's gaze in his article "Seeing Blindness On-Screen: The Blind, Female Gaze." In both the dominance of the "normative" (sighted or hearing) is confirmed by offering a version of disability that emphasizes deficit, partly by divorcing it from the total lived experience of blindness or deafness. In the end, this simulation casts Matlin as someone who is not Deaf; rather, she's different and that difference is constructed as one of deprivation only.

Sympathy often breeds admiration for the disabled person who perseveres in "the face of adversity," a common effect of the "overcoming" narrative arc often applied to disability that is reinforced in Matlin's case by public accounts of her personal life. Her current eighteen-year marriage to Chicago police officer Kevin Grandalski is painted in her autobiography as well as in clip packages on *DWTS* as a kind of Rockwellian "American Dream" in stark contrast to the physically abusive relationship that she shared with William Hurt as a young actress. Matlin has also overcome childhood sexual molestation by a trusted babysitter, beat drug addiction, and established herself as a formidable figure in Hollywood, despite the virtual absence of persons with disabilities in such an image-conscious profession. While none of these events can be causally linked to Matlin's deafness, dominant cultural views of disability that frame the disabled person as victim or hero by virtue of physiological impairment often encourage such linkages in audiences' minds. As a result, these biographical story lines can function to reinforce the persona and narrative arc Valentine describes.

On *DWTS*, Matlin's persona participates in a key element of the hero narrative of disability as a model of individual success achieved through personal strength of character for the purposes of inspiration, which Matlin articulates in the Episode 5 clip package: "My goal this week is to inspire deaf children and show them that anything is possible: they can dance if they want to." Later in the season this positioning of Matlin as the inspirational contestant is reinforced in the clip package that precedes her Mambo routine. It begins with a voice over by Bergeron, who intones that "last Monday Marlee struggled to find the Samba beat," followed by a montage of clips from the previous week's Samba illustrating Matlin's struggles. One of the next shots focuses on the current week's rehearsals of the Mambo. Despite her partner Sanchez's assurances that Matlin is "in perfect hands" given that he is "the Mambo King," she becomes increasingly frustrated as she fumbles on the timing and the choreography. Enter Matlin's long-time friend Henry Winkler who takes Matlin aside and advises, "Okay, no dwelling. So, whoosh [he wipes her forehead clean], [the flawed Samba is] gone. Okay? I know your spirit, Marlee. Your spirit is intense. Your spirit is on fire. There is nothing you cannot do. I don't care what happened last week. These legs will Mambo us into submission." The final shot of the clip package is Matlin in confessional saying, "Henry put everything into perspective for me and helped me realize that *I am who I am* and just dance" (emphasis added, "Episode 11").

Winkler's words are standard fare for encouraging contestants of all kinds in reality shows, but in the context of the show's narrative positioning of Matlin and her response — "I am who I am" — Winkler effectively stands in for the nondisabled viewing audience, giving voice to its desire for the disabled underdog character to complete the tragedy-begets-heroism story arc. When Winkler asks, "Have you made mistakes before?" his question implicitly points to her deafness and its potential impact on function, thereby reminding viewers that Matlin is always a vulnerable figure by virtue of a deficiency (especially on the dance floor) and therefore destined to make mistakes. When he encourages her to "pick yourself up [...] dust yourself off" and warns, "No excuses," he literally reinforces the up-by-your-bootstraps, Horatio Algerian elements of individual initiative that the medical model story arc employs, thereby demanding disabled persons to achieve heroism in the face of adversity and redeeming the deficits of disability. This clip package, then, is set up as a kind of mini-climax, a turning point in Matlin's character arc across her season on *DWTS*. From frustration (with a poor performance of the Samba) to encouragement (by Winkler) to, finally, that "can-do" attitude that enables Matlin's realization that "I am who I am and just dance," this clip package beautifully illustrates the "development" that disabled persons typically go through on television, a development that locates the drama of disability squarely within the individual, absolving the audience of considering the ways in which disability — including Matlin's — is socially, environmentally, and narratively constructed.

The Mambo turned out to be Matlin's final dance after a flawed performance with her partner led to their elimination. The judges' final evaluation reinforced conflicting and ultimately condescending messages about disability inherent in *DWTS'* casting of Matlin. Inaba, apparently unable to reconcile dancing with deafness, implies that Matlin's early success on the show was due to her acting skills — her ability to create story and character — not her apparently solid dance technique. Inaba goes on to suggest that performing the Mambo depends upon a "connection with the music," implying that a deaf person cannot, even in the moments of her successful dancing, be a dancer. Goodman, the show's stickler for precise technique and traditional choreography, doesn't critique Matlin's actual moves as he typically would with nondisabled contestants. Instead, he opts for feel-good empty praise of the kind one gives to token candidates. He claims that Matlin "proved that the only limitations that you have are the ones you put on yourself," refers to her as "a real inspiration to so many people." His only professional critique is atypically vague: "It was just — it looked uncomfortable tonight." Goodman's words sound doubly contrived given his suggestion that Matlin danced without limitation, which ignores the very real lived, material conditions of deafness within *DWTS'* venue that are a component of Matlin's performance experience. To say, as Winkler does, that "there is nothing you cannot do" or, as Goodman put it, that "the only limitations that you have are the ones you put on yourself," is to place the onus for a level playing field and for success and failure squarely on the individual regardless of social or material influence or reality — an inherently conservative construction of any form of disadvantage. At the same time, those claims often also imply that there is only so much that disabled persons can actually do. Achievement is expected; failure is inevitable; inspirational heroism is possible (and desired by the nondisabled).

To this point, my analysis of the cultural and ideological implications of Matlin's performances on *DWTS* might seem to belong to a category of interpretations that disability scholar Tom Shakespeare has termed "overcensorious readings" (165). Given the meager number of representations of deafness in American culture, my critique of *DWTS'* recapitulation of medical model discourses could be seen as "overly critical." To insist on thoughtful and ideologically progressive representations of disability before a substantial visibility has been established may seem misguided and I might well be reminded that "in a culture where deafness has been rendered largely invisible, even flawed representations may be considered preferable to broad disregard" (Valentine 708). Matlin and *DWTS* appear to illustrate this perspective when they combine Matlin's appearance on the show with medical advocacy for the deaf in Mexico. The Episode 5 clip package features Matlin's *DWTS*-sponsored trip to Guadalajara to provide hearing implants for 1,000 patients, which ostensibly enables them to integrate into hearing Mexican society and raises the consciousness of viewers to their plight, albeit by reinforcing a medical model approach to deafness.

To devote my attention only to the ideological conservatism of *DWTS* with regard to its representation of disability is also to ignore the fact that "disability discourses are more complex and multi-faceted than might appear" (Shakespeare 170). After all, Valentine cautions us that disability "narratives are loaded: by the way these dramas are structured, certain interpretations are favored over others. It all depends on the availability of alternatives" (722). To this end, I am not arguing that Matlin's performances on *DWTS* always and only propagate one idea — chiefly medical, dated and condescending — about what constitutes "disability." But following Valentine's lead, I would argue that *DWTS'* representation of

Matlin's performances were ideologically loaded in a conservative direction and that any other alternative cultural meanings produced by those performances were ultimately overshadowed by the more overt and conventional meanings of disability circulating within the dominant nondisabled culture of viewers.

Of course, performances by Matlin in other productions have been ideologically loaded in very different ways, for example in the skit she performed on *Family Guy Presents Seth & Alex's Almost Live Comedy Show.* During this performance, Seth MacFarlane confesses that while he has poked fun at Matlin on a number of occasions, he harbors great admiration for her as an actress, as a *DWTS* contestant, and as a pop singer. Cue Alex Borstein who begins performing a track — Lady Gaga's "Poker Face" — from Matlin's (fictional) upcoming release. As Borstein belts out lyrics in her tone deaf imitation of Matlin, Matlin herself enters and strides confidently to center stage where Borstein stands. Twice Matlin orders Borstein to "Shut up! You're embarrassing yourself!" as a shame-faced Borstein professes her adoration of Matlin's work. Then, Matlin performs an impression of Borstein: "I'm Alex. I'm an arrogant little whore. All I do is not exercise, eat Oreos, and complain that I'm not in more movies. [Wipes fake tears from her eyes in a melodramatic fashion] Here's me walking down the street. [Waddles exaggeratedly]." Following her purposefully mocking imitation, Matlin asks a seemingly shell-shocked Borstein, "How's that? Feel good? Huh?" to which Borstein replies, "No it doesn't, Ms. Matlin" (Downard).

What I find so clever about this particular skit is that it takes to task those critics who might dismiss it as "offensive." Matlin initially stands in for those offended viewers, an alliance that is underscored by the cacophony of applause when Matlin enters from the wings. As the skit continues, though, and as Matlin proceeds to wage her own increasingly offensive assault against the overweight Borstein, the thematic and ideological focus shifts away from disability as a punch line and concentrates on the nature and purpose of comedy. Matlin's participation in this skit, then, is less about "mocking the mockers" (as one commentator put it) than it is about encouraging perhaps a more nuanced understanding of the "complex and multi-faceted" discourses of disability even (perhaps especially) within the world of comedy. Borstein and Matlin invite us to understand that disability has produced a wide range of cultural narratives. Some of those narratives do "replicate [...] pathologizing practices that oppress people" (Chivers and Markotić 9), but others celebrate the unique beauty of disability, and still others challenge the status quo through their own representations. The point, then, is to discourage totalizing and essentialist responses to any form of disability representation. Not all medical discourses are pathologizing, not all academic discourses are liberating, and not all comedic discourses are offensive. It all depends on context, and the availability of "alternatives."

The *Family Guy* skit so brilliantly captures the kind of cultural work that Matlin consistently performs around the topic of disability by offering a telling alternative to her work on *DWTS*. While Matlin has admitted that she dreams of a time when fans might say, "There's Marlee, not, there's the deaf actress" ("Marlee Matlin Quotes"), she also is enough of a realist to acknowledge that, as a society, we have not yet reached that level of understanding where disability is concerned. As Matlin has said, "Every one of us is different in some way, but for those of us who are more different, we have to put more effort into convincing the less different that we can do the same thing they can, just differently" ("Marlee Matlin Quotes"). As a competitor on *DWTS*, Matlin probably did not convince those who are "less different" that someone (like her) who is "more different" can triumph in the worlds of competitive Latin and ballroom dance. After all, she was voted off the program well before the winner of that season's Mirrorball Trophy was announced. Nevertheless, she was respectfully successful: some of her dance performances were superior. And while we have not yet learned to say simply, "There's Marlee," maybe we now can at least say, "There's Marlee, the deaf actress. And, boy, does she cut a mean Viennese Waltz!"

Notes

1. This essay focuses primarily on Marlee Matlin's appearance on *DWTS*. For an insightful consideration of the ways in which Heather Mills' disability was constructed in and through responses by journalists and bloggers, see Margaret Quinlan and Benjamin Bates, "Dances and Discourses of (Dis)Ability: Heather Mills' Embodiment of Disability on *Dancing with the Stars*," *Text and Performance* 28:1–2 (2008): 64–80. Print.

2. Although studies on representations of disability in primetime television are relatively few in number, some important ones have been conducted, especially in relation to Japanese television. See Carol Dillon et al., "Television and Disability," *Journal of Rehabilitation* (Oct. 1980): 67–69. Print; Shinichi Saito and Reiko Ishiyama, "The Invisible Minority: Under-representation of People with Disabilities in Prime-Time TV Dramas in Japan," *Disability & Society* 20.4 (June 2005): 437–451. Print; and Alison Wilde, "Disabling Masculinity: The Isolation of a Captive Audience," *Disability & Society* 19.4 (June 2004): 355–370, Print.

3. The rigor of the rehearsal process has been visually underscored on many occasions as celebrities like Kyle Massey, Kelly Osbourne, and Marie Osmond slim down over the course of their stint on *Dancing with the Stars*. No celebrity transformation, though, has been quite as dramatic as Kirstie Alley's. Alley, who earned second place on the twelfth season of the program, lost 38 inches in her dress size from her debut to her performance on the season finale (Cohen).

4. Davis' reference to the "circus freak show" aligns Mills' appearance on *DWTS* with a long history of popular exploitative displays involving figures like Joseph Merrick (The Elephant Man), Madame Clofullia (The Bearded Lady of Geneva), or Myrtle Corbin (The Four Legged Lady). For comments on the participation of reality television in this tradition and an extended analysis of the freak show in American culture, see Martin Binks, "The Exploitation of Obesity: Why 'Fat TV' Is a National Disgrace," *Duke Health*, Duke University Health System, 16 Apr. 2010, Web, 21 July 2011; Jesse Byrd, "The Black Reality of Reality TV," *The Loop 21*, 14 May 2011, Web, 21 July 2011; Andy Dehnart, "Is A&E's Intervention Exploitative?" *Reality Blurred*, 23 Mar. 2005, Web, 21 July 2011; and Rosemarie Garland-Thomson, *Extraordinary Bodies: Figuring Physical Disability in American Culture and Literature* (New York: Columbia University Press, 1996), Print.

5. The "popularity contest" element of many "call-in-and-vote" reality programs became explicit in a recent episode of the sixth season of *America's Got Talent*. After a Semifinal performance of David Gray's "Babylon" by Dani Shay that left both judges and audience a little unimpressed, Howie Mandel told the young, aspiring singer: "In order to win this competition ... it's kind of a popularity competition on top of talent, and I think you have to choose much more popular, relatable songs" ("Top 48: Round 2"). The next night, Shay was eliminated from the program while another aspiring singer, Daniel Joseph Baker, who during the live show the previous evening had belted out his rendition of the then-popular Lady Gaga cover "The Edge of Glory," progressed to the Top 12 ("Top 48: Round 2 — Elimination").

6. "In this model of disability, the lives of people with disabilities are defined by a label or diagnosis and it is the individual, and not society, who has a problem and needs to be repaired. In other words, the medical model views disability as something that 'belongs' to a person" (Kluth). Often, medical model discourses construct disability as a "disease" rather than an alternative embodiment (Stibbe 22). See also "Medical Model vs. Social Model," *Resources*, Family Violence: Kids as Self Advocates, Web, 27 July 2011, PDF. For a discussion of the social model of disability, in which "disability is viewed as a problem located within society rather than within individuals who happen to have impairment," see: Sally French, "Disability, Impairment, or Something In Between?" *Disabling Barriers — Enabling Environments*, eds. John Swain, et al. (London: Sage, 1993), 17–25, Print.

Works Cited

Belsey, Catherine. *Critical Practice*. London: Routledge, 1980. Print.
Blackmon, Joe. "Dancing with the Stars — Jennie Garth Takes a Fall." *Reality TV Magazine*. She Knows. 1 Oct. 2007. Web. 21 July 2011.
Cheu, Johnson. "Seeing Blindness On-Screen: The Blind, Female Gaze." *The Problem Body: Projecting*

Disability on Film. Eds. Sally Chivers and Nicole Markotić. Columbus: Ohio State University Press, 2010. 67–82. Print.

Chivers, Sally, and Nicole Markotić. Introduction. *The Problem Body: Projecting Disability on Film.* Eds. Chivers and Markotić. Columbus: Ohio State University Press, 2010. 1–21. Print.

Cianci, Christopher C. "Entertainment or Exploitation? Reality Television and the Inadequate Protection of Child Participants Under the Law." *Southern California Interdisciplinary Law Journal* 18 (2009): 363–394. PDF.

Cohen, Sandy. "Kirstie Alley Weight Loss: 38 Inches Since 'Dancing With the Stars' Debut." *HuffPost Entertainment.* The Huffington Post. 24 May 2011. Web. 27 July 2011.

"Dancing with the Stars Most Memorable Moments." *Xfinity.* Comcast. Web. 21 July 2011.

"Dancing with the Stars (U.S. TV Series)." *Wikipedia: The Free Encyclopedia.* Wikimedia Foundation, Inc. 17 July 2011. Web. 21 July 2011.

Davis, Noah. "Dancing with the Stars." *PopMatters.* PopMatters Media. 26 Mar. 2007. Web. 21 July 2011.

De Leon, Kris. "Heather Mills' Leg Sparks Bets for Online Gambling Site." *BuddyTV.* 13 Mar. 2007. Web. 21 July 2011.

Dolan, Jill. *Presence and Desire: Essays on Gender, Sexuality, Performance.* Ann Arbor: University of Michigan Press, 1996. Print.

Donovan. "How Much Do The Stars from Dancing with the Stars Make?" *Homorazzi.* 16 May 2011. Web. 26 July 2011.

Downard, Dave. "Family live lady gaga song." *YouTube.* 9 May 2010. Web. 26 July 2011.

EBRADY. "DWTS Season 11: Dancing With the Stars' Celebrity Salaries Revealed." *FameCrawler.* Babble. 1 Sept. 2010. Web. 27 July 2011.

Free Britney. "Dancing with the Stars: A Bristol Palin Conspiracy." *The Hollywood Gossip.* 3 Nov. 2010. Web. 19 July 2011.

Guthrie, Marissa. "Why Bristol Palin Is Still on 'Dancing With the Stars.'" *The Hollywood Reporter.* The Hollywood Reporter mag. 11 Nov. 2010. Web. 19 July 2011.

Kluth, Paula. "Toward a Social Model of Disability." *Disability Studies for Teachers.* Center on Human Policy. 2006. Web. 25 July 2011. PDF.

"Marlee Matlin Quotes." *Brainy Quote.* BookRags Media Network. Web. 27 July 2011.

Meister, Pam. "Another Reality Show, Another Exploitation of American Life." *Big Hollywood.* Breitbart. 31 Mar. 2009. Web. 21 July 2011.

Rizzo, Monica. "*Dancing* Producer Responds to Voting Controversy." *People.* People Magazine. 19 Nov. 2010. Web. 19 July 2011.

"Sabrina Bryan." *Wikipedia: The Free Encyclopedia.* Wikimedia Foundation, Inc. 18 July 2011. Web. 19 July 2011.

"Season 6, Episode 2." *Dancing with the Stars.* ABC. WTVG, Toledo. 18 Mar. 2008. Television.

"Season 6: Episode 3." *Dancing with the Stars.* ABC. WTVG, Toledo. 24 Mar. 2008. Television.

"Season 6: Episode 5." *Dancing with the Stars.* ABC. WTVG, Toledo. 31 Mar. 2008. Television.

"Season 6: Episode 9." *Dancing with the Stars.* ABC. WTVG, Toledo. 14 Apr. 2008. Television.

"Season 6: Episode 11." *Dancing with the Stars.* ABC. WTVG, Toledo. 21 Apr. 2008. Television.

Shakespeare, Tom. "Art & Lies: Representations of Disability on Film." *Disability Discourse.* Eds. Mairian Corker and Sally French. Buckingham: Open University Press, 1999. 164–172. Print.

Shuter, Rob. "How Much Do Celebs Make on 'Dancing With the Stars?'" *PopEater.* AOL. 4 May 2011. Web. 27 July 2011.

Stibbe, Arran. "Disability, Gender and Power in Japanese Television Drama." *Japan Forum* 16.1 (2004): 21–36. Print.

"Top 48: Round 2." *America's Got Talent.* NBC. WNWO, Toledo. 19 July 2011. Television.

"Top 48: Round 2 — Elimination." *America's Got Talent.* NBC. WNWO, Toledo. 20 July 2011. Television.

Valentine, James. "Disabled Discourse: Hearing Accounts of Deafness Constructed Through Japanese Television and Film." *Disability & Society* 16.5 (2001): 707–721. Print.

PART II: DISABILITY IN PRODUCTION AND RECEPTION

Don't Film Us, We'll Film You

Agency and Self-Representation in the *Joined for Life* Television Documentaries

ELLEN SAMUELS

Abigail and Brittany Hensel are conjoined twins who were born in 1990 in a small town in Minnesota. They were introduced to the world in 1996 with a cover story and photo spread in *Life Magazine*, followed by an additional profile in *Time* and appearances on the television shows *Oprah* and *Good Morning America* (see Miller and Wallis). After gaining worldwide fame through these media appearances, however, the sisters and their parents largely withdrew from public life, despite what they have described as "an avalanche of media requests" (*JL*). "That's not the kind of life we wanted to have," said Patty Hensel, the twins' mother (*JL*).

From that time until 2012, the Hensel twins' primary media appearances consisted of two hour-length televised documentaries, produced by Advanced Medical Productions/Figure 8 Films in collaboration with the Discovery Channel, which originally aired in 2001 and 2006.[1] The documentaries, entitled *Joined for Life* and *Joined for Life: Abby and Brittany Turn Sixteen*, have been described by the sisters and their parents as a calculated choice to create a media presence for the twins which is neither freakish nor exploitative, and over which they can exercise considerable control.[2] Yet the question remains, not only how much actual control the Hensels had over their representation in these documentaries, but also how much of that original intention can be retained in a twenty-first century media environment, in which content is excerpted, reproduced, and shared in a globally proliferative market. These questions can be explored through a close examination of the documentaries as well as their subsequent reproduction and distribution through television and the Internet.

This essay will first consider some of the primary meanings conveyed by the documentaries, historically contextualized in relation to other cultural displays of conjoined twins. This discussion sets the stage for questions of agency and representation: how do the twins, their parents, and the filmmakers express agency in each documentary, and do these expressions exist in productive or disruptive tension with one another? Are these documentaries *reflexive*, in the sense that the production apparatus, such as the cameras, staging, and presence of filmmakers, is made apparent, or *reflective*, in the sense that the narrators speak directly to the viewer about the reasons and conditions for making each film?[3] Finally, what can we conclude about the effect of the documentaries, the ways in which they create, reinforce, and challenge cultural perceptions of extraordinary bodies in general and the Hensel twins in particular? These questions have wide resonances and implications, both in the arena of representational politics and in the ever-changing realm of media studies in the twenty-first century.

Extraordinarily Normal

By far the most emphasized overt message of both *Joined for Life* documentaries is that Abby and Brittany are "normal" and "just like everyone else." In *Joined for Life*, both the narrators and the twins' parents frequently voice these messages, in statements such as "these are just normal eleven-year-old kids," who "have the same hopes and dreams as any other child their age" (*JL*). Similarly, in *Joined for Life 2*, the narrator again states in the film's opening scenes that the Hensels are "perfectly normal teenagers" "whose greatest accomplishment is how normal their lives continue to be" (*JL2*). This insistence on normalcy is of course vividly undercut, not only by the accompanying footage of the twins' unusual body, but also by the simple fact that if the twins *were* truly like everyone else, they would not be the subject of a documentary. Indeed, since Abby and Brittany's bodily non-normativity is the instantiating event of the films, the frequent statements about normalcy are voiced within a representational structure that denies the possibility of their truth.

Of course, the point which the narrators and the Hensel parents are trying to make is not that the girls' shared body is actually "normal," but rather that its non-normativity is not the defining factor of the girls' lives. In that sense, these assertions are borne out by the film's display of the twins engaged in familiar and quotidian activities like getting dressed, going to school, and playing sports. As Alice Dreger suggests with regard to *Face to Face*, a 2000 documentary about conjoined twins Lori and Reba Schappell, by including such everyday matters, "the film does not give the impression that the twins are brave heroes or freaks of nature. If anything, it makes their lives seem remarkably unremarkable. After observing them in their ordinary activities, one realizes that they're typical in every way but the obvious" (130). G. Thomas Couser similarly argues that, in *Face to Face*, "by entering their home to show them in a familiar domestic routine ... the film suggests that [the Schappells'] unobserved lives are not so different as others might imagine" (58).

Yet such portrayals also correspond to an earlier tradition of freak show displays described by Robert Bogdan, in which people with exceptional bodies "tended to be presented as physically normal, or even superior, in all ways except for the particular anomaly that was their alleged reason for fame" (30). These performers often impressed audiences by doing everyday tasks "which one might assume could not be done by a person with that particular disability" (30). Such a mode of presentation certainly encompasses many aspects of the Hensel documentaries, from simple matters such as showing the twins walking, eating, and brushing their hair, to the extended focus in *Joined for Life* on their sports prowess and in *Joined for Life 2* on their successful mastery of driving a car. Thus, I suggest that Couser and Dreger's interpretation of the portrayal of everyday activities as a form of normalization — and thus, humanization — of conjoined twins' radical difference is overly optimistic, although also understandably appealing. Seeing such familiar and routine activities may certainly lead singleton viewers to identify with the twins; however, these viewers may also and simultaneously be consumed with an objectifying wonder at the particular fashion in which the twins accomplish these activities.

Sharon L. Snyder and David T. Mitchell make a slightly different argument in relation to what they call the "new documentary disability cinema":

> The day-to-day details *are the point* because it is at this most basic level of modern existence that bureaucracies have doubted the ability of people with disability to manage their own affairs.... When viewers enter these new disability documentary media landscapes, they discover immediately that routine activities refute the opposition to disabled people's freedom as a denial of the right to pursue lives that are recognizably ordinary [173–174].

Here, Snyder and Mitchell ascribe a particular political efficacy to the depiction of disabled people engaged in everyday activities. Less concerned with how such depictions might normalize their subjects, Snyder and Mitchell argue that these films, through the power of the visual, can provide persuasive evidence to effect policies which support independent living for people with disabilities. Certainly, this makes sense, for example, when films depict people with common disabilities such as spinal cord injury, cerebral palsy, or blindness independently negotiating their daily lives with simple accommodations.[4] Similarly, in the case of the Schappells—who were institutionalized for twenty-four years on the mistaken assumption that their cranial conjoinment was mentally incapacitating—the sight of the sisters grocery shopping, cooking, sight-seeing, working, and performing on stage functions as a powerful negation of such assumptions and their related policy decisions.

However, it is difficult to make a direct analogy between these examples and the portrayals of the Hensels in *Joined for Life*. One key factor in this difference, I suggest, is that not only *what* they do, but *how* they do it, appears to be a more absorbing question in relation to the Hensels compared to the Schappells due to their different bodily configurations. Because Abby and Brittany share one body from the neck down, and each controls one half of that shared body, the question of how the twins coordinate their movements is both mysterious and endlessly fascinating to medical and lay observers. In both documentaries, doctors muse wonderingly on the failure of science to entirely explain how the twins move, and the narrator of *Joined for Life* declares their physical coordination to be "astounding" (*JL*). These comments are overlaid and interspersed with footage of the girls riding their bike and playing softball and basketball to visually reinforce the message that their coordination is at once normal and extraordinary. In *Joined for Life 2*, Patty states early in the film that she would like people to see Abby and Brittany "through the eyes of a child, and just accept what you see," rather than constantly asking: "How do they do this? How do they do that?" (*JL2*). Yet, later in the film, Patty herself engages in repeated speculation about how the twins are able to do certain things like driving and typing in unison when instant messaging. This apparent contradiction suggests that such questions are pervasive and perhaps inevitable. (Certainly they are a preoccupation among my students when I teach about the Hensels.) In fact, one part of the films' appeal appears to be their promise to answer such questions, and in the process transform each viewer into an expert on the twins, a dynamic to which the documentary film is particularly suited: "Aligned with the controlling discourse of the titles or voice-over within the documentary film ... we identify with the 'other' of knowledge, a position of mastery, and are interpellated as members of the community of knowledge" (Cowie 102).[5] By allowing the viewer a kind of intimate mastery over the details of the twins' lives, the documentaries appear to serve an objectifying function that directly opposes the humanizing goals of the Hensels and the filmmakers.

Yet there are also many moments in which individuals in the films disrupt or resist this process. One notable example takes place near the end of *JL2*, when Steven Koop, the orthopedic surgeon who successfully operated on the girls' spines, radically deviates from the film's insistence upon the value of normalcy. He explains:

> I take care of children with unusual issues that often push them out of mainstream everyday life. Many times I'm asked, "What's normal?" I've moved away from doing that kind of arithmetic that tries to quantify how close to normal someone is, because it's filled with biases and perceptions. I've just decided that kids are here. They're presented to me by their family, and the fact that they simply exist already gives them a dignity that is beyond being quantified [*JL2*].

This speech carried particular weight because it is voiced by a member of the medical community, historically charged with the normalization of bodies and — in the case of conjoined twins — generally portrayed as heroic and all-powerful (usually in relation to separation surgeries).[6]

It is even more important to note that Abby and Brittany themselves make no statements in the films about being, or wishing to be, normal or "like everyone else." If they had made such statements on camera, it seems likely that these moments would have been included in the films to complement the narrators' and Hensel parents' frequent assertions in this regard. Instead, Abby and Brittany appear mostly concerned with communicating the particulars of their lives, most of which are indeed "normal," even trivial, in nature. In one of the few moments in either film where the sisters directly address the fact that they are conjoined, toward the end of *Joined for Life*, they read a prepared list of the "Top Ten Questions People Ask," along with their answers. In this scene, concepts of normalcy are implied but never directly addressed. When Brittany reads question number seven, "How do you know when to move your leg or arm to play sports?," she quickly and defiantly answers, "I don't know," and moves on (*JL*).

Aside from these disruptions of the films' normalcy discourse, it is also important to note the films' covert assumption that the social and personal factors that constitute normalcy are obvious and neutral, rather than contingent and suffused with power relationships.[7] While the films' discourses equate being normal with being "like everybody else," since the nineteenth century the norm has departed significantly from the "average" to denote instead a realm of hegemonic and rigidly policed qualities (Davis; Garland-Thomson, *Extraordinary*). There are multiple axes of normalcy which intersect around the twins to enable their extraordinary body to be perceived as their only deviation from social expectations: they are American, Christian, white, economically privileged, and beloved members of a family which includes a mother, father, siblings, and pets. Additionally, the twins possess "the symbolic properties and qualities that define the cute in white supremacist culture (white skin, blond hair, blue eyes)" (Mersh 186). The hidden assumptions of class status and cultural background are deeply naturalized in the documentaries, as seen when the narrator introduces the twins' piano lessons by commenting that "part of a normal childhood is learning how to play a musical instrument" (*JL*).[8] The fact that the Hensels have enough money to pay a seamstress to alter the girls' clothes and to pay two tuitions at their private Lutheran school is clearly key to enabling the girls to be perceived and treated as two individuals "like everyone else." Similarly, the combination of financial security with Patty's educated status as a nurse enabled the Hensels to reject doctors' suggestions of surgical separation and make the decision to raise them at home in privacy.

These observations are not made to grudge Abby and Brittany one iota of the love and comfort with which they have been raised. However, since their films are so widely viewed and understood as representative of modern conjoined experience, it is important to contextualize their relative privilege when compared to many, if not most, other such twins. Some notable twentieth and twenty-first century examples which come to mind include Daisy and Violet Hilton, Yvonne and Yvette McCarthur, Lori and Reba Schappell, and Krista and Tatiana Hogan. The Hilton sisters, born in Brighton, England, in 1908, were abandoned by their horrified mother to midwife Mary Hilton, who made a fortune from exhibiting the twins while keeping them in virtual captivity until they won their freedom in a court case in 1931. After their show business career fizzled, the twins sank into poverty and were working as grocery store clerks when they died at age 61.[9] In 1949, Yvonne and Yvette McCarther were born conjoined at the tops of their heads and kept in Los Angeles General Hospital for nearly two years while doctors evaluated the possibility of separation. In the end, the twins' mother, Willa Jones, an African American garment worker with five older children, was told that separation was impossible and then presented with an enormous hospital bill which she was forced to repay by exhibiting the twins with a traveling circus (Quigley 111; Stumbo, "Sisters" B1, B3). As adults, Yvonne and Yvette's mother kept them in lonely seclusion for years until the twins moved out at age thirty-eight, sparking a brief media flurry which concluded with the sisters' sudden death in 1993 (Stumbo, "Taking" B1; "Siamese" 16). The Schappells' story has a happier ending, as despite being inappropriately institutionalized for twenty-four years, they were able at last to win their release, live independently, and pursue careers (*Face to Face*, Dreger, Couser). Most recently, Tatiana and Krista Hogan have come to public view through a 2010 televised documentary which aired on the CBC (Canada) and the National Geographic Channel (U.K. and U.S.), and a high-profile 2011 article in the *New York Times Magazine* (Dominus). The Hogans, who are also joined at the head, have a more extensive brain connection than other known craniopagus twins, leading to much media fascination with the likelihood that they can share thoughts and see through each other's eyes. The Hogans live in an extended family group in British Columbia that largely survives on public support, and their parents have engaged a talent agent and are reported to be pursuing a reality television show, in part for financial reasons (Dominus). Each of these examples demonstrates how financial pressures and social prejudices often shape the experiences of conjoined twins, such that the Hensels' ability to live a relatively "normal" life is actually quite unusual.

One reason to foreground the constructed nature of normalcy in the portrayals of the Hensels is to understand how these films intervene into the dominant filmic representation of conjoined twins: the separation documentary. José van Dijck has traced the history of filmed separation surgeries nearly to the beginning of moving pictures themselves, with the 1902 recording of a separation surgery performed by Dr. Eugène-Louis Doyen on Radica and Doodica Neik (544).[10] Dreger, Van Dijck, David L. Clark, and Catherine Myser have all critiqued the separation documentary for its privileging of medical expertise over the subjectivity and privacy of the twins whose conjoinment is the occasion for the film itself. Additionally, the fact that such documentaries often involve twins from other countries being brought to the United States or England for separation surgery has been observed to construct a neocolonial relationship in which "pathology" is identified with an "othered cultural group" (Clark and Myser, "Being" 342).

The *Joined for Life* documentaries, then, already constitute a radical break with the dominant mode of representing conjoinment in the modern era. However, I suggest that, if "surgical separation marks the extent to which the medical regime is willing to go to reconstruct the body so that it more closely approximates what is posited as ideal and reiterated as normal" (Clark and Myser, "Being" 350–51), then the rejection of separation in the Hensels' lives and documentaries ironically produces an even more insistent need for normalcy to be constituted by other means. This foundational normalcy is then defined in opposition to disability, or at least to the state of disablement rhetorically contrasted in the films to the twins' remarkable able-bodiedness, most often represented by their participation in sports. In *Joined for Life*, when the narrator raises the question of separation, Patty and Mike respond that they would have pursued surgery if it would have benefited the girls. But, as Patty explains, "to separate them probably would have made them handicapped, would have taken away all their bike-riding, and they would have had a whole artificial half of a body." Mike chimes in: "It probably would have meant being in a wheelchair, just tons of things they wouldn't have been able to do that they're able to do now. I guess, if you have to trade off things, I guess I'd rather do it all than do half of it and not be able to participate" (*JL*). Most of this dialogue is aired over footage of Abby and Brittany playing softball, thus emphasizing the particularly normative realm of sports as the arena in which the girls would not have been able to participate if disabled by separation.[11] The centrality of sports to the twins' construction as physically-able subjects is further signified by Mike's proud observation that "as soon as they started walking they picked up balls and threw them" (*JL*). The girls' school gym teacher and coach then expands their athletic aptitude to encompass the stereotypical role of the heroic overcomer: "With Abby and Brittany, nothing is impossible. You can challenge them to anything and they will do it. They won't let 'no' or 'can't do it' stop 'em" (*JL*). The extent to which disability is cast as the abject other to the twins' physical abilities is also captured in their adult friend Tamara's assertion that "there is not even a disability about 'em; you may as well just knock the word 'dis' right off, because it is the ability" (*JL2*).

Thus the films consistently equate disability with an invalid and artificial existence excluded from social participation — an ironic position for films which are simultaneously invested in the acceptance and normalization of profoundly different bodies. It is also notable that the films' discussions of separation never acknowledge that, judging by previous attempts to separate twins conjoined like Abby and Brittany, there is a very high likelihood that death, not disability, would result from an attempt at separation (Dreger).[12] Disability then becomes the symbolic substitute for death in the films' discourse, and the viewer is enlisted on the side of life through the twins' performance of vital physical ability. This dynamic is at once subversive, in that it requires viewers to redefine their understandings of desirable lives and functional bodies, and reactionary, in that it re-inscribes disability as an abject state that necessarily evokes pity: "They're not two poor little girls, they are up and at 'em, running around just like anybody else is at that age" (*JL*).

The films thus present a double-bind for the disability-conscious viewer who rejects the valorization of able-bodiedness and the implication that a life with impairment is less worth living, but who cannot endorse a medical interventionism that would promote a pseudo-normal appearance of singularity at the expense of health, ability, and even survival. I cannot offer a resolution to this particular conundrum. However, if we adopt Stuart Hall's model of encoding/decoding for understanding how mass media works in the postmodern age, we can see how the contradictory messages encoded in the documentaries may be decoded by different viewers depending upon their particular knowledge-bases and political investments (Hall "Encoding"). Considering the power of the heroic overcoming narrative now embedded in the cultural psyche, one might certainly speculate that the average viewer would decode the films' message about disability to paradoxically conclude at once that while surgery would have negatively impacted the Hensel twins, surgery *should* be pursued in other cases of conjoinment in order to avoid the abject state of disablement presumed to attach to non-normative bodies. This paradox is captured, for example, in the sub-headline from a 2006 puff piece in England's *News of the World* about *Joined for Life 2*: "They Should Have Died at Birth ... Now Two Girls Who Share One Body Have Turned Sixteen" (Basnett and Collin). This article, like the film, at once hyperbolically foregrounds the many things the girls are able to do — "COMPETE! PLAY! TYPE!" — and conveys the message that these accomplishments are a surprising exception to the expected outcomes for conjoined twins: separation or death.

Since the Hensels are both living and unseparated, their status as fully human must be insistently reinforced by the films, not only through the discourses of normalcy discussed above, but also through a related emphasis on individuality. Both films prominently insist that Abby and Brittany are separate and distinct individuals who just happen to share a body. Such a claim is well-merited by many of the sisters' statements and actions, as well as by the examples of other conjoined twins who also generally evince notably different tastes and opinions (Dreger, Quigley, Smith). However, in the case of Abby and Brittany, this claim seems to be pushed harder than usual, even exaggerated at times. This dynamic was notable as early as a 2008 *Life* article, when the twins were eight, whose author supported his point about the twins' individuality by contrasting "Abby's navel baring outfit versus Britty's demure ensemble" (Miller, "Our Summer" 40). Yet the accompanying pictures showed two outfits of shorts and tank tops that were nearly identical except that the top preferred by Abby was about an inch shorter, hardly the radical contrast suggest by the juxtaposition of "navel-baring" and "demure." Again, I make this point not to suggest that the many differences between Abby and Brittany's personalities are not real, but rather to highlight the manner in which discourses *about* the twins appear hyper-invested in claims of individuality which can exceed or exaggerate the real.

A telling moment in *Joined for Life 2* further illustrates this dynamic: Patty's voiced explanation of the girls' different personalities is overlaid onto brief illustrative clips of each sister performing the behaviors under discussion: Patty in voice-over says that Abby likes pink, while a clip plays of Abby choosing a pink shirt, for example. The moment of rupture in this smooth pattern of show-and-tell occurs when Patty is explaining that Abby is the bossier of the two twins: as her voice declares that "Abby bosses Koty [their younger brother]," a clip immediately plays of the twins telling Koty to stop doing something on the computer. But in fact, it is *Brittany* who is speaking, not Abby (*JL2*). An error like this, I suggest, is not merely a sign of carelessness, but also of an editorial drive toward a dichotomous narrative in which the twins always function oppositionally. The documentary drive to present both compelling messages and graspable truths, I suggest, is particularly likely to produce such slippages within its own totalizing narratives: "Claiming to offer the truth about reality, documentary suffers the anxiety of failure and of being found wanting in its answers and in its truths. Its very persuasions are evidence of its own insufficiency" (Cowie 107). Consideration of the films' portrayals of normalcy and individuality, then, inevitably leads to questions about how those portrayals are produced and by whom. Thus, we turn now to consider issues of agency and "truth" in the making of the *Joined for Life* documentaries.

Agency and Authorship

From the beginning of the Hensel twins' emergence into public life in 1996, they have presented a narrative of carefully chosen venues and calculated control over their public appearances. In *Joined for Life*, Patty explains that "when we first ever decided to do the *Life Magazine* story, and we were called [by various media] ... we went with quality TV programs that could educate" (*JL*). Rosemarie Garland-Thomson expands on the significance of venue for the twins' first public appearance: "The choice to introduce the girls in this magazine structured the way people would see and understand them. *Life Magazine* was as far from a sideshow as the family could get" (*Staring* 179). Avoiding a sideshow atmosphere was clearly important to the Hensel parents, who fortunately lack the financial pressures which might induce them to pursue more lucrative, less tasteful venues. They have avoided the talk show and reality television circuit, and have limited the girls' television appearances primarily to reputable news programs such as *Good Morning America* and *Dateline*. The media world's resistance to this decision is signaled in Patty's comment that "I've had TV people come up to me and say that I owe the world more of an explanation regarding Abby and Brittany. I don't owe the world nothing, and Abby and Brittany don't either" (*JL2*).

The *Joined for Life* documentaries, then, are presented as deliberate responses to these media pressures, the products of free choice and self-representation. As the narrator of *Joined for Life* explains, "Now as a family, they've chosen to tell their story. Their goals are simple: to answer the questions and allow the world to meet these incredible individuals" (*JL*). Similarly, the narrator of *Joined for Life 2* describes the Hensel family as refusing most media requests, adding that "instead, they chose to occasionally give the world an update of sorts," in the form of the *Joined for Life* films (*JL2*).

One might question why the Hensels made this choice of controlled yet highly public representation, rather than seeking to preserve their family's privacy as long as possible. Patty explains her reasoning in *Joined for Life*: "The bottom line to all this is so people can understand Brittany and Abby when it's not our own little community any more. People can come up and talk to them and know what to say to them. And it just kind of breaks the ice when people can say, we saw you on TV and you did a good job, or whatever" (*JL*). In the second film, when Abby and Brittany are older and more able to articulate their own purposes, Abby gives a very similar explanation: "We wanted to do this documentary so people wouldn't have to always stare and take pictures cause we don't like when they take pictures — so they just knew who we are and stuff" (*JL2*). Thus, the choice to expose the sisters' private lives on national television is somewhat ironically presented as a means to preserve privacy, so that people won't "stare and take pictures." Indeed, one could argue that the depiction of the twins throughout these two hour-long films serves to de-commodify their images through repetition and accumulation. If such images are widely familiar and easily accessible, there would be presumably less motive for strangers to try to capture them during casual encounters. And if, as the documentaries assert, these films are primarily produced by the twins and their parents, the Hensels crucially retain some level of control over the types of representation available to the wider cultural sphere.

Indeed, the narrator of *Joined for Life* insists that "although we have helped the Hensels tell their story, it is *their* story, complete with their occasional contributions running the camera" (*JL*). During this voiced-over statement, which occurs in the opening minutes of the film, we see a rare glimpse of a cameraman, followed by a shot of the twins themselves using a video camera (Abby is the one actually holding it). Footage shot by the twins is interspersed throughout the first documentary, adding an additional narrative level which arguably provides the twins' own self-representation, a significant rarity in the history of conjoined twins.[13] Of course, this footage has been subject to selection, editing, and even possible staging by the filmmakers, so we cannot naïvely interpret it as a pure expression of agency on the part of Abby and Brittany, however tempting such a construction might be. However, I would also suggest that disregarding the role of the twins as filmic agents and viewing their footage as entirely subjugated to the filmmakers' post-production interventions is a far too simplistic, not to mention disempowering, interpretation.

As Michael Renov explains, the introduction of video technology in the latter twentieth-century transformed and complicated the relationship between documentary filmmakers and subjects, often merging the two through new "capabilities to write *through* the body, to write *as* the body" (185). Renov continues:

> Durable, lightweight, mobile, producing instantaneous results, the video apparatus supplies a dual capability well suited to the essayistic project: it is both screen and mirror, providing the technological grounds for the surveillance of the palpable world, as well as a reflective surface on which to register the self [185–186].

No longer was the camera a bulky apparatus necessarily separated from, and dominant over, its subject. Instead, and particularly in the medium of televised documentaries using the new video technology, filmmakers could carry lightweight cameras themselves, and — as in the case of the Hensels — could share those cameras with their subjects to create multi-layered filmic narratives.[14]

In *Joined for Life*, we see the eleven-year-old twins taking on the authorial role of cinematic directors as they roam with the camera, calling out the classic command "Aaaand action!" to their subjects (*JL*). In this sense, the twins' agency is at once realized and made visible through the layering of their own footage with that of the "official" camera's recordings of them. It is certainly not difficult to separate the two registers, as the girls' footage is shaky, uneven, and punctuated with giggles. Another marked difference, of course, is that while the goal of the official camera is to foreground the twins' body as much as possible, the twins themselves are far more interested in filming the world around them. Their scenes focus on the domestic, even trivial details of their home lives, such as their dog, their bedroom, a detailed tour of their kitchen — "our refrigerator, our island, our stove" — and mock interviews with family members. At one point the twins corner Mike, one of their voices declaring: "Here is my lovely gray-haired father." Mike laughingly responds: "This is gonna be terrible with you guys having a camera around all of us" (*JL*). Similarly, when the girls film Patty and ask her, "What do you think of the new program we are doing?" she tells them, "I think we're gonna have to do a lot of editing" (*JL*). In these cases, we see Abby and Brittany taking on various authoritative documentarian roles — the voice-over narrator, the interviewer, the camera operator — and their parents responding with a humorous uneasiness and perhaps discomfort with that role reversal. We need not read too much into these responses — which of us would be serene about our children filming domestic scenes that could end up on national television? — but it is possible to register a certain tension here between the parents' expressed desire to control the representation of their extraordinary children, and the increasing agency of those children in claiming self-representation.

It is intriguing, in that regard, that the second documentary, filmed when the twins were sixteen, does not incorporate the device of the twins' own camera-eye view. This decision may have been budgetary, or a choice by the twins themselves, or driven by a number of other speculative factors; the result is that *Joined for Life 2* presents a flatter, less multidimensional portrait of the sisters' lives. In particular, one is struck by the absence of the "bedroom monologue" scenes of *Joined for Life*, the several occasions in which Abby and

Brittany spoke directly to a fixed camera mounted near their bed in their shared room. The "private" subjectivity voiced in these scenes is emphasized in the first one, which opens with the twins standing at their bedroom door, calling out, "Mom and Dad, don't come in, or anybody else!" (*JL*). The twins then sit on the corner of their bed, facing the camera, and Brittany narrates in a video-diary mode: "Hi, it's April 16, and we're here at our bedroom. It's the big night before our big tournament at Grand City. I wonder who is going to win? And, [I'm] just really nervous" (*JL*). As in the other footage controlled by the twins, the details of the bedroom monologues tend toward the trivial and minute: The twins tell us about being sick, vent their anger at Patty for not letting them babysit yet, show off Sadie the dog, and sometimes fall into self-conscious silence. Yet, these moments, I argue, seem to come closest to being genuinely self-authored by the twins themselves, and as such, constitute the most unusual and valuable aspect of the films, their nearest approximation of documentary as "disability life writing" (Couser 49). Through "intimate to-camera testimony" and "microsocial narratives" (Corner 263–265), the twins materialize a subjectivity that functions oppositionally to the objectification that usually surrounds extraordinary bodies, and which indeed, can be argued to emerge in many other aspects of the *Joined for Life* films as well.

The tension between multiple layers of representationality and agency is most vividly apparent in a scene from *Joined for Life 2*, when the twins travel outside their familiar community to visit their friend Tamara in Texas. During an outing to meet the Houston Astros, as Abby and Brittany are conversing with several players in the ballpark, they become aware that a stranger on the outskirts of the gathering has trained a videocamera upon them. At once, their faces register disapproval and anger. One of their voices says off-camera, "We hate, absolutely hate when people take pictures of us and try to videocamera us" (*JL2*). The narrator then chimes in to explain that this individual is filming the twins without their permission, and the film cuts to Patty elaborating that such behavior "drives them crazy because they feel like they're being violated" (*JL2*). This scene is intriguingly multi-layered and meta-representational, as the unauthorized filming and the twins' reaction is captured and displayed by another, authorized camera which remains invisible during the scene itself. Again, we see the assertion of control and the right to privacy performed through visual display and deliberate exposures. If "the Hensel twins' emergence from their domestic haven into the wider world was a carefully crafted invitation to stare" (Garland-Thomson, *Staring* 180), the *Joined for Life* films are at once invitations to certain kinds of stares and cautions against others. In this sense, they echo many aspects of the Schappell twins' attitudes portrayed in *Face to Face*, particularly in a scene where Lori tells a stranger not to take her picture, but adds that it is all right to take Reba's picture, since she, as a country singer, is a public figure (*Face to Face*; see also Couser 57, Dreger 133). And, as in *Joined for Life*, Lori and Reba Schappell wield video cameras during parts of their film, thus able to "make others the target of the objectifying gaze — to stare back" (Couser 63). The particularly objectifying aspect of visual, as opposed to verbal, attention is emphasized when Abby remarks, "We don't mind when people ask questions," and Brittany immediately adds, "That's better than taking pictures or being mean about it" (*JL2*). The film places this statement just prior to the trip to Texas, clearly framing our understanding of the subsequent scene of illicit videotaping. Even more strikingly, that scene is immediately followed by an interview snippet in which Abby declares, when discussing possible future careers, that "we might want to go into photography," perhaps in a sly comment on the preceding scene's struggle over the power of visual representation (*JL2*).

Such moments, like the bedroom monologues and the twins' camera-wielding in the first film, suggest that the *Joined for Life* films fit the genre of reflexive documentary, in which the mimetic relationship of representation and reality is disrupted by a conscious display of the film's constructed nature: "In its most paradigmatic form, the reflexive documentary 'prompts the viewer to a heightened consciousness of their relation to the text and of the text's problematic relationship to that which it represents'" (Govaert 247). By including a filmed scene in which the twins reject the right of a stranger to film them, *Joined for Life 2* may provoke viewers to question their own roles as strangers watching a film about the twins' intimate lives. Similarly, the Hensels' explicit discussions of their reasons for making these documentaries foregrounds the films' status as crafted narratives, rather than "unmediated slice[s] of reality" (Govaert 250).[15] Nevertheless, as Charlotte Govaert observes, the presence of reflexive elements in a film does not guarantee that viewers will respond with the assumed level of critical distance. It is likely that for many, even most viewers, the fascination of Abby and Brittany's exceptional bodily configuration, combined with the attraction of their personalities and their presentation as "heroic overcomers," will override any more reflective responses. This appears particularly true for those audience members who may, after viewing the films, take on the role of experts about the Hensels, such as those who comment online to correct others' misapprehensions and to explain aspects of the twins' anatomy: "Reflexivity proves critically in/significant when it merely serves to redefine and to further the accumulation of knowledge" (Minh-ha 104).

Ruptured Representations

The knowledge-effect of the documentaries is one of several concerns which become apparent when we consider the *Joined for Life* films not as isolated, pristine texts, transmitted directly from filmmakers to audiences, but as dynamic and interactive representational encounters in a twenty-first century media context. This final section explores the fragmented reproduction and distribution of the films after their original airings, and the particular importance of this dynamic in relation to the role of medical authority and the portrayal of the twins' surgery in *Joined for Life*.

As noted at the beginning of this chapter, *Joined for Life* originally aired on the Discovery Health Channel in 2001, while *Joined for Life: Abby and Brittany Turn 16* originally aired on The Learning Channel in 2006. Since those original airings, bits and pieces of both films have appeared in subsequent television programs in both the United States and around the world, sometimes as part of formal presentations such as *Extraordinary People: The Twins Who Share a Body*, which aired on BBC Channel 5 in 2007, but more often as informal excerpts in news and public interest programs.[16] It seems clear that the production and distribution companies involved—Advanced Medical Productions, Figure 8 Films, and the Discovery Channel—re-licensed the content to maximize the films' profitability. Outside of this formal re-distribution network, however, even more fragmented bits of the films may be found on YouTube and other video-sharing sites on the Internet, under a variety of titles, captioned or translated into numerous languages, and framed by the idiosyncratic editing choices of individual, presumably unlicensed posters. Thus, it does not appear that the Discovery Channel has exerted its right to control the sharing of the films' content, either by monitoring and removing un-licensed sharing, or limiting sharing to endorsed, advertisement-driven venues such as Vevo.

The question then arises whether this indiscriminate and enthusiastic sharing of the documentaries fulfills the Hensels' expressed goal of enabling the twins to be known and recognized in the wider world, to give a context for their initial encounters with strangers? Or is it actually a fracturing of the documentary's original intentions through the loss of context and the re-framing of these excerpts within multiple modes of enfreakment?

One way to address these questions is by considering the *Joined for Life* films within the larger context of documentaries about conjoined twins, the vast majority of which have centered on separation surgeries. Indeed, issues of distribution have been central to the evolution of the separation documentary since its inception: Dr. Doyen's original footage of his separation of Radica and Doodika in 1902 was sold without his knowledge to an impresario to be shown in coffee houses and fairs. Indeed, while Doyen had embraced the new medium for its potential for medical education, "to his chagrin, his movies ended up in the entertainment domain" (van Dijck 545). Currently, televised separation documentaries are part of the emerging hybrid genre that Jonathan Corner describes as "popular factual entertainment" or documentary as "diversion" (260). Since this genre usually involves "forms that are very high in exchange value, strategically designed for their competitive strength in the television marketplace" (Corner 262), it is understandable, and perhaps inevitable, that separation documentaries lend themselves to multiple and proliferative distributions, thus often subsuming the medical and educational aspects of these films into their sensational and exploitative effects.

However, *Joined for Life* and *Joined for Life 2* are *not* separation documentaries, and thus their distribution does not necessarily reproduce that dynamic. In particular, the fracturing and de-medicalizing of the first film may actually be understood as strengthening the Hensels'—if not the filmmakers'—didactic intentions. In separation documentaries of the past two decades, such as *Katie and Eilish* (1992), *Siamese Twins* (1995), and *The Girl with Eight Limbs* (2007), doctors play a central role as the "heroes" attempting to save children from the presumptively dreadful fate of remaining conjoined (Clark and Meyser, Dreger, van Dijck). The narrative arc of separation films is predetermined, proceeding from the decision whether to pursue surgery, to the surgery itself, to the early days of recovery, with medicine as the primary setting and doctors as the primary actors propelling this narrative forward.

Without the framing structure of separation surgery, the makers of the *Joined for Life* documentaries had to find different narrative arcs to structure the films. On the face of it, their choice was to construct the films around birthdays: *Joined for Life* follows "a year in the life" of Abby and Brittany, from their eleventh to twelfth birthdays, and *Joined for Life 2*, as its subtitle suggests, centers on the twins' sixteenth birthday. However, an unexpected turn in the Hensels' lives during the filming of *Joined for Life* introduced a medical narrative to supplant the purely domestic story of birthdays and daily life. A worsening case of scoliosis affecting the sisters' growth and breathing resulted in their spinal surgery in July 2001.

The presence of a surgical event in the center of the documentary shifts the film's focus away from its supposed goal of showing Abby and Brittany's everyday lives and toward a familiar medical narrative of crisis, intervention, and recovery. That this narrative is constructed, rather than inevitable, and underscored by the placement of the surgery at the exact midpoint of the film, although chronologically it took place about one-third of the way into the events being documented.[17] Thus, the center of the film is dominated by images of doctors and medical technology, displacing the previous domesticity of the twins' home and school lives. The doctors speak against hospital backgrounds, often posed next to light boxes displaying X-rays of the sisters' spines. There is also an extended close-up on the X-rays while the orthopedic surgeon explains the worsening curvature in each girl's spine and the subsequent need for surgery. While the twins themselves are notably absent in these scenes, the display of these X-rayed images "doubly expose[s] the twins' private interior bodies" (van Dijck 550), and substitutes a static and objectifying view for the dynamic, intensely personal vision of the sisters presented in the first half of the film. This objectification is furthered when the film next presents a digital animation superimposed over the X-ray image to demonstrate how the girls' spines will be straightened, attached to metal rods, and covered in bone grafts (*JL*). When these scenes are immediately followed by the surgery itself, the reconstruction of Abby and Brittany into faceless and passive bodies appears complete. According to the usual narrative of separation films, we are now prepared for the real actors — the doctors — to intervene and provide the climactic drama of the surgical attempt.

Yet the surgery scene that follows here, with its familiar close-ups of bright lights, blue-clad personnel, and metal instruments, has an oddly abstract feel. Indeed, while the film implies that these shots are taken during the twins' actual surgery, I suggest it is more likely that they are merely generic set pieces meant to symbolize, not depict, the surgical procedure. It is notable that, unlike most filmed surgical separations, in which shots of the twins' bodies are included and it is clear that the cameras are present in the operating theater itself, the "surgery scene" in *Joined for Life* remains anonymous, nonspecific, and relatively brief. The implication that the filmmakers have been shut out of the actual surgery is strengthened when the next shot is of the *outside* of the door to Abby and Brittany's hospital room. Patty's voice then explains that "Brittany and Abby do not want the camera on them as they are recovering" (*JL*). Indeed, the first glimpse the cameras — and therefore, we — have of the recovering twins is on the day of their discharge from the hospital, as they sit slumped in a wheelchair. Yet even in this moment, the sisters assert control over their representation: Brittany beckons the camera closer, as if she wants to say something, and then covers the lens with her hand, effectively ending the camera's access to their bodies (*JL*). These scenes signal a far greater tension between the agendas and desires of filmmakers, the girls, and the Hensel parents than is seen in the rest of the film. It seems clear that the filmmakers sought greater access to the intimate moments of the twins' surgery and were denied. Again, we can certainly question the extent to which this resistance on the part of the Hensels signals genuine agency and self-representation, as well as whether that agency belongs primarily to the twins or to their parents. At the least, however, we may certainly conclude that the Hensels wielded a significant amount of control over which footage was shot and used, and that this control is both unusual and refreshing in the realm of representations of conjoined twins. If "film spectators arrive at the screen prepared to glimpse the extraordinary body displayed for moments of uninterrupted visual access — a practice shared by clinical assessment rituals associated with the medical gaze" (Snyder and Mitchell 158), then the interruption of this visual access not only realigns the power dynamic between viewer and subject, but also disrupts the pseudo-clinical gaze taken on by the viewer of medical documentary.

When we then move outward to consider issues of distribution and reception, we may actually find that disruption continued. The majority of fragmented excerpts of the *Joined For Life* films found on video-sharing sites do not include the surgery scenes, more often including the quotidian scenes of the sisters in their family, at school, and talking directly to the camera. Thus the constructed narrative arc which centers the surgery does not appear to have survived the transition into the mode Corner describes as "postdocumentary culture," which relocates traditional documentary "as a set of practices, forms, and functions" into multiple levels of digital media access (266).

On the other hand, these hundreds of brief excerpts, which are virtually all taken from one of the *Joined for Life* documentaries, do not present their global viewership with the original films' full representational complexities. If, as Couser argues, the long duration of the documentary *Face to Face* serves to gradually undo the enfreakment of the Schappell twins as the viewer becomes accustomed to seeing their non-normative body (59), the fragmentation of the Hensel films may reinscribe that enfreakment. As Van Dijck observes, "The live freak show never really disappeared, but took on a new cloak: it evolved into medical documentary, the appeal of which is based, to a large extent, on the convergence of medical and media techniques" (538). Those techniques continue to converge in the era of digital media sharing, in which content becomes increasingly separated from its creators' control and intention. In this setting, is it possible to argue for self-representation and agency by any filmic subject, particularly those as historically enfreaked as conjoined twins? Possibly not; yet I suggest it is even more crucial then that we remain alert to those glimpses of agency which appear, however fleetingly, in representations such as the *Joined for Life* films.

Notes

1. *Joined for Life* originally aired on Discovery Health. *Joined for Life: Abby and Brittany Turn 16* originally aired on The Learning Channel (TLC).

2. For brevity, throughout this essay, *Joined for Life* will be cited as *JL* and *Joined for Life: Abby and Brittany Turn 16* will be referred to as *Joined for Life 2* and cited as *JL2*. These citations are to the original, complete documentaries as viewed on DVDs obtained from Advanced Medical Productions/Figure 8 Films in 2010.

3. For discussions of reflexive documentary, see Cowie, Govaert, Minh-ha, and Renov. Many documentary theorists include both direct address by the filmmaker and exposure of the production apparatus within the mode of the reflexive. I have separated the "reflexive" from the "reflective" here to assist with teasing out and differentiating the complex strands of reflexivity (and its failures) in the *Joined for Life* films.

4. For an excellent example of such portrayals, see the 1995 film *When Billy Broke His Head, and Other Tales of Wonder.*

5. Since beginning my research about the Hensels, I often find myself applied to as the holder of such knowledge and note how actively the seductive role of "expert" must be resisted or subversively transformed.

6. For discussion of this portrayal of doctors in separation surgeries, see Dreger, Clark and Myser, and van Dijck.

7. The nonfiction documentary "addresses our *expectations* about the world, and these derive not only from factual or scientific knowledge but also from our knowledge of what is held to be culturally normal for our community" (Cowie 37).

8. As Stuart Hall observes, "It would be more appropriate to define the typical discourse of this medium [TV] not as naturalistic but as *naturalized*: not grounded in nature but producing nature as a sort of guarantee of its truth" ("Rediscovery" 75).

9. For these and additional details on the Hilton twins' lives, see Frost, Jensen, and Pingree.

10. Van Dijck notes that "although the operation was considered a success, Doodica died a week afterwards, while her sister would live for another year before dying (of tuberculosis)" (544).

11. In accordance with this equation of able-bodiedness and athleticism, there is no acknowledgement in either film of the existence of adaptive sports or any other form of accommodation which enables people with different physical abilities to participate in social activities.

12. As is seen for example, in the case of Katie and Eilish Holton, depicted in the 1992 film *Katie and Eilish: Siamese Twins,* and discussed by Clark and Myser in "Fixing."

13. In most scenes, Abby is holding the camera, which is small enough to be carried and used in one hand. To achieve a more accurate and complex version of the twins' own experience, however, the filmmakers

would have needed to give cameras to both girls so that each could film simultaneous footage from her own viewpoint. There is no information in the film as to why this approach was not taken, or whether this was a choice by the filmmakers or the twins themselves (*JL*).

14. Trinh T. Minh-ha, however, argues that the video camera still functions as a structuring authority over the subject: "The lightweight, handheld camera, with its independence of the tripod — the fixed observation post — is extolled for its ability 'to go unnoticed,' because it must be at once mobile and invisible, integrated into the milieu so as to change as little as possible, but also able to put its intrusion to use and provoke people into uttering the 'truth' that they would not otherwise unveil in ordinary situations" (95).

15. According to classic understandings of reflexive documentary, a filmmaker "enters the frame and explains in a direct address to the viewer why she felt compelled to make this film" to "draw attention to the *constructionality* of film [and] cue the audience that the images, although bearing an indexical relationship to the world, are subject to selection (in and pro-camera), order and placement into a certain context" (Govaert 247).

16. The 2007 BBC program is simply *Joined for Life 2* under a new title. Similarly, *Joined for Life* aired in Australia on Channel 2 in 2002 and 2003 under the title *True Stories: Joined for Life*. A search on YouTube will turn up many of these excerpts from news and human interest programs around the world.

17. The film's action supposedly proceeds chronologically from the sisters' eleventh birthday on March 7, 2001, to their twelfth birthday in 2002. The surgery takes place at the beginning of July 2001. Other minor discrepancies in the chronological order can be seen, for example, in scenes of the sisters with braces on their teeth which are shown before the orthodontist visit in which they first get braces (*JL*).

Works Cited

Angier, Natalie. "Joined for Life, and Living Life to the Full." *New York Times* 23 Dec. 1997. Web.

Basnett, Guy, and Robbie Collin. "Just Twin-credible." *News of the World* (England) 31 Dec. 2006. Lexus-Nexus. Web.

Bogdan, Robert. "The Social Construction of Freaks." Garland-Thomson, *Freakery* 23–37. Print.

Clark, David L., and Catherine Myser. "Being Humaned: Medical Documentaries and the Hyperrealization of Conjoined Twins." Garland-Thomson, *Freakery* 338–354. Print.

_____, and _____. "'Fixing' Katie and Eilish: Medical Documentaries and the Subjection of Conjoined Twins." *Literature and Medicine* 17.1 (1998): 45–67. Print.

Corner, John. "Performing the Real: Documentary Diversions." *Television and New Media* 3.3 (2005): 255–269. Print.

Couser, G. Thomas. *Signifying Bodies: Disability in Contemporary Life Writing*. Ann Arbor: University of Michigan Press, 2009. Print.

Cowie, Elizabeth. *Recording Reality, Desiring the Real*. Minneapolis: University of Minnesota Press, 2011. Print.

Davis, Lennard J. *Enforcing Normalcy: Disability, Deafness, and the Body*. New York: Verso, 1995. Print.

Dominus, Susan. "Could Conjoined Twins Share A Mind?" *The New York Times Magazine* 25 May 2011. Web.

Dreger, Alice Domurat. *One of Us: Conjoined Twins and the Future of the Normal*. Cambridge: Harvard University Press, 2004. Print.

Face to Face: The Schappell Twins. Dir. Ellen Weissbrod. A&E, 2000

Frost, Linda, ed. *Conjoined Twins in Black and White*. Madison: University of Wisconsin Press, 2009. Print.

Garland-Thomson, Rosemarie, *Extraordinary Bodies: Figuring Physical Disability in American Literature and Culture*. New York: Columbia University Press, 1997. Print.

_____. *Staring: How We Look*. New York: Oxford University Press, 2008. Print.

_____, ed. *Freakery: Cultural Spectacle of the Extraordinary Body*. New York: New York University Press, 1996. Print.

The Girl with Eight Limbs. National Geographic Channel, 2007.

Govaert, Charlotte. "How Reflexive Documentaries Engage Audiences in Issues of Representation: Apologia for A Reception Study." *Studies in Documentary Film* 1.3 (2007): 245–263. Print.

Hall, Stuart. "Encoding/Decoding." 1980. *Media and Cultural Studies: Keyworks*. Eds. Douglas M. Kellner and Meenakshi Gigi Durham. Oxford: Blackwell, 2001. 166–176. Print.

_____. "The Rediscovery of 'Ideology': Return of the Repressed in Media Studies." *Culture, Society, and the Media*. Eds. Michael Gurevitch, Tony Bennett, James Curran, and Janet Woollacott. London: Routledge, 1982. Print.

Jensen, Dean. *The Lives and Loves of Daisy and Violet Hilton.* Berkeley: Ten Speed Press, 2006. Print.

Joined For Life. Dir. Bill Hayes. Advanced Medical Productions/Discovery Channel, 2001. DVD.

Joined For Life: Abby and Brittany Turn 16. Dir. Rachael Pihlaja. Advanced Medical Productions/Discovery Channel, 2006. DVD.

Katie and Eilish: Siamese Twins. Dir. Mark Galloway. BBC/ITV, 1992.

Merish, Lori. "Cuteness and Commodity Aesthetics: Tom Thumb and Shirley Temple." Garland-Thomson, *Freakery* 185–203. Print.

Miller, Kenneth. "Together Forever." *Life* Apr. 1996: 44–56. Print.

_____. "Our Summer Vacation." *Life* 16 Sep. 1998: 34–40. Print.

Minh-ha, Trinh T. "The Totalizing Quest of Meaning." *Theorizing Documentary.* Ed. Michael Renov. New York: Routledge, 1993. 90–107. Print.

Pingree, Allison. "The 'Exceptions That Prove the Rule': Daisy and Violet Hilton, the 'New Woman,' and the Bonds of Marriage." Garland-Thomson, *Freakery* 173–184. Print.

Quigley, Christine. *Conjoined Twins: An Historical, Biological and Ethical Issues Encyclopedia.* Jefferson, NC: McFarland, 2003.

Renov, Michael. *The Subject of Documentary.* Minneapolis: University of Minnesota Press, 2004. Print.

Siamese Twins. Dir. Jonathan Palfreman. PBS/Nova, 1995.

"Siamese Twins Buried in Specially-Made Casket." *Jet* 22 Feb. 1993: 16–17.

Smith, J. David. *Psychological Profiles of Conjoined Twin: Heredity, Environment, and Identity.* Westport, CT: Praeger, 1988. Print.

Snyder, Sharon L., and David T. Mitchell. *Cultural Locations of Disability.* Chicago: University of Chicago Press, 2006. Print.

Stumbo, Bella. "Sisters in a Singular World." *Washington Post* 27 Aug. 1981, final ed.: B1, B3, B6, B7. Print.

_____. "Taking the Wonderful Plunge." *Washington Post* 10 May 1987, final ed.: F1. Print.

Wallis, Claudia. "The Most Intimate Bond." *Time* 25 Mar. 1996: 60–64. Print.

When Billy Broke His Head and Other Tales of Wonder. Dir. Billy Golfus. Fanlight Productions, 1994.

The Making of 18q-

Parental Advocacy, Disability and the Ethics of Documentary Filmmaking

VERONICA WAIN

To give life to a child is, in my experience, a profound encounter with another human being. To have been home to another living, breathing human who is at once a part of you and separate defies expression in words alone. Giving life to my third child, Allycia, born in 1995 with a rare condition occurring on the 18th chromosome, known as 18q-(deletion)[1], intensified this profound experience as I came to terms with the different path that her life, our family's lives and ultimately my own life would take as a result. As Allycia's mother, my role has expanded beyond that of nurturer and carer to one of advocate as we have navigated our way within the complex medical, political, educational and social milieus that determine so much about what kind of life she can live.

Realizing how markedly our lives and attitudes had changed since Allycia's birth, I felt compelled as a parent and a filmmaker to bring our story, and those of other families whose experiences resonated with ours, to the screen in a bid to raise awareness about 18q- and challenge the way the story of disability continues to be told. I was driven by a lack of awareness about the condition in the wider community, the consistently negative ways in which information was delivered to me concerning my daughter and her needs, and our family's sense of aloneness until finding an international community — a community united by the birth of our children with this condition and shared life experiences.

This essay reflects on the making of the autobiographical documentary *18q-: A Different Kind of Normal*, the specific act of disclosing on film one's experience as a nondisabled parent of a child with a disability, and the ethical considerations particular to the form.

18q- *in Production*

Completed in 2011, *18q-: A Different Kind of Normal*[2] is the first substantial work to explore the lives and experiences of those with genetic anomalies occurring on the 18th chromosome and their families.[3] In making the film, I shot and edited approximately 90 hours of footage using a mini DV over a five-year period in collaboration with a number of professionals in the field.[4] This includes many hours of "on the run" interviews and event

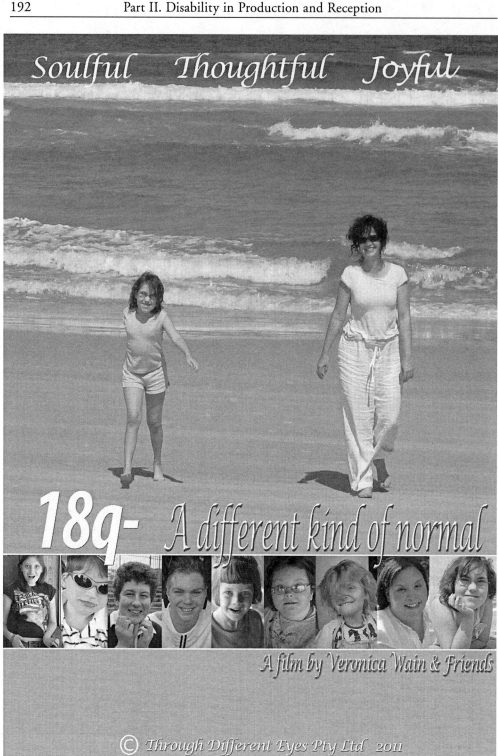

The promotional poster for the autobiographical film *18q-: A Different Kind of Normal* features Allycia and Veronica Wain walking together near their home in Australia above shots of Chromosome 18 community members who participated in the making of the film.

taping at Chromosome 18 Research and Registry conferences Allycia and I attended in Sydney, and Plymouth, Massachusetts. It also includes observational footage of Allycia at school, at play, and in the medical settings she often frequents, as well as footage of our family in our everyday, ordinary lives, interviews with myself, several family members, disability academics and activists, and with the only one of Allycia's physicians who agreed to appear on camera. As is the nature of film, nearly all of this material was necessarily omitted in the final cut, resulting in a feature length documentary of 80 minutes.

From the beginning *18q-* was intended as an advocacy film that aimed to highlight the existence of the condition, explore some of the broader issues facing families with children with congenital disabilities, and articulate the value and meaningfulness of our lives in a bid to challenge the medicalized categorizing and devaluing of persons born with genetic differences. Despite the nature of the film, I was initially a reluctant subject. I had imagined myself as a filmmaker creating a forum for other families and people born with the condition to bring their own stories to the screen. But it became clear from both artistic and advocacy perspectives that the film required the kind of overarching narrative framework that the autobiographical provides. My experiences and those of my family would be the vehicle for exploring the twists and turns inherent in living with a particular disability, and my autobiographical voice-over narration would drive the larger story the film tells of the journey from ignorance to awareness in relation to genetic difference. The film begins before Allycia's birth, weaving our journey with the voices of others in the 18q community, ultimately documenting our embrace of new medical knowledge alongside a systematic unlearning of what "being normal" means and a discovery of community and connection as a means of flourishing in our lives.

From the outset, the film presented a number of production challenges. How could I deliver information about a medical condition in a way that was engaging as well as educative? How could I create a visually engaging piece when my primary format for bringing forth people's stories was going to be "talking heads" style interview footage due to the time and location constraints within conference environments, my only opportunities to access the families I wished to interview? How was I going to interview myself on film given my personal reluctance to be in front of the camera? Through the production process I found a number of answers to these questions: balance interior and exterior footage, use selected editing techniques, include highly stylized animation. But making a documentary that advocates effectively is not only a matter of technical challenges; it is a matter of ethical ones, too.

The Pitfalls of Autobiographical Advocacy: The Cautionary Tale of The Broken Cord

The value of autobiographical texts as advocacy remains contentious within disability scholarship. While Dorothy Atkinson and Jan Walmsley argue in favor of the genre as having the potential to "disrupt inherent power differentials in pursuit of disability research" (203), David Mitchell is critical of autobiographical writers such as Brenda Brueggemann, Georgina Kleege and Michael Bérubé.[5] As he writes in his review of Leonard Kriegel's autobiographical *Flying Solo: Reimagining Manhood, Courage, and Loss*:

> Instead of serving as a corrective to impersonal symbolic literary representations, disability life writing tends toward the gratification of a personal story bereft of community with other disabled people. Even the most renowned disability autobiographers often fall prey to an ethos of

rugged individualism that can further reify the longstanding association of disability with social isolation [311].

In addition to guarding against making a film that perpetuated entrenched ideals of successful exceptionalism and rugged individualism, I found that creating a work that further embedded limited ideologies concerning quality of life outcomes for people with disabilities was a serious risk. Having committed to the production of *18q-* as autobiographical advocacy, Michael Dorris' nonfiction literary memoir *The Broken Cord* provided me with a cautionary model that further guided my approaches to making the film.

Dorris' beautifully written memoir charts his life with his adoptive Sioux son, who was born with Foetal Alcohol Syndrome (FAS), and the seeming hopelessness of his son's life as a result of his physiological condition. The work of advocacy here is to bear witness to the tragic effects of FAS on Dorris' son's life as a powerful call for prevention. However, Dorris' sweeping approach to a solution was perceived as bordering on misogyny with its call for the sterilization of repeat "offenders" and the conditional incarceration of childbearing Native American women. These proposed policies have potentially disturbing cultural precedence in government efforts to control Native American families and reproduction over the last four centuries. Dorris' calls were met with vehement criticism from Native American scholars (Cook-Lynn 83). Criticism of Dorris' work also came from life writing and disability scholar G. Thomas Couser. He views self-representation through autobiography as a potentially powerful retort to ideologies of oppression and segregation in the dominant ableist culture, thereby restoring the voices of those living with disability. However his support for life writing as playing "a crucial role by providing the reading public with mediated access to a kind of diversity that might otherwise remain opaque, exotic, and threatening to them" is qualified. It must also be "properly conceived and carried out" (*Signifying Bodies* 15). Couser reads Dorris' *The Broken Cord* as a work flawed in its conception insofar as it fails to acknowledge the ways in which it participates in eugenic discourse that ultimately dehumanizes people with disabilities (*Vulnerable Subjects* 72).

As a parent advocate, I am in a less problematic position than Dorris because my daughter's difference is not the result of socio-environmental or behavioral impact on maternal health or fetal development, but rather the result of genetic diversity. I did not set out to "solve" the "problem" of being born with Chromosome 18 conditions, but rather to challenge entrenched ideologies of "normal" and what it means to live a valuable life. Pre-natal diagnosis, which is available for chromosome 18, is still delivered primarily, if not exclusively, with medical stories of difference that combine factual information with case studies delivered in a language imbued with a risk mentality. This narrow rhetorical framework has long been critiqued by members of the disability community as leading all too quickly to the belief that persons with disabilities should be prevented from existing when possible, a form of genetic cleansing without a full understanding of the place of genetic difference within our species, as well as a form of contemporary eugenics ideology and practice. [6] This topic deserves a more comprehensive treatment than my film could provide, so *18q-* does not address pre-natal testing and birth decisions. But it does speak to the limits of medically oriented narratives of what it means to live with a genetic difference, and the myth that disability necessarily results in diminished lives, by focusing on the joys and challenges of individuals and families as articulated in their own words. In this sense, *18q-* is not intended to be a "pro-life" film, but a "pro-story" film.

Nevertheless, Dorris' book remained a cautionary model for me in terms of the use of autobiography itself as a parental advocacy genre, particularly in two respects: first, the handling of informed consent with my own child; and second, the importance of moving beyond my own voice to include not only Allycia's voice and editorial perspectives, but those of other members of the 18q- community in developing the film's narrative portrait. Armed with this prior knowledge I determined I would involve Allycia, as well as her peers, both in front of and behind the camera and that I would consult with my family and our Chromosome 18 community with progressive cuts of the film to ensure we were in general agreement with the direction of the work.

While acknowledging that Dorris writes from a place of love, concern, and the desire to prevent further suffering caused by a preventable syndrome, Couser finds that *The Broken Cord* is a troubled work for a number of reasons, not the least for the complex and insufficiently delineated dynamics of informed consent in the memoir's production. Dorris includes a chapter written by his son and states that his son read the manuscript prior to publication and gave his consent for distribution, but these assurances seem undercut by Dorris' own description of his son's inability to make informed decisions.[7]

As a minor, Allycia is subject to many decisions I make on her behalf, as all children are in relation to their parents or legal guardians, including decisions about how much of our personal lives I choose to share for public view and the extent of her participation in these acts. As a parent, this is a daily responsibility. As a director seeking to practice ethical documentary filmmaking, it is sobering and often complex in practice. The notion of obtaining informed consent from Allycia is — to be honest — a difficult one to assess. How do I explain to her the possible ramifications of bringing her story to the screen? That exposing our personal lives could potentially open us up to public criticism, debate and ridicule? These are the realities of our lives in a world that scorns "retards" and challenges the value of supporting people whose contribution to society is seen as wanting and whose existence is evaluated in terms of the tax dollars it takes to offer effective educational opportunities or supported living arrangements. They are also abstract concepts that can be difficult to process cognitively.

Ultimately, I approached my conversations with Allycia about consent and choice in participating in the film in terms of education. I explained that we would make a film showing and telling other people about what it is like to have a Chromosome 18 condition so that more people will know what that means, although some of them may still not understand. I have explained that "we are like teachers." She understands this and has delighted in the filmmaking process, both in front of and behind the camera, along with her peers. It is impossible, however, for me to project into the future to know how Allycia as an adult will come to view the film. At this point in her life she is proud of it and of seeing her new-found friends on screen. I am hopeful she will continue to be proud of herself, her family and her Chromosome 18 community in the future and that this film will facilitate her pride and her ability as an adult to handle the negatively charged counter-narratives about intellectual impairment that she will no doubt encounter.

In making *18q-: A Different Kind of Normal*, I explored the conventions of documentary filmmaking, including those now synonymous with the craft, namely observational, expositional, interactive and reflexive (Nichols). Within these traditions, the self-reflexive mode has emerged alongside the many hybrid forms documentary now exhibits, whereby filmmakers bring stories to the screen with greater transparency regarding the constructed nature of the works, revealing themselves as active participants in or as the subjects of their own films. My film sits primarily within this category as an autobiographical/biographical work aimed at bringing a group of vulnerable individuals' private lives to the screen with the intention of producing an instrument that challenges perceptions of disability in general. But it quickly became clear to me that self-reflexivity was not enough given the context of the "worlds" our stories were to enter. As Angela Aguayo asserts: "It is not enough to visually and aesthetically parade counter-cultural values and images. Activist documentary must leave a footprint in the sphere(s) of politics, opening up spaces for social change" (234).

In seeking to meet Aguayo's challenge and to avoid the potential limitations and problematic representations arising from Dorris' more purely autobiographical approach to advocacy, I also interviewed academics and disability activists for the film with an eye toward including their perspectives as well. In the end, only one of these interviewees succeeded in appearing in the final cut — Ann Greer, an Australian disability activist and parent of two young adults living with disability. Whilst the information gleaned from these interviews "outside" the Chromosome 18 community were invaluable in terms of backgrounding disability theory and experience, the personal touch I wanted to deliver with the film diminished when people were included whose emotional connection was one or more steps removed from those central to the storytelling. Instead, I focused primarily on including multiple perspectives wherever possible to demonstrate the diverse reactions that occur within families when a person of difference arrives in their lives. Does the film "leave a footprint in the spheres of politics, opening up spaces for social change"? In terms of the worlds outside the international 18q community, that will depend in large part on the viewership the film finds, distribution having the impact on influence that it does. But it is my hope that the film also has political efficacy within the 18q community, fostering unity within diversity and functioning as an affirming articulation of community experiences and a resource for advocacy with others.

Ethical Frameworks: Dramatic Encounters, Costs and Benefits

In his work, *Lies, Damn Lies, and Documentaries,* Brian Winston critiques prolific filmmaker Frederick Wiseman's style of observational documentary, exploring the ethical implications of the filmmaker's choices in content, editing and stylistic approach. Wiseman laid bare the political and social dilemmas of institutions in the 1960s, adopting an observational style in his films using only footage and synchronous sound captured from within the walls of the institutions he chose as subjects. These included a mental institution in *Titicut Follies* (1967)[8], a secondary school in *High School* (1968) and a public hospital in *Hospital* (1970). Wiseman relied on the editing process, rather than manipulating the environments or subjects to craft the films into works that challenged the injustices and inequalities of American institutions. By showcasing graphic and disturbing scenes of subjects made vulnerable by virtue of circumstance, and disempowered by those charged with their care, Wiseman created films that placed raw visual and sound footage in front of an audience to allow them to find their own way within the work, rather than using voice-over narration to contextualize or suggest a point of view. While acknowledging the larger attitudinal or policy changes spurred by the attention Wiseman brought to these institutions, Winston is concerned with the subjects themselves, who are captured in their vulnerability and displayed for the public to see in circumstances lacking dignity. He ultimately asks the question of Wiseman's *Titicut Follies*: What good did the film do *for those whom it portrayed*? (85–6).

Thus the question "What good will the film do for my daughter, our family, and the

Chromosome 18 community?" became my ethical touchstone throughout the making of *18q-*. The ends cannot justify the means: collateral damage to those in front of the camera for larger shifts of social consciousness or for the benefit of those who may come later is unsustainable ethical ground. This is a particularly powerful maxim for me because it knits together all three of the advocacy roles in my life: those of parent, 18q community member, and filmmaker. But it is also particularly challenging in practice because of the many choices in filming, editing and narrative representation that arise, requiring the privileging of one role over another — either the parent whose advocacy focus is the family unit, the community member whose advocacy focus is the knitting together of the lives of those touched by an issue, or the filmmaker whose advocacy focus is the educating of an outside audience.

Larry Gross, John Stuart Katz and Jay Ruby's 1988 work, *Image Ethics: The Moral Rights of Subjects in Photographs, Film and Television,* explores the power differentials that exist between artist and subject, the construction of informed consent given these power differentials, and the moral obligations entailed in capturing and reproducing images of subjects in a variety of contexts. I turned to their four-step evaluation as an initial framework for the making of *18q-*:

1. The image maker's commitment to him/herself to produce images which reflect his/her intention to the best of his/her ability.
2. The image maker's responsibility to adhere to the standards of his/her profession and to fulfill his/her commitments to the institutions or individuals who have made the production economically possible.
3. The image maker's obligation to his/her subjects.
4. The image maker's obligation to the audience [6].

Katz's application of these four ethical responsibilities in evaluating Ira Wohl's Academy Award winning documentary *Best Boy* (1979) and its sequel *Best Man: Best Boy and All of Us Twenty Years Later* (1997) provided a more pointed framework for my work, especially given Wohl's familial relationship with the subject of his films — his cousin Philly Wohl, who is intellectually impaired. Ira Wohl's intent in the first film is clear: Philly and his parents are not getting any younger and a future for 52-year-old Philly without parental care is precarious. Establishing suitable living arrangements and support for Philly to ensure his well being is central to the film with the outcome being Ira's intervention in facilitating Philly's eventual relocation to a group home. The second film sees Ira revisit his cousin's life, shows Philly flourishing, and records two significant events orchestrated by Ira: Philly makes his Bat Mitzvah and visits his mother's grave. With Philly's intellectual disability being the driver for Ira's intervention, Katz questions whether Philly really understood the context within which his life was being made public in these films.

Katz's discussion touches not only the conventional power relations between filmmaker and subject, but other dynamics that, to coin Renov's (216–267) term, may be involved in bringing "domestic ethnography" to the screen, especially when a film's subject is intellectually impaired. How do we think about the ethics of filmed advocacy when the advocacy extends to changing a subject's lived situation and filming that change? Filmmaking is the capturing of dramatic circumstance on screen, so how do we consider filmed advocacy that extends to arranging for dramatic encounters, such as Philly's visit to his mother's grave and then capturing his visible distresses on camera? Was this necessary for Philly to experience or for the audience to experience? So too, what were the motivations for Philly's Bat Mitzvah, which was orchestrated by the filmmaker? Do we as filmmaking family members have the right to orchestrate events on behalf of those in our lives living with intellectual impairment? These questions remain even though Philly experienced positive outcomes as a consequence of Ira's interventions. He found a welcoming community and a sense of independence from his aging parents demonstrated on screen by his demeanor and interactions with members of his community in his group-home accommodation. However in retrospect and in my own experience, these ventures in the representations of others present many questions requiring self reflection and an effort to see our lives and those of our subjects, as well as our relationships with them, beyond the world of the film.

With Ira Wohl's films in mind, I chose not to stage any dramatic encounters for the filming of *18q-*. In my interviews, I endeavored to listen closely and watch for non-verbal feedback indicating whether or not interviewees maintained a sense of comfort as a guideline. Distress that I generated as a filmmaker would not be included in the film. This occurred once when my manner of questioning was particularly distressing for a subject and this footage was subsequently omitted. The exchange occurred early in my interview process when my enthusiasm to know more overran a young man by not allowing him enough time to process the information I was communicating to him. As a result, he felt inadequate and reacted to the counterproductive context I had created. I attempted to reconcile with him and ameliorate the negative impact of the situation, but in the end needed to simply leave him be to regain a sense of calm and composure. I was able to speak with him the following day and we were able to move on as members of the same community. However, I learned very quickly that unless I was centered, focused, and sensitive to nonverbal cues during interviews, my desire to empower these individuals and families would be lost in the wave of my own goals as a filmmaker.

I also decided after the first year of the project that I would screen progressive cuts at various intervals during the production and editing process to Chromosome 18 and wider disability community audiences. Screenings took place in 2008 at the Powerhouse in Brisbane and in New Zealand. The Brisbane screening was hosted by Rick Guidotti with invitations extended to a number of disability groups in Queensland. More than 100 guests attended to offer feedback. Allycia, Rick and I took questions from the audience at the conclusion. The New Zealand screening took place at a Chromosome 18 conference for families with physician members of the San Antonio, Texas, Chromosome 18 Research and Registry Society in attendance. The film was given the go ahead by all attendees. These screenings were critical in helping me to ensure that my work was ethically and accurately reflecting the themes and issues that face us as a small unknown community and establish whether the challenges and circumstances my own family faces in the film resonated within our wider disability and nondisabled communities in Australia and would be useful to a wider audience. Those screenings provided valuable feedback, confirming rather than prompting alteration of the film's content and presentation. In the end, it was easier to be a community member filmmaker than a parent filmmaker because — as Ira Wohl's relationship with Philly demonstrates — family relationships entail prior familiarity and more complex patterns of relational experiences, responsibilities and desires.

With my two eldest children, Adam (age 18 at the time) and Kristina (age 17), who were born without differences on their 18th chromosomes, these lines were perhaps hardest to draw and the ethics of my own choices most challenged. Midway through the film a sequence occurs where my family — my three children and I — are sharing a Mother's Day breakfast they prepared for me. My son Adam's discomfort in front to the camera becomes crystal clear when he states: "This is my home; it's private, not for the whole world to see."

He is a private person by nature and while he supported the intent of the project, he clearly would have preferred me to turn the camera off. Would I have turned it off if Allycia expressed this feeling instead of Adam? If Adam had been younger rather than older? If I had been filming someone else's child?

Those answers and their implications may be clear in retrospect. But at the time I had a personal desire to show that he was an active member of our family, especially since he had already chosen not to appear on camera in a personal interview, as Kristina did. Prior screenings of the film had prompted audiences to ask: where's Adam? Why was he not included? It became about how as a parent rather than a filmmaker I wanted to see my son and our family portrayed. I discussed the reasons I wanted to include his appearance in the Mother's Day sequence with Adam. He understood my motivations and gave permission for its inclusion. But I have little doubt that had I been a filmmaker outside the family, he would not have allowed this intrusion into his private life. So I am left with the knowledge that my son did it for me. He graciously allowed his need for privacy and sense of what is appropriate to show on screen to be put aside. This experience made me aware that these encounters have the potential to damage family relationships if as filmmakers — or as family members — our desire for our work to be crafted in a particular way usurps our regard for the close relationships we have in our personal lives and the perspectives of those we love.

Kristina, also supportive of the project, is more outgoing by nature and agreed to be interviewed. She became distressed on camera, though, as she recounted the confusion she felt at not having me or her new baby sister around shortly after Allycia's birth when Allycia suffered heart failure and an extended hospital stay. Following the interview Kristina agreed that the experience was cathartic. It enabled her to revisit a particularly painful time in her life and give voice to her experiences now that she is a young adult, including the grief and confusion she felt during the early years of her childhood. These were difficult times for her and she has said that the public disclosure of them has been powerful in allowing her to leave the sadness of those years behind and move forward in her life. And thus, this footage appears in the film. My experience behind the camera during the interview was somewhat different.

As Kristina spoke on camera, I chose to maintain my distance when she broke down and cried, giving her time to regain her composure, rather than holding her as I would have, had a camera not been perched between us. When I look back upon that moment, knowing that I had become the filmmaker across the table from Kristina rather than her mother, it does not sit comfortably with me. My commitment as a filmmaker to producing powerful shots, my knowledge that this happens if you continue to hold the camera, allow emotion to sweep over the subject, and see where it takes you, seemed to override my parental impulse to forget the film and comfort my daughter. Whilst these experiences with Adam and Kristina may not be especially striking, they were invaluable experiences for me in terms of examining my own ethics and values. I believe I now have a far greater level of self awareness within my professional practice than I did prior to making the film. In spite of this newfound knowledge — or perhaps because of it — the tension I experienced in juggling the dual roles of mother and filmmaker became disconcerting.

In terms of my relationship with Allycia as a parent filmmaker, my most ethically challenging moment of filming and editing came not with Allycia herself, but with my father. As I recount Allycia's medical history in voice-over narration, the film leads the viewer from the hospital where she was born to an interview with my father and me, exposing the strained relationship we experienced as a result of his religious beliefs surrounding Allycia's conception, subsequent health issues and intellectual impairment. My father had agreed to be interviewed and be honest about his beliefs and I did not wish to disrespect him on screen. On the other hand, I wanted to document the effect that religious beliefs towards people with genetic differences can have and the possible consequences of these ideologies between family members. Seeing the footage, I realized the capacity of the editing process to evoke further isolation and estrangement between the two of us, which could impact the loving relationship he had developed over the years with Allycia. I was also mindful of not wanting to expose Allycia at the age she was at the time of the film's release to the knowledge that her grandfather saw her birth and subsequent condition as a result of sin. So I edited with family bonds and parental responsibility forefront in my mind. As a result, this sequence in the film does not reflect the tremendous emotional impact that we experienced in our family as a result of my father's religiosity. The balance of "truth telling" in this film was tempered by my knowledge once again of the need to preserve relationships beyond the film.

In the context of parental advocacy filmmaking, I propose a fifth criteria that must be added to Katz's four, particularly when filming minors with differing intellectual capacities: the image maker's responsibility to sustain, or certainly to do no harm, to the child's relationships with family members and community members, or to the child's own sense of self in relation to others. Protecting and encouraging all of these relationships falls under the larger umbrella of a parent's responsibility to ensure their child's future as an adult, which doesn't end when you pick up the camera or examine raw footage. We often think of filming as the moment in which subjects are most vulnerable. But the choices made in the editing process often have greater potential for empowering — or not — those who chose to be a part of the work. This process is little understood by those outside filmmaking and is least transparent. It is the moment, I discovered, in which we most need to keep in mind the lives of participants, particularly children, beyond the release of the film. As for being a parent filmmaker, ours is still a very close family, with intimate, honest exchanges and whilst I am happy with the final piece and believe I have delivered on the aims I set out to achieve, I have no desire to film any of my children again. I am now content to leave my filmmaker role at our front door.

Parental Film Advocacy: Documentary and Community

> *Without the formation of counter-publics, activist documentary has little hope of achieving and sustaining the process of social change [...] How counter-publics or social movements create change from or with activist documentary is a complicated process involving much more than a documentary screening.*
>
> — Angela Jean Aguayo (225)

Prior to making *18q-* I had very little knowledge about our wider, international Chromosome 18 community. Allycia and I attended our first annual family conference for members of the Chromosome 18 Registry and Research Society in conjunction with the filming of *18q-,* and segments of the conference appear in the film. The society is an international parent-founded advocacy organization based in the United States, which was a long journey from our home in Australia. I met many of the conference participants who appear on camera and many more with whom I spoke for the first time at the conference, only hours before our interviews, although I had prior contact with some via the group's list serve. Through our attendance and the filming process, this community became more important in my life and in Allycia's. Joining it added a third advocacy role to parent and filmmaker: that of community member.

It appeared that my goals in making this film would naturally align with those I hoped to represent. However, we are a diverse community from a multitude of countries, cultures, and backgrounds, so it did not necessarily hold that we all wanted the "same" things for our children, and our children are themselves diverse with their own perspectives. I was afforded much trust as personal information, beliefs and values, and deeply emotional experiences were disclosed with the hope that I would deliver a piece worthy of them. A worthy work for me, which I discussed with the participants, meant delivering a piece that brought our children and experiences to the attention of an unknowing public with dignity. This did not necessarily mean a "positive" piece by way of presenting only the "good" things about our lives, but rather addressing some of the many challenges and offering various perspectives in meeting those challenges, as well as the joys and delights that living with intellectual impairment can bring.

The close connections forged at this conference, which brought trust and access to the participants in the film, also meant that my relationships within our now expanded community were potentially at stake, a position quite different from that of an "outside" filmmaker with no other connection to the topic or the people it touches. If I misrepresented my family or the other individuals and families in ways that were contrary to what we collectively might agree upon as appropriate advocacy and truth telling, I may have succeeded in further isolating myself from my loved ones and a community that will in the future be an important part of Allycia's life. To this end I sought frameworks and guidance from other filmmakers' works and theorists in the field of ethical representation within image making and documentary film.

Two works, *99 Balloons*[9] (1997) and *Including Samuel*[10] (2009), released during the making of *18q-: A Different Kind of Normal*, became models for me of best practice in parental advocacy filmmaking, particularly when framed within emergent content creation, production, and distribution methods that Aguayo describes as the "third wave of the activist documentary impulse which began percolating in the 1990s" (231). The approaches used by the parent filmmakers in the distribution of these works and the ways in which they have approached challenges intrinsic to social change demonstrate in the best sense what Aguayo means when she writes that "activist documentary should be defined in terms of its function in the process of social change and by the manner in which the camera is utilized as a tool of social justice" (223).

99 Balloons, a six-minute parents' video tribute to their baby Eliot, born with an anomaly on the 18th chromosome (trisomy 18),[11] which was broadcast on YouTube and showcased on Oprah in 2009, has now led to the founding of two non-profit organisations.[12] *Including Samuel*, an award-winning documentary film by photojournalist and parent of a son with cerebral palsy, Dan Habib, addresses issues of inclusivity in education and demonstrates the impact a parent's documentary film can have in mobilizing social change when the focus of the work is directed towards specific action. This film, which can be ordered with accompanying resource materials for educational programs, has reached a broad national audience within the U.S. and an international audience through the Internet. These films align with the new modes of production, distribution, and accessing of social media networks that have also inspired and enabled the youth-led campaign I am Norm.[13]

Strategies like those employed by the parent creators of *99 Balloons* and *Including Samuel* have resulted in the emergence of a number of other non-profit organizations now mobilizing in pursuit of effecting social change in a variety of areas, including supporting children with special needs in remaining with their families rather than being institutionalized, promoting full inclusion of children and adults with disabilities in all levels of education, and changing nondisabled public assumptions about people with genetic and physiological differences. These examples demonstrate what can be achieved when film content is created with a clear intention to effect real change, is ethically produced, is informed by disability aware perspectives, and reflects an understanding of the many public and private arenas involved in impacting the lives of people with disability. The standard set by these two parental advocacy projects has given me an extremely high bar to which to aspire. Their practices also resonate with filmmaker Peter Broderick's new independent distribution models for films[14] and may well be a worthy case for researchers, such as Aguayo, concerned with monitoring and evaluating the impact of the new technological environment and its capacity to bring about shifts in public perceptions and policy creation.

In spite of the lengthy time my film took to create, the challenges of distribution and of translating its release into real change, I remained committed to the project because I believed that the work could be of benefit to new parents of children born with Chromosome 18 anomalies and hopefully effect change in the medical and education sectors by providing vivid alternate life stories and documentary depictions of the potential of persons labeled intellectually impaired to live vibrant lives. My faith in this goal was strengthened during the process as I continued to learn so much more about the diversity of our children's conditions and lives and to delight in their unique personalities. It is also my hope that the participants in particular, and the whole Chromosome 18 community by extension, will benefit from the film, because it has given them the opportunity to voice their experiences and forge a presence where previously they remained unseen and unheard. The film was first and foremost created for other families to share with their friends, medical and health providers and educators, to challenge the way that living with disability is communicated and explore a different kind of normal. Since its release, the DVD has been used by some parents as a tool for advocacy when their situation is not fully understood. I also hope that it is and continues to be a tool for Chromosome 18 community strength and cohesion as a counter-public within our larger worlds.

Notes

1. Refer to the Chromosome 18 Registry and Research Society at www.chromosome18.org for a full explanation of the variations of the 18th chromosome that produce different conditions.

2. *18q-: A Different Kind of Normal* has screened at The Powerhouse in Brisbane and a number of disability-related events. It is available for purchase by contacting the filmmaker at veronica_wain@yahoo.com.au. A trailer can be viewed at the film's website: www.18q-adifferentkindofnormal.com.

3. The Chromosome 18 Registry and Research Society website carries a number of video clips of parents sharing their experiences, many of which can also be found on YouTube. The best known is *99 Balloons*, a short film made by the parents of Eliot, who was born with Trisomy 18 and lived for 99 days. See www.chromosome18.org.

4. In particular filmmakers Martha Goddard and Kathryn Westbrook, editors Tfer Mader and Nicole Bourke, camera assistant Jan Keilland, and Rick Guidotti of Positive Exposure in New York, who became both a persona in the film and an artistic contributor. Rick's portraits of people with genetic differences challenge entrenched ideas of beauty endemic to his own profession as to society as a whole. His work can be seen at www.positiveexposure.org.

5. See Brenda Brueggemann, *Lend Me Your Ear: Rhetorical Constructions of Deafness* (Washington, DC: Gallaudet University Press, 1999); Georgina Kleege, *Sight Unseen* (New Haven: Yale University Press, 1999); and Michael Bérubé, *Life As We Know It: A Father, a Family, and an Exceptional Child* (New York: First Vintage Books, 1998).

6. Marsha Saxton, a disability activist born with spina bifida, states in her essay "Disability Rights and Selective Abortion": "The message at the heart of widespread selective abortion on the basis of prenatal diagnosis is the greatest insult: some of us are 'too flawed' at our very DNA core to exist, unworthy of being born. This message is painful to confront. It seems tempting to take on easier battles or even just to give in. But fighting for this issue, our right and worthiness to be born, is the fundamental challenge to disability oppression; it underpins our most basic claim to justice and equality: We are indeed worthy of being born, we are worth the help and expense, and we know it!"

7. Following the death of his son, Michael Dorris wrote an essay entitled "The Power of Love" that was published in his collection *Paper Trail: Essays* in 1994. He writes about his son's consent for the memoir *Broken Cord* saying he was "passively agreeable to this idea, just as he would have been if I had proposed we move to Mars, eat only peanut butter, or go live in a cave" (114).

8. See Barry Keith Grant, "Ethnography in the First Person: Frederick Wiseman's *Titicut Follies*" in Barry Keith Grant and Jeannette Sloniowski's *Documenting the Documentary: Close Readings of Documentary Film and Video* (238–253).

9. View the film at http://vimeo.com/1992220.

10. Additional information on this film and an extended trailer can be viewed at www.includingsamuel.com or the DVD can be purchased from the Institute on Disability Bookstore online at www.iodbookstore.org.

11. The genetic effects of Trisomy 18 are similar to my daughter's but differ significantly in physical and intellectual manifestation. See www.chromosome18.org for further information on the variations that occur on the 18th chromosome.

12. Information on these two organizations, Ecess and TEAMworks, is available at www.99balloons.org.

13. I am Norm is available at www.iamnorm.org.

14. Peter Broderick's "Welcome to the New World of Distribution" is posted at www.peterbroderick.com and first appeared in *Indiewire*, 16–17 Sept. 2008.

Works Cited

"Against the Odds." *The Oprah Winfrey Show*. 27 Oct. 2008. Television.
Aguayo, Angela Jean. *Documentary Film/Video and Social Change: A Rhetorical Investigation of Dissent*. Diss., University of Texas at Austin. Ann Arbor: UMI, 2005. Print.
Atkinson, Dorothy, and Jan Walmsley. "Using Autobiographical Approaches with People with Learning Difficulties." *Disability & Society* 14: 2 (1999): 203–216. Web. 15 Dec. 2007.
Best Boy. Dir. Ira Wohl. Only Child Motion Pictures, 1979. Film.
Best Man: Best Boy and All of Us Twenty Years Later. Dir. Ira Wohl. Only Child Motion Pictures, 1997. Film.
Brueggemann, Brenda. *Lend Me Your Ear: Rhetorical Constructions of Deafness*. Washington DC: Gallaudet University Press, 1999. Print.
Dorris, Michael. *The Broken Cord*. New York: Harper Perennial, 1990. Print.
_____. "The Power of Love." *Paper Trail: Essays*. New York: HarperCollins, 1994. Print.
Cook-Lynn, Elizabeth. *Anti-Indianism in Modern America: A Voice From Tatekeya's Earth* Champaign: University of Illinois Press, 2001. Print.
Couser, G. Thomas. *Signifying Bodies: Disability in Contemporary Life Writing*. Ann Arbor: University of Michigan Press, 2009. Print.
_____. *Vulnerable Subjects: Ethics and Life Writing*. Ithaca: Cornell University Press, 2004. Print.
18q- A Different Kind of Normal. Dir. Veronica Wain. Through Different Eyes, 2011. Film.
Grant, Barry Keith, and Jeannette Sloniowski, eds. *Documenting the Documentary: Close Readings of Documentary Film and Video*. Detroit: Wayne State University Press, 1998. Print.
Gross, Larry P., John Stuart Katz and Jay Ruby, eds. *Image Ethics*. New York: Oxford University Press, 1991. Print.
High School. Dir. Frederick Wiseman. Osti Productions, 1968. Film.
Hospital. Dir. Frederick Wiseman. Osti Productions, 1970. Film.
Including Samuel. Dir. Dan Habib. *The Including Samuel Project*. The Institute on Disability at the University of New Hampshire. 3 Aug 2009. Web. 3 Aug 2012. Film.
Kleege, Georgina. *Sight Unseen*. New Haven: Yale University Press, 1999. Print.
Kriegel, Leonard. *Flying Solo: Reimagining Manhood, Courage, and Loss*. Boston: Beacon Press, 1998. Print.
Mitchell, David T. "Body Solitaire: The Singular Subject of Disability Autobiography." *American Quarterly* 52.2 (June 2000): 311–315. Web. 13 Sept. 2007.

Nicols, Bill. *Introduction to Documentary.* Bloomington: Indiana University Press, 2001. Print.

99 Balloons: A Tribute to Eliot. Dir. Matt Mooney. *chromosome18.org.* Chromosome 18 Registration and Research Society 3 Apr. 2007. Web. Nov. 2008. Film.

Renov, Michael. *The Subject of Documentary.* Minneapolis: University Minnesota Press, 2001. Print.

Saxton, Marsha. "Disability Rights and Selective Abortion." *Abortion Wars, A Half Century of Struggle: 1950 to 2000.* Ed. Rickie Solinger. Berkeley: University of California Press, 1998. Print.

Titicut Follies. Dir. Frederick Wiseman. Zipporah Films, 1967. Film.

Winston, Brian. *Lies, Damn Lies, and Documentaries.* London: British Film Institute, 2000. Print.

Overcoming the Need to "Overcome"

Challenging Disability Narratives in *The Miracle*

TERRI THROWER

I first encountered *The Miracle* (2007)[1] at a preview party/fundraiser hosted by the star of the film, my friend Tekki Lomnicki,[2] and director Jeffrey Jon Smith. They had invited several dozen people to see the trailer and raise funds to complete the movie. As we ate hors d'oeuvres and sipped wine, an activist friend in the Chicago disability community leaned over to me and whispered something disapproving about the film's title conjuring ideas of "curing" or "fixing" disability in some way. But Tekki, whose experience is the basis of the film, was standing in the room, still 3'5" tall with crutches. Obviously no actual miracle had occurred. *The Miracle* looked to be a purely "inspirational" or "overcoming" tale in which a disabled protagonist somehow learns to accept herself despite her embodiment and does such a good job of being a positive individual role model that she inspires the nondisabled around her.

Many disabled people find the idea of "miracle" in relation to disability troubling. For me, it brings up a variety of "failures" I internalized as a disabled child: failure to be "normal," failure to be "fixed" by doctors, failure to be healed in church. It recalls stories of disabled people being accosted on the street by strangers telling them to "get right with God." Notions of miracles and cures perpetuate barriers between disabled people and the rest of society, rendering us unacceptable as we are. To many disabled people, "miracle" and "cure" are offensive terms.

So, I could see my activist friend's point about the title. What were we about to see? Was *The Miracle* going to repel the disabled activists and artists in the room? Would the title alone deter disabled audiences once the film was released? Although Lomnicki's work is generally lauded within the Chicago disability community where she writes and stages performance pieces, the film's director appeared[3] nondisabled. The few scenes shown from the trailer left me wondering what to expect. Would the director take Lomnicki's story down a stereotypical path in order to make a movie that appeases or satisfies audience presumptions?

After seeing *The Miracle*, I realized that leading viewers to believe this was going to be an inspirational, "overcoming disability" story is exactly what the filmmakers intended. As it turned out, the title enabled the reveal of a different kind of miracle: the challenging

205

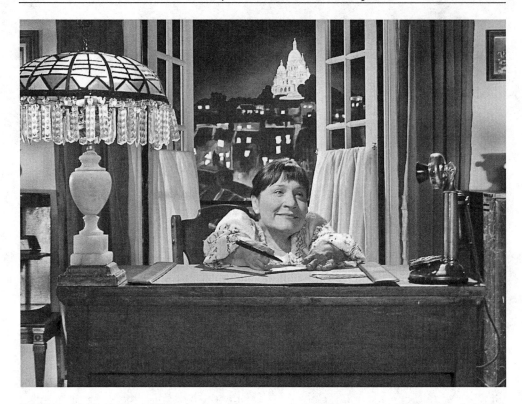

Tekki Lomnicki plays herself in a romantic dream sequence in Jeffrey Jon Smith's *The Miracle* (2007). Notice the placement of the camera at her eye level.

of typical disability film narratives, particularly the prevailing overcoming narrative so preva-lent in conventional films. This essay explores the ways in which *The Miracle* overcomes the "overcoming" narrative of disability, developing representations of disability that tell a different kind of disability story.

The "Overcoming" Narrative

Narratives about actual miracles and cures are passé these days, not to mention phys-iologically unrealistic. Twenty-first century disability portrayals in film and television have moved on to ostensibly more realistic overcoming narratives, ones that involve personal tri-umph over individual tragedy. As Simi Linton discusses in her essay "Reassigning Meaning," the phrase "overcoming a disability" usually refers to a person with a disability who "seems competent and successful" as a result of individual initiative and assimilation (165). That is, disability is no longer a hindrance through the person's "sheer strength or willpower." Overcoming discourse by definition focuses on how individuals manage to cope with obsta-cles on their own. "What is overcome is the social stigma of having a disability" (Linton 163, emphasis in original).

In her article "Narratives of Disability and the Movement from Deficiency to Differ-ence" (2009), Caroline Gray utilizes a cultural sociological approach to explain three pre-vailing disability narratives: assimilation, hyphenation, and multiculturalism. Simply put, assimilation narratives are the "miraculous cures" in which disability is eliminated, hyphen-

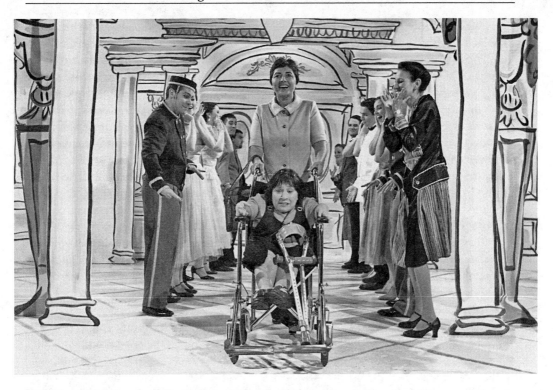

Tekki Lomnicki plays herself with Rula Sirhan Gardenier as her mother alongside cast members in a fantasy musical number in Jeffrey Jon Smith's *The Miracle* (2007).

ation narratives are stories of "overcoming" a disability, and multicultural narratives value disability as difference. The assimilation narrative, which Gray believes to be the most dominant of the three, "always rests on this desire to find 'the cure,' as it appears to offer the only suitable societal response to supposedly deficient disabled bodies" (324). By eliminating disability, physical bodies can be restored to their "natural" states.

In Gray's hyphenation narrative, overcoming is required for social inclusion. This is accomplished through "attempt[s] to heroically overcome his or her disability by adopting a positive attitude" (325). Overcoming or hyphenation grants social inclusion as long as the person demonstrates the right attitude and the desire to be as normal possible. The deficient disabled body can be overlooked if it is conquered by an appropriate state of mind. Gray writes: "Being 'just like everybody else' means that the disabled individual must appear to reject pity and instead insist that others simply see him or her as leading an essentially normal life" (325). Linton calls this "demand that you be plucky and resolute" while overcoming your defective body "a wish fulfillment" generated from outside the disability community (165). You know you've "overcome" when you hear something like, "I just don't think of you as disabled." *What about Hidden DisA?* ^ *BS*

Embedded within the overcoming narrative and Gray's three cultural sociological modes are what Tobin Siebers terms the "ideology of ability" (111). This ideology defines what it means to be human by representing ability as "normative" (111). Gray's multicultural narrative upholds ability as normative as it attempts to move disability towards a "different kind of ability" (326). For Gray, multicultural narratives have the most potential to change societal attitudes about disability because they value differences, making aspects of disabilities into new kinds of abilities. Yet they ultimately do little to move "disability," and therefore disabled people, away from a devalued status in society.

Portrayals of overcoming are structured to separate the person with the disabled body from their disabled body in order to emphasize the human spirit. Tanya Titchkosky, in "Overcoming: Abled-Disabled and other Acts of Normative Violence" (2007), explains that "human-interest" stories make "common, repetitive, and frequent" appearances. The routine mass media depiction of "overcoming as a 'human-interest story' makes humanness interesting by working to exclude anything called disability from the nature of humanity." In its exclusion, disability cannot be perceived as "an ordinary and common fate of all." Instead, it is a triumph for the "universally human" spirit over tremendous adversity. As Titchkosky states, "The overcoming story proceeds by depicting an individual feature or trait as an enabling universally human *force*, such as courageous perseverance, reasoned tenacity, positive attitude, or sheer will" (Titchkosky 181, emphasis in original).

Siebers points out in his essay "Disability as Masquerade" that many human-interest stories exaggerate disability for the able-bodied public in the service of reaffirming and reinforcing the supremacy of ability. To achieve its dramatic story arc, the human-interest story must demonstrate its "protagonist's metamorphosis from nonhuman to human being" (111). Siebers explains:

> Human-interest stories display voyeuristically the physical or mental disability of their heroes, making the defect emphatically present, often exaggerating it, then wiping it away by reporting how it has been overcome, how the heroes are "normal," despite the powerful odds against them. At other times, a [human-interest] story will work so hard to make its protagonist "normal" that it pictures the disabled person possessing talents and abilities only dreamed about by able-bodied people. In other words, the hero is — simultaneously and incoherently —"cripple" and "supercripple" [111].

Human-interest stories, like many film and television portrayals of disability, lack any realistic representation of the experience. And because disability is so misunderstood and misrepresented, it is a simple matter to "conflate pathology with claims of exceptional talent" (Siebers, 113). Exceptional or "super" ability seems to come directly from disability; it is *because* of disability, not in spite of it.

A few Hollywood "human-interest" films from the recent past exemplify Siebers' and Titchkosky's points. "Cripple/supercripple" heroes — individuals who have overcome their disabilities, achieved amazing feats and seem to possess abilities beyond most people — have shown up in such films as *Blindsight, Soul Surfer, Murderball,* and *Temple Grandin.*[4] *Blindsight* (2006) is about six blind teens from Tibet who scale Mount Everest with their blind mountaineer guide Erik Weihenmayer. *Soul Surfer* (2011) retells the story of teen Bethany Hamilton who loses an arm to a shark attack and returns to competitive surfing anyway. *Murderball* (2005) features the collective personal stories of stars on the United States quadriplegic rugby team, and the HBO biopic *Temple Grandin* (2010), starring Claire Danes in the lead role, depicts the success of a livestock scientist with Asperger's. These films ultimately downplay the realistic aspects of living with disability, enabling the overcoming narrative to represent these characters as larger than life on screen. The enforced invisibilities and devaluation of real daily life remains because none of these films addresses the larger systemic dynamics that create and naturalize the narrative pressure of overcoming.[5] They simply encourage its internalization. And as Simi Linton has pointed out, "when disabled people internalize the demand to "overcome" rather than demand social change, they shoulder the same kind of exhausting and self-defeating "Super Mom" burden that feminists have analyzed" (165).

Ultimately, "normal" becomes unattainable for people with visible impairments, so long as "normal" is a category that includes only those with physiological appearances perceived to be standard, and not the full range of human embodiment.[6] What is presumed to be left are "abnormal" bodies that cause self-imposed psychological obstacles that require finding inner strength to handle. This means that disabled persons must learn to adjust physically, emotionally, and psychologically to their own unique situations. But the successfully adjusted disabled person of popular imagination is simply the flip-side of the unsuccessfully adjusted one. They are born of the same paradigm. Paul Longmore explains:

> These "real-life" stories of striving and courage seem the antithesis of the bitter and self-pitying "cripples" in dramas of adjustment, but both stem from the same perception of the nature of disability: disability is primarily a problem of emotional coping, of personal acceptance. It is not a problem of social stigma and discrimination. It is a matter of individuals not only overcoming the physical impairments of their own bodies but, more important, the emotional consequences of such impairments. Both fictional and nonfictional stories convey the message that success or failure in living with a disability results almost solely from the emotional choices, courage, and character of the individual [Longmore, 139].

For disabled people, the responsibility to cheerfully, independently, triumphantly, and *individually* overcome their conditions removes any opportunity for conceptions of civil rights. It is an inherently limiting narrative. For the nondisabled, the overcoming narrative presents a recurring challenge to achieve by self-making: "If someone so tragically 'crippled' can overcome the obstacles confronting them, think what you, without such a 'handicap,' can do" (Longmore, 139). The overcoming narrative of disability turns out to be restrictive for disabled and nondisabled alike: it precludes opportunities for social change for everyone.

Growing Up with Klara

In one of Shirley Temple's most beloved films, *Heidi* (1937), the pseudonymous Swiss heroine becomes the companion of another little girl, Klara Sesemann (Marcia Mae Jones), who uses a wheelchair. Bubbly, optimistic Heidi gets Klara to walk again with the power of positive attitude alone. Generations of North American television viewers watched Heidi and Klara in reruns through the 1970s. The film has long been a children's classic and a classic example of the disability cure narrative. In *Cinema of Isolation*, Martin Norden contends that *Heidi* presents physical disability in a "simplistic and facile way" (135). Paul Longmore observes that the depiction of Klara is typical, especially for films from that period. Disabled characters in such films "lack insight about themselves and other people, and require emotional education, usually by a nondisabled character. In the end, nondisabled persons supply the solution: they compel the disabled individuals to confront themselves" (Longmore, 138). At the end of the movie when Klara walks through the miracle of Heidi's intervention, she delivers the blissful lines: "I'll be normal! Normal!"

Lomnicki remembers the film vividly: "*Heidi* was one of my favorite movies as a kid," (Lomnicki and Smith). She related to the character in the wheelchair. "[Klara was] a girl like me who can't walk like other kids. Then I was impressed that she walked at the end and was also hoping that there would be a miraculous cure for me someday" (Lomnicki). She drew from her memories of Klara in the development of her solo performance piece *Thanksgiving*, first performed in 1996 at the Blue Rider Theater in Chicago, Illinois. *Thanksgiving* takes the audience inside Tekki's autobiographical experience through the theatrical articulation of her fantasies, thoughts, and prayers. The following scene from *Thanksgiving* takes up her adolescent desire for a miracle, channeling Klara's famous lines:

> In my fantasy my family takes a cruise ship to France and then rides donkeys (like Jesus did on Palm Sunday) into the village of Lourdes. At the gates of the grotto we are greeted by monks who lift me from my wheelchair and into one of those cane wheelchairs like Bette Davis had in *Whatever Happened to Baby Jane* [1962]. And these are no ordinary monks ... they look like David Cassidy, Paul McCartney and Mickey Dolenz of the Monkees. These monks wheel me to the grotto where I kneel in front of the statue of the Blessed Mother with my brothers on either side like altar boys. "Blessed Mother, please heal me. And if you do, I promise I'll become a nun." Suddenly I feel stronger and take a few tentative steps, then I start to walk, then run to my parents *(Drop crutches)* like Heidi at the end of the movie.
> *(CHANT OUT "I'll be normal")*
> Of course in this fantasy I am also two feet taller and have breasts. But for one reason or another Lourdes was put on the back burner. My mother sent away for Lourdes holy water that came in a plastic bottle shaped like the Virgin Mary and the top was a blue screw off crown [Lomnicki, *Thanksgiving*, unpublished script].

Like *Thanksgiving,* Lomnicki's subsequent works, *Blurred Vision* (2006), which recalls her first twelve years of life in the hospital while doctors tried to "fix" her twisted legs, and *Clothing Optional* (2008), which reflects her experience at a nudist camp, interrogate the assumptions of "normal" and the power structures, desires, and body images "normal" generates. Her approach is not radical—this is not divisive "in your face" theater—rather, Lomnicki uses humor to build a bridge between disability and able-bodiedness, excelling in her performance work at melting away differences and moving disabled and nondisabled audience members to a common ground. Both of these pieces focus on themes of "normality" and acceptance, but in the end Lomnicki never concludes that she herself as a mobility impaired little person needs to change. She explains:

> I wish to work against the idea that in order to be whole, functioning individuals, people with disabilities have to be cured or look like everybody else. In my work I like to reveal myself to people, crutches, short stature, emotional scars and all. It took me a long time to accept myself and stop striving to be "cured" or "normal" and I like to put that in my work [Lomnicki].

Instead of reinforcing the ideas of disability assimilation, the audience comes away from her work with altered ideas of what is acceptable, including disability. Her subtle and mildly political theater work appeals to nondisabled audiences and winks knowingly at disability culture.

Cinematic and Performance Models

The Miracle came about after *Thanksgiving* stirred the visual imagination of Jeffrey Jon Smith. Friends since 1981 and a fan of her work, Smith knew he could collaborate with Lomnicki on a film version of the piece, produced as a film project at Columbia College in Chicago. *The Miracle* "more or less follows the storyline of the performance piece, but most of what happens on screen was not in the original, and is fiction" (Smith). Smith used *Thanksgiving* as a "taking off point for a fictional fantasia on Tekki's real life story." He added three key elements to transform it into a cinematic piece: (1) the priest as Tekki's "talk-to" and stand-in for the audience, (2) several fantasy sequences not in the play, and (3) making the conflict between Tekki and her mother "the spine of the story." For the third element, Smith penned several original dramatic scenes, two of which are fiction, to develop the narrative of their relationship (Smith).

Both personally and professionally, Smith and Lomnicki were excited about the opportunity to collaborate on the project. "[Smith] saw it as an advance toward expressing a personal aesthetic by adapting the work of another person, and as a chance to make a film with an unconventional heroine at its center" (Smith). Lomnicki saw the collaboration with a director who understood her work as an opportunity to "get my story out there to a wider range of people" (Lomnicki and Smith). It was also a way to use the medium to expand and articulate the message of her performance piece:

> It illustrates things that I only mention in passing ... in my original piece my dad says, "Give her a ball glove, throw her a ball. She'll catch it like the boys. Can do anything the boys do, if you don't baby her." ... From that one line, Jeff created an entire baseball scene with me playing [Lomnicki].

Of course, adapting the performance piece into a short (29-minute) film was not without its problems. Smith reports that the screenplay "wrote itself," but challenges emerged during pre-production, production, and post-production. "Because of the range and the variety of the scenes, the number of people involved (more than 100 people worked on the film), the expense, and the scope, it was like undertaking a military campaign on a weekend getaway budget" (Smith). The aesthetic vision was also ambitious. "She's theater," Smith says of Lomnicki, so he wanted to expand her performance without slipping into a dry documentary or biographical style, which would represent neither her lived experiences nor her artistic expression of them. He also wanted the film to draw from the film genres he loves most, musicals and classic Hollywood films in which the dialogue is matched with action and evocative *mise-en-scène* (Lomnicki and Smith). Smith's underlying concept for *The Miracle* is expressed in the film through hyperbole, theatricality, and an Avant-garde visual style. Smith explains:

> Memory, when it's reconstructed, is not a documentary of what really happened in your life. It's a fabrication put together from bits and pieces, not only from the event that happened, but movies you've seen, and books you've read, and [it's] something different when you remember it. And so I wanted to give [the film] a feeling that was constructed and somewhat artificial [...] hence the theatricality and sort of the quotes around a lot of the scenes that makes it look ... presentational rather than representational [Lomnicki and Smith].

In developing *The Miracle*, Smith and Lomnicki drew on their perspectives of several major films that feature protagonists with physical disabilities. In terms of casting, they considered the precedent of *My Left Foot* (1989), which gained Daniel Day-Lewis a Best Actor Oscar for his portrayal of Christy Brown, the son of an Irish family disabled by cerebral palsy, and led to many other Hollywood projects with disabled protagonists. Lewis' performance is widely credited as nuanced, three-dimensional, realistic, and powerful. However, as a nondisabled actor his casting participates in what Tobin Siebers has called "disability drag," a form of disability masquerade that occurs when nondisabled actors play disabled characters. These actors' performances, like drag queen performances, make visible the stigma of disability on screen. But they also function to reassure audiences that the disability they're watching is not real: the actor will return to able-bodiedness when the film is over. This dynamic arguably obscures "both the existence and permanence of disability" (Siebers, 116), adding to its invisibility. Lomnicki expressed concern with the way in which nondisabled actors transforming themselves into disabled characters has become a standard path to the Academy Awards. "I mean it bothers me that [Christy Brown] was played by a nondisabled person. I'm more militant now and would rather see a real disabled person in a role" (Lomnicki and Smith). Smith agreed, "using a non-disabled actor — I see that as a form of blackface, and completely unacceptable in this day and age" (Smith).

In *The Station Agent* (2003), a much-loved film of Lomnicki's, a disabled actor leads the cast. Dwarf actor Peter Dinklage plays the film's main character, Finbar, who inherits a station house along railroad tracks in a small New Jersey town. Finbar, who wants to be left alone, is unable to avoid the well-meaning locals he encounters. Dinklage's body is prevalent in the film, but not emphasized with visual tricks or juxtapositions. Though the role was not written for an actor with a disability, the film incorporates realistic experiences surrounding Dinklage's size and physical abilities. Lomnicki explained that for her, the film works because

> It showed the day-to-day life of a little person without striving to make him "special" or a "hero." Some of the things that happened to him mirrored my life, like a clerk at the grocery store or Walgreen's not seeing me at the counter, or someone screaming when they are not expecting me to be around a corner. I like to do the same in my work, [to] just show the things that happen to me, funny or not [Lomnicki].

The Station Agent makes visible and explicit what I call the "everyday freak show" phenomenon. Strangers stare at Finbar, teenagers make fun of him, a librarian screams when she first sees him, but he responds only mildly to these instances that tend to happen to me (and many disabled people) every day. The disabled person is not the actual spectacle — either in the film or in life — rather it is the reactions of others that both enfreak the person they are viewing and become freakish in their own right. While disability is actually tangential to the plot in *The Station Agent*, it is central to *The Miracle*. For both of these films, though, the characters' common humanity, not their physical differences, is most vital and ultimately most prominent. In both films, "freakishness" becomes not an aspect or element of character to be overcome, but an arbitrarily superimposed designation of little value that artificially divides characters — and people — from one another. Smith wanted his audience "to feel what [Tekki] felt: that these differences are essentially imaginary. I wanted these differences for the audience to melt away. Humanity is what links everybody" (Lomnicki and Smith).

> There's a thing that happens when minorities of any kind are represented in mainstream films. It happened for a long time with gay people, with African American people. The thing that makes them different from other people is the subject of the film. It's about how they overcome being different, and many times, like with gay people, it ends in death. It ends in suicide or misery because, of course, they never should have been that way to begin with [...] Everything's about explaining to supposedly a non-gay, non African American, or nondisabled audience why it's okay to be that way. I didn't want to do that [Lomnicki and Smith].

The Miracle

The Miracle uses familiar religious imagery and dominant disability tropes in order to engage with dominant disability narratives. In particular, the film overturns the overcoming narrative in six specific ways. First, the filmmakers committed to casting a disabled actor to play the role of a disabled character. Second, the film makes Tekki's character rather than her disability central to the narrative through: (a) camera shots that frame her viewpoint as central, and (b) presenting Tekki's disabled body as a "given" — without exaggeration, sentimentality, or explanation. Third, the film resists indulging in Tekki's emotional "adjustment," coping skills, or positive attitude or courage in the face of adversity. Fourth, the film does not valorize either impairment or "super abilities." However, it does play with these ideas during some of the fantasy sequences as a means of presenting new possibilities for disability storytelling. Fifth, *The Miracle* explores the idea that mother and daughter have internalized the desire for a normative body, placing social perception rather than physiological difference at the heart of the characters' narrative arc. Finally, the film takes the viewer from an expectation of a disability overcoming narrative to a deep engagement in a more universal relationship narrative that is informed by disability — one of many possible contexts in which the dynamic of social expectation and parental disappointment or acceptance could play out.

Tekki's Character as Central to the Narrative

To illustrate how the film makes Tekki's character central, I'll describe the opening frames, which provide a sense of the film's engagement with religious and disability imagery. *The Miracle* opens with a camera shot of a large church steeple then pans down to the sidewalk outside its entrance. Pedestrians mill around, parting to reveal a dwarf woman (Tekki Lomnicki) on crutches staring up at the church. The bells are ringing as the woman goes inside, struggling momentarily with the heavy wooden door. The next shot is the back of the woman's body as she stops at a large basin of holy water and dips in her hand. She then moves deeper into the church; the camera angles up and the music swells.[7] The title appears against the iconic arches and spires, directing our imaginations toward a miracle of faith, one that the film suggests will likely be enacted upon this disabled woman. Focusing on her two-footed gait, which alternates with her metal crutches on the tile floor as the woman walks, the camera slowly pans to her face. She stops near the front of the church, and we see that the camera is level with her height, which is also level with the church pews on either side of her. Here, the director provides a visual reference of her physical viewpoint, which he maintains throughout the film. The woman continues to walk, then stops while the camera closes in on her face. We follow her gaze up and right to a statue of the Virgin Mary. Her facial expression toward the sculpture is almost reproachful, as if some great disappointment is directed there. Looking away from the statue, the woman makes the sign of the cross and starts to walk again until she reaches the confessional. She tells the priest, "I dishonored my mother." From there, the rest of the story is told through flashbacks.

As Martin Norden has observed, mainstream cinematic practices have tended to isolate disabled characters, reducing them to "objects of spectacle" both on the screen through camera angles and in society through plot lines. Film audiences in particular are situated with an "able-bodied point of view" that the camera provides (Norden, 1). Knowing that the spectacle of her body would be in play for able-bodied audiences, Smith chose to align the audience's eye-line with Tekki's, placing both viewer and viewed on the same plane, thereby eliding a difference of physicality with a lack of difference in visual perspective. In fact, whenever Tekki appears on screen, the camera captures her from her level, not from the visual perspective of a person of "standard" stature. Smith identifies this practice as a key strategy in shifting the focus of the film from Tekki's character's physicality to her perceptions and to ours: "I knew it was unavoidable that Tekki's difference from people would be in their mind when they were watching, but I didn't want the film to be about how she copes with being disabled ... I wanted it to be *a given*" (Lomnicki and Smith, my emphasis). By portraying Tekki's body realistically and without reserve in multiple shots, while at the same time undercutting voyeuristic difference through aligned visual perspective, *The Miracle* shifts the audience toward Tekki's character's experience, rather than placing her in a position of viewed "other."

The first "miracle" of *The Miracle* is Tekki's birth. This sequence is set in a hospital and shot in black and white,[8] evoking years past. "I was born on a September morning, something like this one," the little woman says to the priest in voiceover, "but I arrived with legs twisted like a soft pretzel, not breathing" (*The Miracle*). The nurse, Sister Mary Thecla, baptizes the newborn with holy water, naming her after Saint Mary Thecla, a teenaged saint who defied death. "God, please give this baby a happy death," says Sister Thecla, and the baby starts to cry. She rushes baby Mary Thecla, later shortened to Tekki, to her parents. Tekki's mother (Rula Gardenier) takes one look at her first-born child and says, "It's okay. I'll take her to Lourdes."

This is the first time of only a few when Tekki's disabling condition is mentioned. A second time is when Tekki refers to her first twelve years of life spent in a hospital while doctors tried to fix her twisted legs. Both of these references acknowledge Tekki's disabled body, but do so as a matter of fact. These minimal references, without sentimentality or exaggeration — like the way her body and viewpoint are framed by the film — present disability as routine aspects of Tekki's character. Lourdes, on the other hand, is significant in a different way. The mention of Lourdes, a French town famous for the appearance of the Virgin Mary and for the disabled who have been miraculously healed there, along with the film's title and the opening scenes inside the church, encourages the viewer to assume that the narrative arc of the film will end in *the* miracle: Tekki's healing because disability, not character, is assumed to be central. By literalizing this expectation, the film can work with it more effectively by bringing it to the forefront of our consciousness as viewers and then overturning it.

The Resistance to Emotional Adjustment as a Developmental Trajectory

As *The Miracle* unfolds, it resists indulging in Tekki's emotional adjustment, coping, or positive attitude in the face of adversity. On the contrary, many of the scenes between Tekki and her mother revolve around parent-teen arguments in which disability is just another characteristic, like age, personality or behavior, over which battles about boundaries, rules and safety are fought. For example, in the exchange below, a teenaged Tekki intentionally pushes her mother's buttons, while her mother reveals her irrational overprotectiveness:

> MOM: You know I'd never try to hold you back from what you want to do, but this theater thing. It's just not safe.
> TEKKI: Mom, it's perfectly safe!
> MOM: These musicals, these plays whatever, they were not written...
> TEKKI: For who? For cripples?
> MOM: No. You don't know what I think.
> TEKKI: (Yelling) How am I supposed to fit in?
> MOM: Pray the rosary. The Blessed Mother will never let you down. She's never let me down.
> TEKKI: Not even when I was born? [*The Miracle*].

Mom walks away without answering. Tekki's final line is intentionally hurtful and shifts the focus to the roots of their misunderstanding and Tekki's social "dishonor." Calling herself a "cripple" is an attack on her mother's sensibilities, while it also calls attention to the hyper-visibility and paradoxical silence surrounding the stigma of disability, which both characters feel acutely.

In another scene, Tekki applies to go to college in Paris. An argument between mother and daughter about safety and independence ensues when Tekki is told she can't go to Paris if her mother can't be there to take care of her.

> Tekki: You just don't want me to be happy!
> Mom: You are happy, right here with your family. Happy and safe!
> Tekki: I'm sick and tired of being safe! You treat me like I'm going to break if I do anything [*The Miracle*].

But Tekki does go to Paris where she gains a sense of freedom. Her negative outbursts in these arguments are notably not about self-pity; rather they reflect her unhappiness about being so overly dependent and protected. Once in Paris, however, she becomes a more relaxed and contented heroine, which has more to do with growing up from sheltered teen to adult woman than putting on a brave face about disability.

The Refusal to Valorize Either Impairment or Super Abilities

The film takes up the representation of inability and "super abilities," which are so often paired in overcoming narratives, through a fantasy sequence featuring Tekki as a Little League baseball player. In this scene she appears to be 10 years old and is playing centerfield on a Little League team, crutches and all. The announcer names each player by position, and when "Lomnicki" is called, Tekki grabs her crotch in a stereotypical tough, irreverent athlete gesture. After the pitch, the batter hits a high fly ball straight to centerfield. It looks like it's going to "go all the way," the announcer exclaims, as the camera follows Tekki in slow motion. She runs, glove in hand, further out in centerfield. She stops, turns, and falls backward onto the ground. She looks up, and just at the right amazing moment, the ball lands in her glove. This fantasy pokes fun at overcoming narratives that provide the heroine with an unrealistic social triumph that redeems disability, but it also aligns Tekki with the audience insofar as dreams of success on the ball field are prototypical of American childhood, regardless of actual ability. The scene also points to the ways in which the social structures of this prototypical American childhood, in organizations like Little League, also delimit the opportunities of children with disabilities and the shape the public view of them. Why isn't there such a thing as integrated Little League for all kids?

The Exploration of the Internalization of a Desire for the Normative Body

To illustrate one of the ways in which *The Miracle* promotes the idea that mother and daughter have internalized the desire for a normative body, we must return to Lourdes. After some time in Paris, Tekki invites her mother to visit her in France, and they journey together to Lourdes. From the beginning, the film makes this journey a central part of their relationship, thematically powerful from the moment of Tekki's birth. "And once we're there, maybe your, maybe *our* prayers will be answered," Tekki writes to her mother in the film. Once in Lourdes, however, Tekki becomes irritable. Her mother is "deliriously happy" as they tour "Disneyland for Catholics," as Tekki puts it. "What's next," she asks, "a musical number?" Sure enough, her frustration is comically articulated through a whimsical musical number that begins during their cab ride to the hotel when the cab driver breaks into song.[9]

The hotel staff joins in with robust singing, dancing, and cartoonish, faux Broadway sets. It is a surprising, funny, imaginative, and completely over the top scene of the bizarre and uplifting. Meanwhile, Tekki's character is not amused. The song the characters sing is sweet and romantic, claiming the sexual, even reproductive space for our heroine. It also serves to lighten the tension of being at Lourdes. This is what the film has been building up to. This is the moment we've all been waiting for: the miracle of Lourdes' healing that promises to change every aspect of Tekki's adult womanhood.

When the number is over and they arrive at the little inn in Lourdes, Tekki's face registers dread. Preparing to go to the shrine, Tekki's anxiety becomes evident, intensifying with every move that her mother makes. Each sound — the clasp of Mom's purse, the sound as she slips on her shoes — reverberates for both the audience and for Tekki. She looks terrified, and we feel her internal tension as the inevitable disappointment, the failure to change, looms. The two women exit their hotel room in silence. The last shot, once they leave the room, is of the closed door. The screen fades to black until images of Tekki's life slowly flash across the screen: bottles of holy water, a photo of the Blessed Mother and Child, a yellow rose petal. Sound bites from earlier in the film accompany the images: Tekki being named after a saint, her mother telling her she "never wants to hold her back," and Tekki yelling, "How am I supposed to fit in?"

The scene at the shrine is quiet and quick. Tekki soaks one foot in the water of a pool. Her face is solemn. Her legs are unchanged. The moment is decisive, with it the film audience and characters alike released from the strictures of the miracle cure narrative. It releases us, too, from the limits of the overcoming narrative. There is no overcoming. There is simply Tekki with the body she has always had and the many desires for her life that she has already expressed and that she is already capable of pursuing. But the release cannot occur without concomitant realization — the realization of the ways in which this narrative has shaped our assumptions not simply about our relationship to disability, but about our relationship to the expectations of others, especially those we love. Ultimately, Tekki must face her fear that she is a disappointment to her mother, the fear that has fueled her resentment and frustration. It is a fear common to child-parent bonds, with or without disability.

In the final scene of the Lourdes journey, Tekki and her mother return to their hotel room. Her mother enters first, slowly followed by Tekki. They do not look at one another. Tekki has stopped in the doorway, hesitating. She enters and closes the door, watching her mother take off her shoes and prepare to pray. Her mother kneels at the bed, and Tekki lifts her eyes. Then she takes a deep breath and steps forward towards her mother. Tekki tearfully, with great anguish, says:

> TEKKI: I'm sorry Mom! I'm sorry I wasn't healed.
> (Her mother slowly gets up turning to her daughter, and sits on the bed.)
> TEKKI: I'm sorry there was no miracle.
> MOM: Miracle? Tekki, I didn't come here to pray for that. I came to give thanks for you, as you are. You're my miracle.

In overcoming narratives, the disabled character typically must overcome his or her physical limitations by overcoming his or her psychological ones. In *The Miracle*, Tekki has apparently long accepted herself for who she is. She struggles instead with the fear that others, particularly those she is closest to, do not truly accept her in the way that she accepts herself, that those she loves wish she were different in ways she cannot change. Lomnicki's performance in *The Miracle* of this "core conflict" is moving. Her character's anxiety and fear are palpable. This is also the only scene in the film that is not fictionalized. Lomnicki recalls:

It was Thanksgiving Day [...] we were at Lourdes [...] and I was so thankful. I was only 18 and I got it, you know, I really got it that my mom didn't want me to change...she was just thankful for the way I am [... I was] thankful that our issue had been resolved. So that's why it was called *Thanksgiving* [Lomnicki and Smith].

For Smith, "there's a moment where the world comes clear," when we realize that we have been perceiving it through the lens of our socially internalized fears and fantasies (Lomnicki and Smith). *The Miracle* is more than just a lightning bolt moment between one mother and child. Their misunderstanding is mirrored in common misperceptions and misrepresentations by a nondisabled society, often rejecting disabled people as they are. When film audiences are situated with an able-bodied perspective, when disabled characters are isolated rather than integrated, and when the ubiquitous overcoming narrative remains unchallenged, disability remains restrictive, unacceptable and misunderstood. Conversely, Films like *The Miracle*, which present new potential for representing and constructing disability narratives, create hopeful possibilities for all of us. As Sally Chivers and Nicole Markotić write in *The Problem Body: Projecting Disability on Film*:

[T]here are many ways of living with disability. Narrative film presents some of those ways. How experience is represented textually and how that representation is projected onto and via audiences are both central aspects of the experience itself. That is, the *representation* of disability does not exist separate from disability itself. Accordingly, we propose that — disabled or not — when "we" all watch a film, we all participate in disability discourse [4].

Notes

1. See themiraclemovie.com for information on purchasing a copy of *The Miracle* on DVD.
2. In the interest of full disclosure, I have worked as a member of the board for Tellin' Tales Theater whose artistic director is Lomnicki. In addition, Lomnicki's solo piece, *Blurred Vision*, and interviews with her about it are included in my dissertation research.
3. Jeffrey Jon Smith is not "visibly" disabled, nor does he identify as a disabled person. He does, however, identify as a person with depression: "Though not considered an official disability, I have struggled with clinical depression since I was 12. That's 51 years and counting as of this writing. That, plus my sexuality and commitment to the arts, has made me instinctively take the part of the underdogs, the outsiders, and the dreamers" (email correspondence, July 2011).
4. Both *Temple Grandin* and *Soul Surfer* utilize Siebers' concept of disability drag and both heroines require assistance from able-bodied relatives for emotional adjustments. In *Blindsight*, however, this assistance is provided by supercrip Erik Weihenmayer, despite paternalistic concern from the teens' blind teacher. The athletes of *Murderball* need to overcome their diminished masculinity (due to disability) through heterosexual pairings with able-bodied women. In all of these films, a form of "super ability" replaces disability.
5. Siebers (99–100) discusses social invisibility as inherent in the often hyper-visibility of disability, race, and queerness. As he observes, "Society has a general tendency to repress the complex embodiment of difference" (100).
6. Linton explains that "passing," can be a viable option for people with both visible and non-apparent disabilities (166–167). Yet, passing often takes an emotional (and sometimes physical) toll. Linton's concept of passing in relation to disability, and Siebers' understanding of passing, visibility, and invisibility (96–97 and 100) is derived from race, gender, and sexuality studies. Linton describes the repercussions of shame and self-loathing that result from passing, often at the hands of families who want their disabled children to appear as normal as possible.
7. According to Smith, "All the music in the film ... was original, and was composed and performed (digitally) by Adgio Hutchings (Smith, email interview).
8. The camera used for filming *The Miracle* was an Arriflex SR2, a 16mm camera using Kodak Super16 mm film. The entire film was shot in color, and "digitally altered to black and white in post-production. We shot on film rather than HD because of my belief that film is still better able to convey a sense of fantasy, of the magical" (Smith).

9. The song is "Mimi," by Richard Rodger and Lorenz Hart, which the filmmakers licensed from Sony / ATV music. Chevalier first performed this song in the classic film musical *Love Me Tonight* (1932).

Works Cited

Blindsight. Dir. Lucy Walker. Image Entertainment, 2006. Film.
Chivers, Sally, and Nicole Markotić, eds. *The Problem Body: Projecting Disability on Film*. Columbus: Ohio State University Press, 2010. Print.
Gray, Caroline. "Narratives of Disability and the Movement from Deficiency to Difference." *Cultural Sociology* 3:2 (2009): 317–332. Web. 5 Mar. 2011.
Linton, Simi. "Reassigning Meaning." *The Disability Studies Reader: Second Edition*. Lennard J. Davis, Ed. New York: Routledge, 2006: 161–72. Print.
Lomnicki, Tekki. "Blurred Vision." 2006. Performance.
_____. "Clothing Optional." 2008. Performance.
_____. Message to the author. July 2011. Email.
_____. "Thanksgiving." Unpublished script.
Lomnicki, Tekki, and Jeffrey Jon Smith. Personal Interview. Jan. 2011.
Longmore, Paul K. *Why I Burned My Book and Other Essays on Disability*. Philadelphia: Temple University Press, 2003. Print.
Murderball. Dirs. Dana A. Shapiro and Henry A. Rubin. Velocity/Thinkfilm, 2005. Film.
Norden, Martin, E. *Cinema of Isolation: A History of Physical Disability in the Movies*. New Brunswick: Rutgers University Press, 1994. Print.
Siebers, Tobin. *Disability Theory*. Ann Arbor: University Michigan Press, 2008. Print.
Smith, Jeffrey Jon. Message to the author. July 2011. Email.
Soul Surfer. Dir. Sean McNamara. Enticing Entertainment, 2011. Film.
Temple Grandin. Dir. Mick Jackson. Perf. Claire Danes. HBO Home Video, 2010. Film.
The Miracle. Dir. Jeffrey Jon Smith. Perf. Tekki Lomnicki. Letterboxed, 2007. Film.
Titchkosky, Tanya. *Reading and Writing Disability Differently: The Textured Life of Embodiment*. Toronto: University Toronto Press, 2007. Print.

Born on the Fourth of July

Production and Assessment
of a Turbulent Text

MARTIN F. NORDEN

After a delay of nearly a dozen years, the film adaptation of Ron Kovic's autobiography, the like-titled *Born on the Fourth of July,* finally appeared on the U.S. cultural scene in late December 1989 and in many other countries soon thereafter. One of the most famous films to feature a disabled character, *Born* is distinguished by the fact that two Vietnam War veterans were largely responsible for its making: director and co-screenwriter Oliver Stone, who was injured in the war but recovered from his wounds and co-screenwriter Ron Kovic, who was paralyzed from the mid-chest down after a bullet severed his spinal cord and whose book served as the basis for the film. It is a complicated text; on the one hand, the film seeks to present its disabled veteran in multi-dimensional terms and show the profound changes in his way of thinking about war and personal loss, yet on the other it indulges in rather ham-handed mythmaking and exhibits a widespread disregard for historical accuracy in its attempt to locate its lead character within a "heroic" narrative framework. With the awareness that *Born* is among the exceptionally small group of disability-themed feature films to have a person with a disability (PWD) among its principal creators, this chapter explores this film's tortuous production history, mixed reception, and thematic preoccupations. I argue that *Born on the Fourth of July* is best understood in terms of its place within the context of other disability themed films, most notably the disabled Vietnam veteran film mini-genre of which it is a conspicuous part, and a range of post–World War II productions that stressed the importance of PWDs "overcoming" their impairments.

The essentials of Ron Kovic's historical narrative — his upbringing in Massapequa, New York, enlistment in the Marines, severe wounding in Vietnam in early 1968, return to the U.S., and antiwar activities — are reasonably well known (e.g., Fuchs; Kovic, *Born*; Moss) and do not require detailing here. Our inquiry begins instead with Kovic's struggle to write his autobiography in the 1970s and his growing interest in movies as a complementary means of conveying his life story.

The years 1968 and 1969 were critical to Kovic's evolution from war supporter to antiwar activist, and by 1969 he had begun speaking out against the Vietnam War. Around that same period, he decided to write a memoir that would focus on his upbringing and his

Vietnam and postwar experiences. He found the writing process painful and agonizing. Living in Santa Monica, California, at the time, Kovic frequently and restlessly moved about. He often dropped in on friends in the middle of the night unannounced, "always carrying the manuscript with me and always frightened, desperately needing to escape the demons that were closing in on me," as he put it (Kovic, "Introduction" 7).

In the midst of his struggles to write the book, Kovic found encouragement from an unanticipated source: Waldo Salt, a Hollywood screenwriter who wanted to interview him for a film currently in development. Salt, who had been blacklisted in the 1950s for his leftist views but whose stock had risen due to his scripts for *Midnight Cowboy* in 1969 and *Serpico* in 1973, had been recruited by producers Jerome Hellman, Jane Fonda, and Bruce Gilbert to develop a screenplay about a disabled Vietnam veteran who becomes an antiwar activist. To Salt's credit, he wanted to make the narrative as veritable as possible and ended up spending more than a year and $50,000 of his own money interviewing disabled Vietnam veterans around the country. One such vet he had targeted was Kovic, whose antiwar activities had been receiving considerable news coverage; for example, Kovic was a key figure in *Operation Last Patrol,* a 1972 documentary film that chronicled the cross-country journey of Vietnam Veterans Against the War to the Republican National Convention in Miami Beach to protest U.S. policies and the Nixon presidency.

Though Salt's original agenda was to interview Kovic in the hope of gleaning material for his script, the two formed a bond that went beyond a basic interviewer-interviewee relationship. Indeed, Salt became a mentor and something of a parental figure for Kovic. As producer Jerome Hellman remembered it: "Ron was floundering and looking for a way out of his own problems. He frequently stayed at Salt's suite at the Chateau Marmont [Hotel in Los Angeles] and got emotional as well as literary support from him" (qtd. in Collier 253). Kovic would later explicitly thank Salt when his book was published, calling him "my friend Waldo — a child at sixty — who gave me courage with his eyes and love with his wisdom" (Kovic, *Born* 5). The high-profile activist impressed Salt and the producers with his insights and passions, and they reciprocated by lining him up as a technical advisor for their film, a project later known as *Coming Home.*

With Salt's encouragement, Kovic wrote a draft of his autobiography in the fall of 1974 in a little under two months and continued to refine it and add chapters over the next year and a half. He was in touch with Salt throughout much of 1975 and into 1976 and initially had no movie plans; he mainly wanted to exorcise his demons through the writing process and publish a deeply cautionary account of his experiences.

Kovic eventually completed his autobiography, now titled *Born on the Fourth of July* (Kovic and his country were coincidentally "born" on the same day of the year), and arranged with his agent to have it excerpted in *Playboy*'s July 1976 issue and then published as a complete book by McGraw-Hill in mid–August of that year. In between those two publishing events, Kovic made a dramatic appearance at the Democratic National Convention, held on July 12–15 in New York City's Madison Square Garden. Taking the podium on the convention's last evening to second the symbolic nomination of draft resister Fritz Efaw for vice president, Kovic seized the opportunity to condemn the conflict that left him, in his words, "with legs that would not stand, a body that would not feel and a pain and anguish that would never leave me" (qtd. in Cannon A16). He could not help but be aware that his primetime speech, which would be seen and heard by millions, could serve as a means of promoting his forthcoming autobiography; in fact, he commenced his speech with the stark, free-verse epigram that begins the book:

> I am the living death
> The memorial day on wheels
> I am your Yankee Doodle dandy
> Your John Wayne come home
> Your fourth of July firecracker
> Exploding in the grave

Kovic's speech garnered an enormous amount of attention as did the book itself, and it did not take long for people in the entertainment industry to approach him about a possible movie deal. Within weeks of the book's publication, actor Al Pacino expressed interest. "Al saw a television clip of me addressing the Democratic National Convention in 1976 while he was in Paris," said Kovic. "The book had just been published. He read it and when he got back to New York he told me that he wanted to make the movie" (qtd. in Buckley C10). Pacino, who stated he had received offers to star in the as-yet-unmade Vietnam-themed projects *Coming Home* and *Apocalypse Now* but declined them, claimed he was drawn to the possibility of playing Kovic because of the book's focus on what he described as "one person struggling" against a society by turns hostile and indifferent (qtd. in Grant B6).

Martin Bregman, who had produced Pacino's starring vehicles *Serpico* in 1973 and *Dog Day Afternoon* in 1975, saw the potential for Pacino, too, and contacted Kovic's agent. The movie negotiations occurred mainly in Sept. 1976 — right on the heels of the book's publication — and, to the dismay of Waldo Salt and the *Coming Home* producers, Kovic withdrew from their project. Kovic, who had worked with the film-minded Salt for months and had famously claimed that movies such as *Sands of Iwo Jima* (1949) and *To Hell and Back* (1955) had strongly influenced him as a youth, could clearly see the movie possibilities in his life story. Though he was careful not to knock *Coming Home* — "It's an important film, but a completely different film than *Born on the Fourth of July*," he said (qtd. in Buckley C10) — Kovic believed there was little point to serving as a mere consultant on a film when his own story could take center stage.

By October, Kovic had sold the screen rights to Bregman's company, Artists Entertainment Complex, for $150,000 plus a percentage (Dickey 114). With Pacino slated to star, Bregman hoped to get production underway in 1977. Kovic was elated: "It looks like a million-dollar proposition," he enthused (qtd. in Dickey 114).

A number of delays ensued, however, one of which concerned the completion of a viable script. A draft was hastily put together, perhaps by someone working directly with Kovic, but, as the veteran noted, "the first screenplay was unacceptable to both Bregman and Pacino. The next screenwriter who came along was Oliver Stone. Oliver was simply a screenwriter at the time — that is how we met" (qtd. in "Not a Pretty" 68). That 1977 encounter proved auspicious. Stone, whose father was friends with Bregman, was not well known in Hollywood at the time and had only a few film credits to his name, mainly a short documentary titled *Last Year in Vietnam* (1971) and a horror cheapie called *Seizure* (1974), both of which he wrote and directed. However, Stone, like Kovic, was a Vietnam War veteran who had been wounded in the war, and the two formed a special connection that would last many years. With Kovic's help, Stone began crafting a screenplay based on the autobiography.

Another delay arose from Bregman's difficulty in finding a director. The producer initially wanted William Friedkin, best known for the hugely successful 1973 horrorfest *The Exorcist,* but he was unavailable and what followed was a long string of failed negotiations.

Bregman discovered that seasoned directors were skittish about the project. "We couldn't get a director, and I approached everyone in town," he remembered. "It was just me and a young unknown writer named Oliver Stone" (qtd. in Dutka 39).

Meanwhile, the press announced in early 1977 that Bregman had struck a deal with Paramount Pictures to distribute the film in the U.S. and presumably provide upfront funding with which to make the film (Grant B6). Paramount had distributed *Serpico* in 1973 as well as the first two *Godfather* movies in 1972 and 1974, and the company seemed an obvious choice for handling yet another movie starring the bankable Pacino. Unfortunately, however, Kovic inadvertently befouled that financial relationship. He had commenced a nationwide book tour in mid–July 1977 to promote the new Pocket Books paperback edition of his autobiography, but Pocket Books shut the tour down the following month after Kovic publicly criticized the firm's corporate parent, Gulf+Western. "I went to Vietnam to make the rich richer in this country," he said while on the tour and specifically tagged G+W as a corporation that financially benefited from his wartime sacrifices (qtd. in Long 4). As it happened, G+W was also the parent company for Paramount. Though it is unlikely that a single public utterance would have soured the deal, Kovic's commentary certainly did not help matters, and Bregman soon found himself having to search for a new financial partner.

The delays stretched into 1978 while Bregman scrambled to find new funding sources for *Born,* but things were looking up; Stone completed a screenplay early that year, Bregman hired longtime television-director-turned-film-director Daniel Petrie after a lengthy search, Pacino was still in place to play Kovic, and all signs indicated that the film would finally go into production in mid–1978. Kovic could not help but be delighted. "Here I am, the crippled war veteran who fought with everybody to bring the war to an end and get justice for the servicemen who were cheated out of their youth and their bodies, living the American dream," he said in May 1978. "I have a nice apartment, a girlfriend, a new car, a best-selling book, and now Al Pacino is going to do my story on the screen. I mean, who wouldn't want to have Al Pacino play his life in a movie? Incredible" (qtd. in Fanucchi SG1). Poignantly, he underscored a kinship between himself and other principals involved in the production. "Oliver was wounded in Vietnam five days before I was, in January 1968," he said, "so we understand each other. Dan Petrie, who is directing — he also did *The Betsy*—was wounded in action in World War II. Marty Bregman, the producer, had polio as a child and walks with a brace" (qtd. in Buckley C10).[1]

Behind the scenes, however, the financial situation was becoming increasingly shaky. *Coming Home,* the film to which Kovic had once been attached as a consultant, had opened in mid–Feb. 1978, and some controversy ensued because of Jane Fonda's connection with it as co-producer and co-star. For many, Fonda was and still is a vilified figure for visiting Hanoi in 1972, making a series of radio broadcasts condemning U.S. policy, and posing for pictures atop a North Vietnamese anti-aircraft battery. In all likelihood, studios and other potential funding sources were wary of getting involved with another film that not only featured the less-than-commercially-promising topic of a disabled Vietnam vet who becomes a war protester but also had a politically contentious person associated with it.

Though Bregman eventually reached an agreement with Orion Pictures to distribute the film on its completion, he was unable to find an American studio willing to provide pre-production funding. With deadlines looming (his representatives were then scouting and securing venues in New York City, Long Island, and Georgia's Jekyll Island for location shooting), Bregman looked overseas and began negotiating with German investors in the hope of securing the necessary funds to bankroll the production.

Shooting was scheduled to begin in Puerto Vallarta, Mexico, in late June 1978 when disaster struck; the film's funding arrangement with the overseas investors fell through a mere four days before the start of principal photography. The deal's collapse effectively pulled the plug on the project.

Stone, still early in his moviemaking career, was devastated by the news. In retrospect, he characterized it as his "bitterest disappointment" as a filmmaker (qtd. in Johnston C28). "Al got cold feet and went on to do *And Justice For All*," he said. "Ron became crazed. Marty was in for $1 million of his own. I just gave up at the thought that a studio wouldn't make a $6 million film — not a lot for one starring Al Pacino — because they considered it too tough, too realistic. It was a heartbreaker for everyone involved" (qtd. in Dutka 39). Though he wielded no clout back then, Stone believed in the project strongly enough to make a promise to Kovic. "If I ever get my opportunity, if I'm ever able to break through as a director, I'll come back for you, Ronnie," he said (qtd. in Seidenberg 56).

Unbeknownst to all concerned, Stone was already on a path that would lead him to such a breakthrough. He had written the screenplay for *Midnight Express,* a film released in the U.S. in October 1978, and his script won him an Oscar early the following year. That success led to other assignments, such as the scripts for such varied films as *Conan the Barbarian* (1982) and *Scarface* (1983), before he hit it big with *Platoon* in 1986 and again with *Wall Street* in 1987. Written and directed by Stone and produced by his new colleague Kitman Ho, *Platoon* and *Wall Street* placed Stone squarely on the Hollywood map. They gave him the influence he needed to make just about any film he wanted. In a development almost unheard of in the movie business, he elected to revive a film that had been on the slagheap of abandoned projects for a decade. That film was, of course, *Born on the Fourth of July.*

Stone proposed the project to Tom Pollock, the new president of Universal Pictures. Pollock, who knew Stone well (he had handled Stone's movie dealings as his attorney at one point), was receptive. "I realized that it was one of the great unmade screenplays of the past 15 years," said Pollock. "I told Stone we'd be interested if he could do it real cheap" (qtd. in Dutka 39).

Stone and producing partner Ho agreed to make the movie for $14 million — a modest figure by Hollywood standards — but delays ensued as concerns continued to be raised about the project's commercial viability. New funding did not come through until a big-name star was signed and, furthermore, agreed to work for a deferred salary. That star turned out to be Tom Cruise, who had impressed Stone with his work ethic and intensity. His background, similar to Kovic's, was also a plus. According to Kovic, Stone "felt very strongly about Tom portraying my life. He felt that Tom and I had a lot of similarities, our Catholic, working-class upbringing, and our determination to do the very best at whatever we did" (qtd. in "Not a Pretty" 68).

With a marquee performer onboard, Stone and Kovic began collaborating on a thorough rewrite of Stone's 1978 script. Kovic served this time as a full-fledged co-screenwriter (he was to have received story credit but not screenplay credit on the aborted film), and he and Stone completed their revision in August 1988. Filming took place over a 65-day period in late 1988 and early 1989 in the Dallas area and the Philippines. Following some reshooting in Los Angeles in the summer of 1989 and the requisite post-production work, the long-delayed *Born on the Fourth of July* finally debuted in American theaters in December 1989, in time for Oscar consideration that year.

Many critics and audiences took the film at face value — at least, at first — and praised

it for its forthrightness and emotional wallop. One of its champions, Roger Ebert, unequivocally stated that *Born* was "one of the best movies of the year" and asserted that it "steps
correctly in the opening moments and then never steps wrongly. It is easy to think of a
thousand traps that Stone, Kovic and Cruise could have fallen into, but they fall into none
of them" (Ebert). Vincent Canby of the *New York Times* was especially lavish in his praise
for Tom Cruise's work in the film, calling *Born* "a film of enormous visceral power with, in
the central role, a performance by Tom Cruise that defines everything that is best about the
movie.... Watching his Ron Kovic, as he comes to terms with a reality for which he was
completely unprepared, is both harrowing and inspiring" (C15). In addition to receiving
such critical accolades, the film was nominated for, and won, numerous awards. Most
notably, Stone won an Oscar and top honors from the Directors Guild of America for his
directorial work on the film. *Born* scored particularly well with the Hollywood Foreign Press
Association, winning Golden Globe movie awards for director, screenplay, performance by
an actor, and drama. To the relief of all who were involved in the production process, it
mopped up at the box office, earning more than $230 million on a budget of $14 million.

   The critical responses to *Born* were by no means uniform, however, with a number of
reviewers, such as *Newsweek*'s David Ansen and *Commonweal*'s Christian Appy, condemning
the film's pageant-like qualities, heavy-handedness, and flatly drawn, symbolic characters.
One of the most vocal critics was the *New Yorker*'s Pauline Kael, who mocked Kovic's youthful naïveté about war and argued that "wherever you look in this movie, people are representative figures rather than people, and the falseness starts during the opening credits."
She also opined that "Stone's movie yells at you for two hours and twenty-five minutes.
Stone tells you and he shows you at the same time; everything is swollen with meaning"
(122).

   A different type of negative criticism began surfacing in the ensuing weeks, as other
observers began raising broader questions about the film's historical accuracy. Richard Eilert,
who was seriously injured in Vietnam while serving with the 26th Marine regiment, wrote
a *Washington Post* op-ed piece bluntly titled "*Born on the Fourth*: It's a Lie" in which he
lashed out at what he termed the "inherent dishonesty in Stone's depiction of those who
served." Discussing both *Born* and Stone's earlier film *Platoon,* Eilert suggested that they
"are laced with enough fact to make the stories difficult to refute, while at they same time
they are saturated with so much hateful negativism that in the end the proper term to
describe them is probably 'propaganda' or 'disinformation'" (A25).

   Writing for the *Washington Times,* Diana West took the criticism a step further by outlining numerous specific differences between the historical record and the events and people
depicted in the Stone/Kovic film. Among the scenes she cited were the Syracuse police riot
(in actuality, there was no rioting, no Kovic, and no Abbie Hoffman; it was just a peaceful
protest), Kovic's encounter with the Wilson family in Venus, Georgia (it occurred only in
Kovic's mind; in fact, there is no such municipality as "Venus, Georgia"), and the riot
outside the Republican National Convention (it simply did not happen, though Kovic in
his book described a similar run-in with the police outside Richard Nixon's campaign head-
quarters in Los Angeles). West also pointedly noted that neither Stone nor Kovic nor their
publicity people were willing to respond in any meaningful way to questions about the
film's accuracy (West E1).

   In retrospect, it is not difficult to see what Stone and Kovic hoped to accomplish with
their revised screenplay — a "revisionist" work in several senses — and subsequent film. They
had learned hard lessons from the 1978 *Born* debacle and were determined to minimize the

possibility of box-office failure for their resurrected film. With the awareness that movies, unlike books, are multi-million-dollar investments and therefore require a certain amount of caution in their planning and execution, Stone and Kovic rearranged historical events, and invented a few new ones, to create a smoothly flowing narrative that followed the classic three-act paradigm that has governed many a Hollywood film. This conservative and time-tested structure, famously identified by the dean of screenwriting teachers, Syd Field (20–30), generally looks like this:

Act I (the Set-Up): A sympathetic Protagonist is introduced and shown in his/her typical day-to-day life.

Plot Point I: A major event turns the Protagonist's life upside down, and the story spins in a new direction.

Act II (the Confrontation): The Protagonist spends a huge amount of time reacting, often in ineffectual ways, to his/her new and bewildering set of circumstances.

Plot Point II: The Protagonist experiences an epiphany and decides to pursue major action to rectify the situation, often ending up in greater jeopardy as a result of that decision.

Act III (the Resolution): The Protagonist draws on inner resources and usually triumphs over the crisis, and a sense of restored order prevails.

The extent to which Stone and Kovic consciously followed this structure as they went about their revision is unknown; there is no question, however, that it solidly undergirds their film. Here in very general terms is the way that *Born* unfolds:

The film's first act — the Set-up — starts with Kovic's childhood in Massapequa, New York, and continues through his high school years, enlistment in the Marine Corps, and eventual arrival in Vietnam as a "grunt." The story's first major turning point — the first Plot Point, in Hollywood parlance — occurs about forty minutes into the film when Kovic is seriously wounded during his second Vietnam tour of duty.

The hefty second act — the Confrontation — depicts Kovic's horrendous experiences in a Bronx V.A. hospital and many other events in his new life as a disabled person. Its numerous scenes illustrate such incidents as his conflicts with family members (especially his mother), a visit to his girlfriend at Syracuse University where he becomes caught up in a police riot, his growing disillusionment with the war, a traumatic trip to Mexico to visit brothels that cater to wounded veterans, and an emotional encounter with the family of a young Georgia man named Wilson whom he believes he accidentally killed in Vietnam.

The film's brief and highly elliptical third act — its Resolution — begins with a second Plot Point that signals the completion of Kovic's evolution from passive victim to action-taking war protester; he is among the leaders of a massive antiwar demonstration outside the 1972 Republican National Convention. Once inside the convention hall, he gives an impromptu, disruptive speech and security guards quickly hustle him out into the parking lot. Dumped out of his wheelchair and beaten, Kovic nevertheless rallies his fellow protesters, telling them "we're gonna take the hall back, you hear that?" and urging them to "fall out — let's move." They stream toward the convention hall, and the film concludes with a scene set four years later as a triumphant Kovic wheels himself toward the speakers' platform of the 1976 Democratic National Convention to deliver a speech.

In electing to structure their screenplay and eventual film in traditional three-act terms, Stone and Kovic created a linearity and closure that's largely lacking in the book. The autobiography, unlike the film, begins and ends with scenes in Vietnam and frequently jumps about in time, its fragmentation accentuated by odd shifts between first- and third-person accounts of Kovic's experiences; the film, on the other hand, is conventionally straightforward. In addition, Kovic's appearance at the Democratic convention, which of course is not included in the book since it had not happened yet, endows the film with a sense of healing and resolution that's absent in the book (Shor 384). Needless to say, the filmmakers' decision to follow the three-act structure had a profound impact on the way the life experiences of its disabled lead character would be represented.

As a means of better understanding the implications of the filmmakers' commercially minded "repackaging" of Kovic's young adulthood for mainstream audiences, I propose at this juncture to examine *Born* within the context of other disability themed films with which it shares some connections. Two sets of films are especially apropos: other films about disabled veterans (Vietnam-related ones in particular; *Born*'s peer films, in a sense), and a group of films that flourished during the decades immediately following World War II. Such an approach will, I hope, shed further light on the workings and agenda of this problematic movie text.

Generally speaking, the Hollywood representations of disabled war veterans have taken two highly divergent forms: (1) exploitive treatments of vets who appear able-bodied but exhibit pronounced symptoms of Post-Traumatic Stress Disorder which in the movies usually translates as psychopathic behavior, and (2) reasonably sympathetic portraits of vets whose bodily differences are highly visible (e.g., missing limbs, wheelchair usage) and who struggle to be reabsorbed into mainstream society. Hollywood filmmakers have reserved some of their most compelling PWD representations for the veterans in this latter category, and *Born on the Fourth of July* is very much a part of that trend (Norden, "Bitterness" 96).

Born is among a handful of fairly high-profile films stretching from the late 1970s to the mid–1990s that centered on disabled Vietnam veterans, and it is worth comparing it briefly to these other films to gain a better sense of what it does and does not accomplish. It is similar to two disabled Vietnam vet films that preceded it — *Coming Home* (1978) and *Cutter's Way* (1981) — and two others that followed it — *Scent of a Woman* (1992) and *Forrest Gump* (1994) — in that all five films bestow the privileged status of white heterosexuality on their veterans and initially depict them as rage-filled, directionless, suicidal, substance abusers who often turn to prostitutes for sexual gratification. Following in the tradition of the disabled-veteran films that appeared in the wake of the Korean War, such as *The Eternal Sea* (1955), *The Wings of Eagles* (1957), and *Bad Day at Black Rock* (1955), which present their disabled vets returning to wartime duty or engaging in some other heroic activity, all five of the Vietnam vet films noted above show their characters eventually channeling their pent-up energy and rage to some larger purpose.[2]

For all its similarity to other disabled Vietnam veteran films, *Born* differs in at least two prime respects. The first is its lack of a politically naïve "enabler" who is arguably meant to represent the general U.S. population as a whole. *Coming Home, Cutter's Way, Scent of a Woman,* and *Forrest Gump* heavily imply that their embittered veterans are utterly rudderless and would remain so were it not for the intervention of certain well-meaning, able-bodied figures. These rather ingenuous characters are, in order, Sally Hyde (Jane Fonda), Rich Bone (Jeff Bridges), Charlie Simms (Chris O'Donnell), and Forrest Gump (Tom Hanks). Perhaps symbolizing America's uncommitted Vietnam War-era populace, they serve as foils to the disabled vets and help them redirect their anger to some larger purpose. They are politically neutral at first but eventually come around to the vets' way of thinking and directly or indirectly assist them with their newfound quests. The films unsubtly suggest that the wounded veterans absolutely need these "innocents" to help them emerge from their depressive funk and be able to claim any kind of heroic status.

Importantly, no such character exists in *Born on the Fourth of July*. The closest is Kovic's fictional girlfriend Donna (Kyra Sedgwick), but she differs in two key ways: she is hardly politically neutral (in fact, the film suggests that it is her activism that pulls Kovic into the tumultuous world of anti–Vietnam War protests), and she disappears about an hour and a half into the 144-minute film.[3] Unlike the disabled veterans of *Coming Home, Cutter's Way, Scent of a Woman*, and *Forrest Gump*, Kovic essentially moves through his postwar life receiving little if any help. People are hostile, indifferent, or ineffective in their dealings with him, or they simply fall away from him until the collective action that marks the beginning of the relatively brief third act. Tellingly, the film presents his fellow protesters in this final act as a mostly undifferentiated mass; Kovic is the only distinct figure — and, by implication, the only character of any importance — to emerge from their numbers.

The second difference that sets *Born* apart from its peer films is its narrative point of attack. *Born* is unique among the quintet of films noted above in that it presents numerous scenes depicting its disabled veteran's childhood and young adulthood years before his service in Vietnam. In contrast, all of the other films initially show their veterans as adults; in fact, the narratives of *Coming Home, Cutter's Way,* and *Scent of a Woman* commence after their wounded vets have been discharged. By showing significant portions of Kovic's pre- and post-disablement life, *Born* reflects its filmmakers' desire to examine in detail the physical adjustment and political evolution of its protagonist.

Tom Cruise's Kovic — a person "struck down" by a disabling circumstance only to make a long, difficult, and lonely but ultimately triumphant comeback — is reminiscent of characters who populated disability-themed films during the late 1940s and intermittently for decades thereafter, the so-termed "Civilian Superstars" (Norden, *Cinema* 187–205). Many such films were based, if flimsily, on the experiences of actual high-achieving people. They include *The Stratton Story* (1949), about professional baseball player Monty Stratton who lost a leg in a hunting accident; *Interrupted Melody* (1955), focusing on opera singer Marjorie Lawrence King and her bout with polio; *Night and Day* (1946), about Cole Porter before and after his serious horseback-riding accident; and *With a Song in My Heart* (1952), which depicts pop singer Jane Froman's life after her plane-crash injury. One of the last films in this tradition, *The Other Side of the Mountain* (1975), examined the life of Olympic skiing hopeful Jill Kinmont before and after her debilitating accident.

There are key differences between *Born* and this set of films, of course. For example, the disabled figures in these older films — civilians, all — were already reasonably well known in their respective fields before their disabling injuries or illnesses occurred. Their movies position them as larger-than-life figures, and there's a strong sense that the drive that got them to the tops of their professions would also see them through their physical difficulties. Kovic certainly had his ambitions, too — "I wanted to be a hero," he wrote of his high-school self (Kovic, *Born* 63) — but he does not rise to the peak of his "profession" as a gung-ho-Marine-turned-antiwar-activist until after his injury and his profound changes in thinking about war, his country, and personal sacrifice.

Despite such differences, *Born* is a distinct throwback to the Civilian Superstar type of film. The film's much-criticized mythic qualities — enhanced by occasional slow-motion cinematography, "God's Eye" high-angle shots, and John Williams' majestic musical score — serve to set Kovic apart from everyone around him and, in a sense, cast him in the larger-than-life terms characteristic of the Civilian Superstars. As presented in the film, the evolving

Ron Kovic is not at all ordinary; simply put, he is as extraordinary as any figure in the Civilian Superstar tradition, perhaps more so, since the filmmakers took pains to suggest that he is also emblematic of his country.[4] He is a world-famous antiwar protester, a masculinist fantasy-figure who aggressively reclaims his lost manhood, and a symbol of America, all rolled into one.

Born is also regressive in that it borrows heavily from the "medical-model" way of thinking about disability. This retrograde paradigm, which had its movie heyday during the 1940s and '50s with the Civilian Superstar films noted above and numerous productions that explored the readjustment problems of World War II disabled veterans,[5] conceptualizes disability mainly in pathological problem-to-be-overcome terms and places the burden of "overcoming" solidly on the shoulders of the individual. Films informed by the medical model imply that the only things newly disabled people need for a successful readjustment are the proper strength of character and support from family, friends, and colleagues. Societally created problems such as prejudice, discrimination, unemployment, and access magically disappear — if they were ever present in the first place — in the worlds represented in these films.[6] Given that Kovic did not identify with the disability rights movement and tended to contextualize disability in medical and rehabilitative terms ("Not a Pretty" 68), the appearance of this perspective in *Born* is hardly surprising. In fact, the loneliness and isolation that often accompanied the Civilian Superstars on their heroic way back to the pinnacles of their professions are, if anything, accentuated in *Born*; the network of supportive family and friends so essential in the Civilian Superstar and World War II disabled-vet films is mostly an illusion in the Stone/Kovic film. Kovic is about as isolated as a person can get until the film's final act, making his Superstar-like triumph all the more dramatic and unusual. It is a solitary Kovic victorious against the rest of the world, or so the filmmakers would have us believe.

The kinship between *Born* and the Civilian Superstar films is especially conspicuous in *Born*'s final scene, in which Kovic is about to address the 1976 Democratic National Convention. This conclusion bears more than a passing resemblance to the ending of one of the most famous of Civilian Superstar movies, 1960's *Sunrise at Campobello*. This film, based on Dore Schary's 1958 Broadway hit about Franklin Roosevelt and his pre-presidential struggles with paralysis, concludes as FDR is about to give a nominating speech on behalf of Al Smith at the 1924 Democratic National Convention. In both films, the venue is New York's Madison Square Garden,[7] and, in both cases, the films conclude before we actually hear the speeches.[8] The purported intent behind each speech (the nomination of Al Smith for president; a seconding of the nomination of Fritz Efaw for vice president) is not nearly as important as what the speeches represent about the main characters. In *Sunrise*'s case, it is to show that FDR had returned to the national political scene, and the film even shows him walking to the lectern as "proof" of his comeback; in *Born*'s case, it is to create the impression that Kovic received a hero's welcome and has, in a sense, returned "home."[9]

To conclude, *Born on the Fourth of July* followed a convoluted developmental path before finally arriving in movie theaters in late 1989. The initial attempt to produce the film had resulted in utter failure and, when Universal Pictures greenlit the film a decade later, Oliver Stone and Ron Kovic were determined that history would not repeat itself. In their desire to maximize *Born*'s commercial appeal, the filmmakers in effect compromised the film by relying on a well-worn narrative framework, introducing numerous historical inaccuracies and borrowing from the antiquated medical-model way of conceptualizing disability.

It would be a mistake to assume, however, that *Born* is without its virtues. Among other things, it frequently invites the audience to share its disabled veteran's perspective, illustrates some of the issues of access that PWDs face on a daily basis, explodes the myth that PWDs are asexual, and features an ageless message about the absurdities and cruelties of war. Though it takes many liberties in its representation and sequencing of events, the film admirably captures the spirit of the times and exhibits an undeniably powerful emotional "truth." Indeed, one of its most significant achievements is its ability to draw viewers into the life of Kovic and the emotions he experiences. Had the filmmakers been more circumspect in their fictionalization of history and minimized their reliance on outdated ideas about movie storytelling and disability, they might have created a film of truly timeless proportions.

Notes

1. Released in February 1978, *The Betsy* is hardly a cinematic masterpiece; it does, however, feature a prominent wheelchair-using character played by Laurence Olivier.

2. Unlike the other movie representations of disabled veterans noted in this chapter, *Forrest Gump*'s Dan Taylor is a secondary character and does not engage in heroic acts but is instead associated with heroic imagery. For more discussion, see Norden, "Bitterness" 107.

3. The film uses the image of Donna only two more times in the film, and both instances are extremely brief: as a fragment of a reverie-like flashback in the film's final minutes, and in the end credits. Donna, incidentally, is very loosely based on Connie Panzarino, who attended the same high school as Kovic — she watched his wrestling matches from afar, just as Donna does in the movie — and developed a close relationship with him after his return from Vietnam. A huge difference is that Panzarino bore a neuromuscular disorder (Amytonia Congenita, now known as Spinal Muscular Atrophy Type III) and used a wheelchair most of her life, whereas Donna is represented as able-bodied. In other words, the filmmakers completely effaced the Kovic girlfriend's disability identity factor. For more about Panzarino and her relationship with Kovic, see Panzarino, Goldman, and Kovic, *Born* 5.

4. Perhaps to deflect criticism of their loose handling of historical events, the filmmakers insisted in interviews at the time that the movie was about Kovic *as* America. For a summary of their views, see Norden, "Bitterness" 101.

5. Among the many movies in this tradition are *Pride of the Marines* (1945), *The Best Years of Our Lives* (1946), *The Men* (1950), and *Bright Victory* (1951). For discussions of them, see Norden, *Cinema* 160–68, 176–83.

6. To Stone and Kovic's credit, though, *Born* does pay some attention to problems of access. For example, it shows that Kovic's family members have modified their house in Massapequa to accommodate his use of a wheelchair, and its scenes set in Syracuse illustrate his difficulty maneuvering his chair along streets and sidewalks due to the lack of curb cuts.

7. In fact, the 1976 convention was the first held in Madison Square Garden by the Democrats since the 1924 convention.

8. The screenplay that Stone and Kovic completed in 1988 actually has Kovic delivering a portion of the speech consisting of the "I am the living death" poem noted earlier and a few additional lines. As director, Stone evidently concluded that the darkly worded speech ran counter to the sense of uplift, closure, and healing he and Kovic were trying to create and jettisoned it. The film simply concludes with a shot of Kovic wheeling away from the camera in slow motion toward the speakers' platform while a rendition of "You're a Grand Old Flag" plays on the soundtrack. See Stone and Kovic 140. At the time of this writing, the script was available as a download from http://www.dailyscript.com.

9. Kovic was quite aware of the *Sunrise at Campobello* narrative, even asking his mother to bring him a copy of the playscript during his post-disablement stay at the Bronx V.A. hospital. See Kovic, *Born* 37.

Works Cited

Ansen, David. "Bringing It All Back Home." Rev. of *Born on the Fourth of July. Newsweek* 25 Dec. 1989: 74. Print.

Appy, Christian. "Vietnam According to Oliver Stone." Rev. of *Born on the Fourth of July. Commonweal* 23 Mar. 1990: 187. Print.

Born on the Fourth of July. Dir. Oliver Stone. Perf. Tom Cruise. Universal Pictures, 1989. Film.

Buckley, Tom. "At the Movies." *New York Times* 23 June 1978: C10. Print.

Canby, Vincent. "How an All-American Boy Went to War and Lost His Faith." Rev. of *Born on the Fourth of July. New York Times* 20 Dec. 1989: C15–16. Print.

Cannon, Lou. "Georgian Seeks a Health Program, Overhaul of Taxes." *Washington Post* 16 July 1976: A16. Print.

Collier, Peter. *The Fondas: A Hollywood Dynasty.* New York: G. P. Putnam's Sons, 1991. Print.

Dickey, Christopher. "Bookmakers." *Washington Post* 10 Oct. 1976: 114. Print.

Dutka, Elaine. "The Latest Exorcism of Oliver Stone." *Los Angeles Times* 17 Dec. 1989, calendar sec.: 38–39, 112. Print.

Ebert, Roger. Rev. of *Born on the Fourth of July. Chicago Sun-Times* 20 Dec. 1989. Print.

Eilert, Richard. "*Born on the Fourth*: It's a Lie." *Washington Post* 6 Feb. 1990: A25. Print.

Fannuchi, Kenneth. "Celebrity Status Was Won With a Bullet." *Los Angeles Times* 14 May 1978: SG1. Print.

Field, Syd. *Screenplay: The Foundations of Screenwriting*, rev. ed. New York: Delta Trade Paperbacks, 2005. Print.

Fuchs, Regula. *Remembering Viet Nam: Gustav Hasford, Ron Kovic, Tim O'Brien and the Fabrication of American Cultural Memory.* Bern: Peter Lang, 2010. Print.

Goldman, Ari L. "Peace, with Honor." *New York Times* 29 Aug. 1976, Long Island sec.: 1, 20–21. Print.

Grant, Lee. "Film Clips." *Los Angeles Times* 5 Mar. 1977: B6. Print.

Johnston, Laurie. "Oliver Stone Reflects on His Frightening Movie." *New York Times* 24 Apr. 1981: C28. Print.

Kael, Pauline. "Potency." Rev. of *Born on the Fourth of July. New Yorker* 22 Jan. 1990: 122–24. Print.

Kovic, Ron. *Born on the Fourth of July.* New York: Pocket Books, 1977. Print.

_____. "Introduction." *Born on the Fourth of July.* New York: Akashic Books, 2005. Print.

Long, Lauren. "Antiwar Author Hits Book Firm." *Boston Globe* 14 Aug. 1977: 4. Print.

McCombs, Philip A. "Ron Kovic: 'I Am Your Yankee Doodle Dandy.'" *Washington Post* 10 Aug. 1976: B1. Print.

Moss, Nathaniel. *Ron Kovic: Antiwar Activist.* New York: Chelsea House, 1993. Print.

Norden, Martin F. "Bitterness, Rage, and Redemption: Hollywood Constructs the Disabled Vietnam Veteran." *Disabled Veterans in History.* Ed. David Gerber. Ann Arbor: University of Michigan Press, 2000. 96–114. Print.

_____. *The Cinema of Isolation: A History of Physical Disability in the Movies.* New Brunswick: Rutgers University Press, 1994. Print. "Not a Pretty Picture." *Accent on Living* Spring 1990: 68+. Print.

Panzarino, Connie. *The Me in the Mirror.* Seattle: Seal Press, 1994. Print.

Seidenberg, Robert. "To Hell and Back." *American Film* Jan. 1990: 28–31, 56. Print.

Shor, Fran. "Transcending the Myths of Patriotic Militarized Masculinity: Armoring, Wounding, and Transfiguration in Ron Kovic's *Born on the Fourth of July.*" *Journal of Men's Studies* 8 (2000): 375–85. Print.

Stone, Oliver, and Ron Kovic. *Born on the Fourth of July.* Screenplay. Aug. 1988. Author's collection. Print.

West, Diana. "Does *Born on the Fourth of July* Lie?" *Washington Times* 23 Feb. 1990: E1. Print.

Deafness as Peripeteia

"Beethoven" and *Immortal Beloved*

DAWNE C. MCCANCE

Bernard Rose's *Immortal Beloved* (1994) has been universally panned by critics (Janet Maslin is the only exception I can find) for its falsification of biographical details. Yet it serves as a good model of the role that Beethoven's deafness has been made to play in interpretations of his life and work. As Lewis Lockwood points out in his review of *Immortal Beloved*, "Film Biography as Travesty," since the nineteenth century Beethoven biographers have latched onto his deafness as a *peripeteia*, a crisis or turning point, through which a life drama unfolds and a destiny manifests (Young-Bruehl 196). Deafness-as-crisis now belongs to an enduring myth that has all-but overtaken Beethoven's legacy: the idea that the composer was destined to become a musical and national hero until, by the third or late period of his life and work, his emerging deafness became a *peripeteia*. In Beethoven mythology, this *peripeteia* works in two opposing ways: first, as the turning point that triggers the fall of the hero and his music; second, as the turning point that triggers the final rise of the hero as Beethoven, faced with deafness, not only liberates music but also overcomes his disability. Either way, deafness becomes the stuff of which the Beethoven drama is made — and Rose's film drama is no exception. I will approach this use of Beethoven's deafness as a case study of some of the pitfalls involved in collapsing work (music, painting, writing) into "life" (biography), especially when, in the interests of a good story, disability is taken to be the interpretive biographical or musicological key.

The Hero Myth

On Sunday, 12 November 1989, as the Berlin Wall began coming down and crowds of East Germans flocked into West Berlin, the Berlin Philharmonic Orchestra staged a concert to which all East German citizens were invited — a performance of Beethoven's music. In *Beethoven in German Politics, 1870–1989*, David B. Dennis asks why, for so many German people, there was no better way to celebrate that day than with the music of Ludwig van Beethoven. Tracing the history of Beethoven's politicization as an image or ideal that has been put to "extra-musical" uses since the unification of Germany in the nineteenth century, Dennis observes that "the emphasis is inevitably on Beethoven as a man who overcame tremendous personal adversity. The most exploitable aspect of the Beethoven story for politicians is his struggle to create" (19). At the center of this story is Beethoven's deafness: "the miracle of music created by an artist unable to hear provides a keystone for picturing Beethoven as a man of monumental will" (19).

Like Dennis, Scott Burnham considers "struggle" to be essential to the "heroic style" that he says Beethoven's music epitomizes, particularly during the middle period, and that accounts in large part for the music's profound and lasting appeal. In *Beethoven Hero,* Burnham draws on a long tradition of critics, some of whom never actually use the words "hero" or "heroism" in interpreting Beethoven's music (see Stanley 468), but who nonetheless appeal to certain elements of Beethoven's music as "heroic" in style. This perceived heroism is not limited to the few, Burnham notes, but is considered to be universal. It "embraces all individualities, [engaging] each of us at a deeply personal level, and yet [engaging] us all in roughly the same way" and thus as involving us in "struggle and eventual triumph as an index of man's [*sic*] greatness" (xiv). Yet, Beethoven's music has also been assumed to allude to some great men in particular, "heroes" such as Napoleon, for example. The first forty-five bars of Beethoven's *Eroica* Symphony have been understood to represent morning on the battlefield before the fighting begins, the hero Napoleon about to arrive (5). Not the least, Burnham points out, the special hero represented by Beethoven's heroic style is Beethoven himself, the man who liberated music from its eighteenth century conventions, "singlehandedly bringing music into a new age by giving it a transcendent voice equal to Western man's most cherished values" (xvi).

Burnham's study is important as an introduction to, and endorsement of, the Beethoven hero-myth, which portrays the composer as "the quintessential artist-hero" (xvi). Despite his deafness, he was able to access the realm of the pure "idea," the realm from which, in the Western tradition overall, deaf humans have been barred.[1] There is another, tragic version of the Beethoven myth in which the composer appears as a Promethean figure. According to this view, the Promethean artist serves "as a firebringer from the gods to man," and yet, is finally "rejected by that society he is bound to serve" (Plantinga 16). The Promethean figure, "flattering in a way to the composer," no doubt "also placed upon him a special burden to prove worthy of his calling" (16). As I will discuss below, part of the attraction of the Prometheus myth for Beethoven's critics is its accommodation of the composer's deafness as key — both to his heroic greatness, and to the burden of a disability to which, as his life and music progressed, he succumbed.

Immortal Beloved plays into the Beethoven myth right from its opening scenes, which depict the composer's 1827 funeral in full heroic mode with his coffin being carried through the crowded streets of Vienna. Still, these opening scenes represent one of "a few moments of emotional truth" in the movie (Lockwood 193). The actual funeral event drew a throng of ten thousand — some have estimated two or three times that number — into the streets to witness the great procession and to hear Beethoven's funeral oration, written by Franz Grillparzer and delivered by Heinrich Anschütz (Solomon *Beethoven*, 383). Sustaining its sense of a monumental event and introducing its first major distortion of facts, the film's funeral procession and burial scenes alternate with shots of Beethoven's former secretary and confidante Anton Schindler (Jeroen Krabbé) reading the funeral oration.

Rose's choice to focus on Schindler at the outset quickly establishes the major structural role he plays in the film as the character who determines to discover the identity of Beethoven's "Immortal Beloved." But the film's portrait of the historical Schindler (1795–1864) as the composer's loyal servant dedicated to discovering the truth about his life is fundamentally falsified. In Lewis Lockwood's words, Rose's Schindler is "one of the marvelous unwitting ironies of this movie, whose makers probably do not know that Schindler has recently been unmasked for the forgeries he made in a number of Beethoven's conversation books, including false entries that put him in a favorable light or tended to lend support to some of his pet theories about Beethoven's works" (193). After Beethoven's death, Schindler removed many of the important documents left in Beethoven's lodgings, converting them into his private property, altering them at will, and finally selling most of the collection to the King of Prussia in 1845 for a large sum of money and a lifetime annuity. Schindler also wrote an infamous Beethoven biography that "largely shaped the nineteenth-century conception of the composer" (Solomon *Beethoven*, x).

Decades later, Schindler's unreliable portrait of Beethoven was seriously challenged, and the main outlines of the composer's life faithfully reconstructed with the publication of the first three volumes of Thayer's Beethoven biography between 1866 and 1879. Discovery of Schindler's forgeries had to wait until the 20th century. Despite Thayer's early challenges and subsequent revelations, Schindler's version of Beethoven has "continued to exert its influence in our own time" (Solomon *Beethoven*, x). Rose's film is an obvious case in point: whether for lack of research or out of indifference to the historical record, *Immortal Beloved* proceeds as if Schindler's version of Beethoven had never been debunked. The film even standardizes Schindler's own conflicting versions, which he published between 1840 and 1860, of the identity of the "Immortal Beloved," the unnamed woman to whom Beethoven wrote a passionate love letter dated July 6 or 7 of an unstated year.

Rose's Schindler is not without dramatic and mythological purpose. Ultimately, the role Rose has the fictionalized Schindler play in *Immortal Beloved* is crucial to the film's rendering of the composer's deafness as *peripeteia*. Directly following the funeral oration, the film shows Schindler combing through the composer's belongings (claiming to have the authority to do so) and discovering Beethoven's letter to the unnamed Immortal Beloved. Determined to uncover the mystery woman's identity, he sets out on a search that takes him to three candidates. Rose uses the voices of these three women, in conversation with Schindler, to narrate flashback scenes of Beethoven's life, such that, as the quest to find the mystery woman proceeds, viewers of the film are increasingly supplied with essential segments of the composer's biography, his growing deafness, and its devastating effects on his life. Schindler's search for the Immortal Beloved thus turns out to be a chronicle of Beethoven's ever-deepening fall into deafness, and the film, in line with the Beethoven criticism I outline below, subsumes his life and music to his disability.

The Hero's Fall

In her essays "Wagner, Deafness, and the Reception of Beethoven's Late Style," and "'Late,' Last, and Least: On Being Beethoven's Quartet in F Major, Op. 135," Kristin Knittel examines Beethoven's early critics — among them Aléxandre Oulibicheff, Joseph Fröhlich, Adolph Bernhard Marx, François-Joseph Fétis, Ludwig Rellstab, Wilhelm von Lenz, and Henri Blanchard — all of whom, she demonstrates, were preoccupied with Beethoven's auditory impairment. Knittel does not address the validity of these critics' biographical "facts" or their understanding of the composer's actual hearing loss itself, but focuses rather on the role deafness plays in their narratives of Beethoven. Each appealed to it in one way or another: to excuse compositional anomalies; to testify to the composer's faulty or failed memory of sound; to explain Beethoven's depressed or altered psychological state; to suggest that the great man had lost his will; to raise the possibility that he was not only deaf but

also mad ("Wagner" 51–58). Convinced of the effects of his disability on his late composi-
tions, they "refrained from suggesting that Beethoven's reputation should be based on these
last pieces alone" (59). They "apologized for them" (59) and for the most part agreed that
the composer's music could be divided into "three styles," with the works of the second or
middle period constituting his greatest achievement (60). For them, the composer's deafness
constituted a musicological, biographical and narrative fall that eventually made it impossible
for him to fulfill his heroic calling.

Marx, for example, who was a proponent of the Beethoven hero myth (Burnham),
invokes the composer's deafness as an "excuse or explanation" ("Late" 18) for the "growling
motif" that appears in bar 142 of Quartet in F Major, Op. 135." He asks whether the motif
"might have burrowed its way into [Beethoven's] spirit with its buzzing, perhaps from the
diseased auditory nerves" (qtd. in Knittel, 18). Oulibicheff, also a proponent of the Beethoven
hero myth (Burnham), was "outraged that Beethoven will force us to listen to his 'non-
music,' or, as he calls it, 'the *chimère du poète*'—'the negation of music itself'" (18–19). He
makes the case that as Beethoven's deafness worsened, his dissonances increasingly lost their
aesthetic character, and by the time of his late work, the composer's ear gave him cause to
forget that "others did not hear as he did" (19). Knittel notes that even the generally favorable
Wilhelm von Lenz writes that given his deafness, Beethoven "was not the same person, let
alone the same composer, that he had been" (19). Despite other differences of opinion, von
Lenz and Oulibicheff agree that "Beethoven forgot the experience of sound" (20).

Whereas these earlier critics saw deafness as an unmitigated fall, the final tragic, downward trajectory in an otherwise heroic life, later critics saw his deafness as evidence of that
very heroism. They cast Beethoven's deafness as an integral part of a larger Romantic plot
in which he struggles against a range of setbacks — pain and suffering, life disappointments,
and ultimately the most tragic loss imaginable for a great musician, his hearing — yet overcomes all of these in order to write great music" (16). In this second dominant narrative,
deafness is the key to Beethoven's fall *and* his most glorious rise. As Knittel notes, the subsequent "elevation of the late style hinged upon the creation of a new Beethoven, a genius
who, far from losing control or creating inadequate pieces, continued to surpass himself"
("Wagner" 60).

It was Richard Wagner who created this new Beethoven heroic myth with his 1870
essay *Beethoven*. For Wagner, Beethoven's deafness is not the key to his demise, but the key
to the apotheosis of his genius and the greatness of his spirit, a spirit that is unmistakably
that of the German nation itself (19). Attempting to elucidate it, Wagner avoids dealing
with "the essential substance of Beethoven's music" in favor of "riveting" his attention on
"the personal Beethoven" (20), as if the composer's "inner" spirit could be known from
details of his "outer" life. Chief among the personal details of interest to Wagner is
Beethoven's deafness. "A musician sans ears!— Can one conceive an eyeless painter?" (23).
With this question, Wagner invokes the blind seer Tiresias:

> His fellow is the deaf musician who now, untroubled by life's uproar, but listens to his inner
> harmonies, now from his depths but speaks to that world — for it has nothing more to tell him.
> So is genius freed from all outside it, at home forever with and in itself [23].

Like other representations of Beethoven's deafness, Wagner's is not without an ulterior
narrative agenda. Nicholas Vazsonyi suggests that we can read Wagner's essay as an exercise
in self-marketing that, together with his fantasized autobiographical essay *Pilgrimage to
Beethoven*, skillfully created "the shelf space and potential demand for a new product"—

that product being "'Beethoven'—as created by Wagner," which in the *Pilgrimage* is essentially endorsed by "Beethoven" himself (204).[2] For all its hyperbole, however, the influence of Wagner's *Beethoven* cannot be dismissed, especially for the ways in which it appropriates Beethoven's deafness—which Wagner saw as insulating Beethoven from "life's uproar." In Wagner's view, as Knittel puts it, "deafness afforded Beethoven protection" ("Wagner" 67). It enabled the "holy one" to retreat from "the hell of an existence filled with fearful discords" into "the paradise of his early harmony" (Wagner *Beethoven*, 26). And as Knittel adds, "Beethoven's ability to dwell in his inner world depended on severing his ties to the world of Appearance; it followed that those works Beethoven composed when he had entirely lost his hearing thus constituted his greatest achievements. His personal tragedy became a triumph for art" (67).

In *Beethoven*, Wagner casts the composer's deafness as "liberating," and claims that his third and latest style represented the height of his genius (24). He subsequently "abandoned his radical position on the composer's deafness and embraced a diametrically opposed view" only three years after publication of this essay (Knittel "Wagner," 25ff, 75). Yet Wagner's "liberation" version of Beethoven's deafness remains highly influential. Contemporary accounts such as Scott Burnham's are indicative of the power and longevity of the holy-hero-genius myth that such "liberation" produces.

We can see Wagner's enduring legacy in other landmark works, such as Theodor Adorno's *Beethoven* essay, a classic in the history of metaphysics, written to mark the centenary of the composer's birth, which romanticizes deafness in the name of "Beethoven," "the Genius of Music" and his "almost savage independence his whole life through: a stupendous sense-of-self, supported by the proudest spirit" (Knittel "'Late,'"; 19, 17). Adorno's *Beethoven* is not a single, coherent treatise on Beethoven's music, but a large number of fragments, notes that Adorno wrote to himself during the course of his never-completed Beethoven project. After Adorno's death, Rolf Tiedemann drew these notes together with additional materials, publishing the result in 1993 as Adorno's *Beethoven: The Philosophy of Music*.[3] Despite its complicated composition, it is a "treasure trove" (Spitzer 44) of Adorno's philosophical and musicological views on the composer. In it Adorno assimilates Beethoven's life and music to Hegelian philosophy. In fragments 24 and 25, for example, Adorno writes: "In a similar sense to that in which there is only Hegelian philosophy, in the history of western music there is only Beethoven," and "The will, the energy that sets form in motion in Beethoven, is always the *whole*, the Hegelian *World Spirit*" (Hegel 10).[4]

According to Hegel in his *Aesthetics*, hearing is the most ideal sense. It is "more ideal than sight" because it is more thoroughly interiorized, spiritualized, more "adequate to the inner life" (890–91). In idealized "hearing," the physical, "sensual" ear *disappears*, as it were, in favor of "presence," of the "inner life" of spirit—a motif that is essential to the heroic Beethoven myth of deafness-as-apotheosis. For Hegel, therefore, music plumbs "the depth of a person's inner life, as such; it is the art of the soul and is directly addressed to the soul" (891). For Adorno, following Hegel's view of idealized hearing, the "incomparable greatness and stature of Beethoven's work" (29) was by no means diminished by his deafness. On the contrary, as Adorno writes in Fragment 75: "It is conceivable that Beethoven actually *wanted* to go deaf—because he had already had a taste of the sensuous side of music as it is blared from our loudspeakers today" (31).[5]

In contrast to Wagner and Adorno, *Immortal Beloved* does not portray Beethoven's deafness as the apotheosis of his genius, the triumph of spirit over the merely physical dimensions of music, or of the deaf Beethoven over sensory sound. Quite the opposite,

Rose portrays Beethoven's deafness as the tragic fall earlier critics Marx and Oulibicheff claimed it to be. He gives us deafness as the key to the myth of Beethoven-as-Prometheus. Rose develops this portrayal by having Schindler visit and interview three women, each of whom the historical Beethoven actually knew and each of whom the fictionalized character of Schindler suspects may be the mysterious Immortal Beloved. Through these interviews, Schindler documents the progression of Beethoven's deafness and its devastating effects on his personal and artistic life.

The first candidate is the young and beautiful Countess Giulietta Guicciardi (Valeri Golino), who was a piano student of Beethoven's the year he composed his piano sonata Op. 27, the Moonlight Sonata. In a letter written in November 1801, Beethoven refers to the sixteen-year-old Countess as "a dear charming girl" with whom he was in love (Cooper "The Beethoven," 16). As Maynard Solomon puts it, Beethoven "had settled his affections" upon her, although the Countess herself, while she was flirting with Beethoven and delighting in her control over him, was actually more seriously involved with another composer, Count Wenzel Robert Gallenberg, with whom she had been intimate since 1800, and whom she married in 1803 (Solomon *Beethoven*, 196). After her marriage, the Countess and her husband left Vienna for Naples where they made their home (211). Scholarly evidence on the possible identity of Beethoven's Immortal Beloved eliminates Giulietta. At the time that Beethoven wrote to his Immortal Beloved in Karlsbad (dated July 6–7, later determined to be in the year 1812), the countess was living in Naples and firmly attached to another man. Nor was she known to be anywhere near Prague, where Beethoven implied that he and his beloved met immediately preceding his writing of the letter (211).

Nevertheless, Rose uses Giulietta to establish an inseparable link between deafness and a number of other psycho-social disorders on which the film elaborates in later sequences. In what has become one of the signature scenes of the film, Beethoven sits at a piano in the Guicciardi residence, preparing to play the Moonlight Sonata while Giulietta and her father hide in an alcove and listen. Before beginning, Beethoven lowers his head and rests it on the piano case so as to "hear" (feel the vibrations of) the notes he is about to play. The gesture discloses his deafness to Giulietta, who emerges weeping from her cover, approaching Beethoven from behind. In Lockwood's words: "Then suddenly the secret of his deafness is shockingly revealed when Giulietta taps him on the shoulder and unleashes his celebrated rage" (194). Discovered as deaf, he flies out of the Guicciardi residence in an uncontrollable fit of temper — the hearing-impaired hero, already on his way to some serious disability-related psycho-pathologies. This scene contradicts historical documentation that Beethoven's hearing loss was gradual in onset and not profound during his early and middle periods, certainly not in 1801. Rose uses the Guicciardi scene to depict that the composer's downfall-by-deafness was well underway by then, to generate a melodramatic story arc that is a vivid example of "Beethoven" characterization in the service of the Beethoven myth.

By the time Schindler arrives by coach in Hungary to interview his second candidate, Countess Anna Maria Erdödy (Isabella Rosellini), pathos has set in. Erdödy was a "most useful and valued" friend to Beethoven (Thayer-Forbes 415). But, "It is doubtful that there was any romantic element in [Beethoven's] relationship with the countess, whom he called his 'father confessor' (*Beichtvater*) and who was his advisor in personal and business affairs" (Solomon *Beethoven*, 201). Moreover, historical timing eliminates her as a candidate for the Immortal Beloved. While there is no evidence of how or when Beethoven's friendship with Erdödy began (Thayer 415), Rose chooses to make their first meeting into another "disclosure" scene. At the height of a public concert, the now-seriously-hearing-impaired Beethoven becomes disoriented, incapable of continuing at the piano or of leading the accompanying orchestra, his deafness exposed to an audience that is shocked, perplexed, possibly mocking. Erdödy, an audience member unknown to Beethoven, rises from her seat, walks elegantly forward, takes the arm of the humiliated and dazed composer, and leads him from the room. According to this now-fictional Erdödy, the two forge a friendship across the barrier of Beethoven's advanced deafness in which they converse through writing rather than speech. She tries to ameliorate his behavior, which has deteriorated *as a consequence of his deafness*, including his increasing displays of mistrust, volatile anger, and self-absorption, and his recourse to a brothel for physical intimacy. The film reinforces the disability-related melodramatic pathos of the Erdödy sequence by emphasizing the countess' brave suffering with her own physical impairment — a limp gained as a result of trauma. Historically, of course, these sequences are implausible, not the least because Beethoven's deafness is exaggerated in them. Beethoven and Erdödy's first meeting would have occurred between 1803 and 1808, a period in which his deafness and decline were not well underway.

Little is known of the early life of Schindler's third candidate, Johanna Reiss (Johanna Ter Steege), who was the daughter of Anton Reiss, a successful Viennese upholsterer. She married Beethoven's brother, Caspar Carl, on May 25, 1806, apparently without objection from Beethoven, and gave birth to their only son Karl less than four months later. Beethoven attributed the premature birth to his brother's immorality and folly (see Solomon "Beethoven" 299). Solomon represents Johanna as a lucid, capable, and intelligent woman, probably subjected to violent abuse by Caspar Carl, and at times also a peacemaker between him and his brother (300–01). There was conflict between the Beethoven brothers, but no lasting estrangement (299) and no single feud led to Caspar Carl's death. On at least one occasion Beethoven worked with Johanna to help Caspar Carl out of an economic emergency and "even claimed that he had acted as her protector during their marriage" (301–02). After Caspar Carl's death, Solomon suggests, Beethoven developed "a number of delusions," including that he began to believe that he *was* the physical father of Karl — perhaps even that he was married to Johanna (304). These "fantasies" can be seen as Beethoven's way of "contending with — or warding off— his desire" for Johanna, Solomon ventures. They constitute a "complex ruse that he unconsciously employed in order to remain enmeshed with his brother's widow" (305). Whether this was the case or not, Johanna may well have had special significance for the composer. He had a charged relationship with her as she became the "woman whom the real Beethoven despised more than any other" (Lockwood 193). In the end, she was also present at Beethoven's deathbed and funeral.

In keeping with the film's pattern of using the three candidates for the Immortal Beloved as vehicles for depicting the deaf hero's tragic fall, Rose alters the historical record with Johanna, using her to depict the tragic finale of Beethoven's fall and to construct a love story that increases its pathos. Through Johanna's conversation with Schindler and through the flashback scenes that this conversation narrates, Rose charts Beethoven's radical change from the vibrant young composer who gazes upon and seduces the beautiful Johanna in her father's upholstery establishment, to the frustrated, belligerent, isolated, disoriented, aging *deaf* man. In *Immortal Beloved*, Beethoven opposes his brother's marriage to Johanna, calling her a "whore" in another instance of his uncontrollable rage, brought on by his deafness (depicted to be profound in 1806). Believing he is Karl's biological father, he wrestles custody of Karl from Johanna after her husband's death, determined to make Karl into a great musician. Flashbacks of bitter legal guardianship proceedings show the humiliating spectacle of Karl publicly confirming Beethoven's inability to hear or understand Karl and his music, which provides another opportunity for the depiction of Beethoven's deafness-induced isolation and anger.

The film reveals Johanna to be the mystery woman who traveled to Karlsbad on July 6 or 7, 1812, to meet her lover Beethoven, although the historical Johanna was in fact in jail at the time (Solomon *Beethoven*, 300). Rose parallels shots of the cloaked Johanna's arrival in Karlsbad on a stormy night with shots of Beethoven pushing his delayed carriage, which had become mired in mud. Tragically, Johanna remains unaware of a letter Beethoven had sent ahead, which the hotel matron had delivered to her room on a silver tray, tucked underneath a napkin. Believing that Beethoven has jilted her, Johanna leaves. Arriving and finding himself alone, Beethoven believes the same and becomes violently distraught. The misunderstanding creates a lifelong enmity between the two. In the final deathbed scenes, which reveal an enfeebled Beethoven aged far beyond his fifty-six years, the fallen hero's deafness is foregrounded as he attempts to communicate one last time with Johanna, but can do so only by writing. Viewed in the context of the film's earlier flashbacks to the side-effects of Beethoven's deafness—isolation, depression, anxiety, bouts of uncontrollable rage if not madness, and not the least, aberrant sexual behavior—the closing scenes may well be "pure moonshine" (Lockwood 194). But they do belong nonetheless to the hero story, as Rose wants to tell it, a story in which deafness is rendered as the cause of the composer's creative downfall.

After Beethoven's death, as the film tells it, Johanna confesses to Schindler that she is the Immortal Beloved. Schindler ends their conversation by giving Johanna the letter. Reading it for the first time and realizing what happened that night, she sits gasping and sobbing at an open window as Schindler leaves. Her heartbreak renders the film's closing all the more poignant. Shots of Johanna at Beethoven's tombstone leave viewers with a tragic sense of what the destiny of this hero, free of deafness and its side-effects, might have been.

What Deafness?

No medical consensus is evident as to the type of deafness from which Beethoven suffered (Eadie 115–16). Nevertheless, this has not stopped generations of "musicologically-inclined physicians" from proposing diagnostic theories. While the medical histories of famous composers have improved in recent decades (Saffle 77), the literature on Beethoven is still replete with diagnostic oddities that serve various versions of the Beethoven myth. In Fragment 75 of his *Beethoven*, Adorno champions the theory of Julius Bahle (derived from the speculative reports of Romain Rolland and a Dr. Morage) that the composer's deafness was a result of his "immense inner concentration, his incessant auditory seeking and grasping," which led to "congestion of the blood in the inner ear and auditory centers, caused by overstrain of the organ through excessive concentration" (qtd. in Adorno 31). With this diagnosis, Adorno writes that "Beethoven had sacrificed himself on the altar of deafness in order 'to draw nearer than others to God, and from that vantage point to spread the divine radiance among mankind'" (31–32). Although Adorno's novel version of the Beethoven myth is well served by the diagnoses he cites, it is curious that he considers it to be medically credible. Beyond Adorno, others have suggested that Beethoven's deafness came and went, that it was at least in part contrived, or that it did not exist at all. Few if any critics who take it for granted that Beethoven was deaf, from whatever cause, demonstrate a good understanding of, or interest in, what the disability actually entails—a gap that contributes decisively to the Beethoven myth, including Bernard Rose's portrayal of it in *Immortal Beloved*.

Beethoven's deafness, neither an illness nor a disease, deserves far better critical and medical analysis than it has received. In light of current medical knowledge, one might wish for more rigorous assessment on the part of "musicologically-inclined physicians" (Saffle and Saffle 77). In their 1993 evaluation of many works on Beethoven's medical history, Michael and Jeffrey Saffle point out that the "single disorder" theory was prevalent among physicians until recently (85). The "single disorder" theory links Beethoven's deafness to the myriad of physical and psychological maladies he is claimed to have suffered, from diarrhea to promiscuity, such that deafness emerges as a key to understanding an overarching pathology. It still appears today, for example, in psychiatrist François Martin Mai's 2007 study, *Diagnosing Genius: The Life and Death of Beethoven.* Mai's book has been faulted for its musicological weaknesses, its biographical errors, and its inadequate coverage of the composer's illnesses (see Cooper "Review"). These errors and omissions allow Mai to make a number of mythologically potent connections between deafness and mental illness. Mai's contention that Beethoven suffered from bi-polarity, depression and solitude paints a picture of the composer in which hearing loss is intimately tied to a dissolute lifestyle, alcohol use, and psychiatric disorders. Clara Marvin suggests that Mai reminds us of "how often greatly creative personalities have endured serious physio- or psycho-pathologies and yet produced astounding work" (258). Yet epidemiologist and infectious disease specialist Philip A. Mackowiak contests Mai's theory that Beethoven's supposedly derelict lifestyle and his overuse of alcohol caused otosclerosis and the shriveling of his auditory nerves. As he states, "If papillary necrosis is associated with alcoholic liver disease or otosclerosis ever destroys the auditory nerves, the hepatologists and otolaryngologists with whom I consulted in writing this review are unaware of such connections" (391).

In one of the most recent Beethoven medical studies, *Beethoven in Person: His Deafness, Illnesses and Death,* gastroenterologist Peter J. Davies outlines twenty-one proposed causes of Beethoven's deafness that were published between 1816 and 1996, ultimately concluding that inflammation of the labyrinth was the likely cause of Beethoven's hearing loss. But this has not proved persuasive. As neurologist Mervyn Eadie argues, the labyrinthitis that was evident to the naked eye at Beethoven's autopsy was probably an acute condition of recent onset, something that would not explain progressive bilateral deafness (115). Cochlear failure, he ventures, is a better diagnostic guess — but only a guess, since confirmation of cochlear pathology "would have required microscopic examination of the inner ears while they remained intact in their bony surrounds," a procedure unavailable at the time of Beethoven's death (115–16).

Alexander Wheelock Thayer, although not a medical man himself, seems to me to have offered one of the least dubious, most succinct and plausible diagnoses yet, and despite the early date at which it was written, one that has withstood the test of time. In his famous biography of Beethoven, Thayer states quite simply that "the composer's loss of hearing was due to nerve- or perceptive-type deafness rather than to a conductive or bone type of hearing loss such as otosclerosis" (252). Nerve deafness is progressive, gradually limiting the pitch range of one's hearing. Hence the impossibility, as in Beethoven's case, of hearing a flute or stringed instrument before losing all hearing of speech sounds, particularly lower pitch speech sounds. With its gradual onset, nerve deafness often affords one an opportunity to develop (intentionally or not) lip reading skills (hence, perhaps, Beethoven's ability to converse with some people, particularly those whose mouths and speech patterns he knew well).

Nerve deafness is also consistent with the tinnitus symptoms from which Beethoven suffered (Morgenstern). And it accounts for some of the problems Beethoven had with such "hearing aids" as ear trumpets (Ealy), which both hasten residual hearing loss and contribute nothing to speech discrimination. They augment volume only, which often serves only to "blur" speech sounds, generating louder volumes that can induce the severe ear pain he experienced often enough. Ealy notes that a resonance device was of some use to Beethoven. This suggests, as some of his biographers have noted, that Beethoven may have relied significantly upon vibrations to "hear." One who suffers from nerve deafness can certainly continue to compose, play, and "listen" to his or her piano music, as Beethoven did himself, no doubt, through the perception of vibrations in relation to acoustic memory. It seems unlikely to me, as some of his early critics proposed, that one ever really loses "the memory of sound."[6]

Immortal Beloved appears to endorse the "single order" theory, depicting Beethoven's deafness as an all-encompassing disability associated with a range of aberrant behavioral and psychological features. "I think he is going mad," Karl tells Schindler in the film, with reference to Beethoven. Rose gives viewers a bleak picture of the years Karl spends with Beethoven, focusing on the composer's escalating physical and psychological decline as extreme, laden with pathos, and tied inextricably to his deafness. In these segments and throughout the film, Beethoven's deafness is always central, portrayed as the source of his frustration and that of those dealing with him. Yet, what deafness is this? Because Rose does not discriminate one type of deafness from another, presenting Beethoven's deafness as an amalgam, the film is medically, factually and narratively inconsistent in its representation of deafness.

Rose depicts against reliable documentation that by 1801, when he was tutoring Countess Giulietta, Beethoven was already profoundly deaf and suffering from (deafness-related) serious psychopathologies. But this depiction of Beethoven's hearing loss as catastrophic this early in the storyline and in Beethoven's life contradicts the film's larger narrative of the hero's progressive decline. Subsequent scenes with Countess Erdödy and flashbacks involving Johanna attempt to construct this progressive decline until Beethoven's pounding heartbeat is all that breaks his unremitting silence. In a climactic montage Rose even extends the arc of deafness back to the beginning of Beethoven's life by adding a shot of his abusive father boxing his ears, suggesting a medically and historically unfounded etiology for Beethoven's deafness in his childhood. It seems that Rose wants to have it both ways: deafness as sudden catastrophic onset and deafness as progressive hearing loss.

Moreover, in *Immortal Beloved,* deafness delivers such an immediate and absolute insularity that it omits many of the adaptations or learned skills that Beethoven might have employed as his hearing gradually faded, such as lip reading or any connection to his composed or performed music. On the other hand, Beethoven's deafness apparently requires a gradual resort to chalkboards and conversation books. Like the film's vacillations in its depiction of deafness, its extremes in the depiction of Beethoven's character in the service of the hero myth are also difficult to reconcile. The stark portrait Rose presents of the person Beethoven became as a result of his deafness, the aging, near-mad composer — abandoned, drunk and disoriented, assailed by a gang, and left to sleep on the street — contrasts without explanation with the film's opening scenes of the hero's great funeral procession. To acknowledge these inconsistencies, however, is to contest the dramatic-decline elements on which the film depends.

Conclusion

For more than 100 years one Beethoven biographer after another proposed a theory on the identity of the Immortal Beloved. In 1972, Maynard Solomon "in a brilliant piece of detective work, reconsidered the known facts, dated the letter unequivocally to the year

1812, and, to the satisfaction of almost everyone, settled the identity question: the woman in question was Antonie Brentano, wife of Franz and sister-in-law of Clemens and Bettina" (Lockwood 192). Indeed, Solomon's *Beethoven* includes a full chapter on the solution to the riddle of the Immortal Beloved. A few years before the first edition of this biography appeared, he also published an essay giving "New Light on Beethoven's Letter to an Unknown Woman." The case now seems to have been closed for more than forty years: Antonie Brentano remains the sole possibility. Antonie Brentano, however, does not appear in Rose's film.

My point is not so much to fault Rose's research on the identity of the Immortal Beloved, or the creative license through which, with Johanna, he may have achieved better dramatic effect. Rather, I suggest that the identity of the mystery woman is really incidental to his film. For *Immortal Beloved* is a disability drama, a film that has more to do with representing deafness than with attending to Beethoven's music or known details of his life. Like Richard Wagner, we might say, Rose neglects Beethoven's life and music in favor of the Beethoven myth. As much as Wagner, Rose idealizes the hero-figure, accentuating his decline by making deafness central to both aspects of this Promethean story — the heroism and the fall. The film's appropriation of disability is unfortunate, although not atypical in Beethoven studies. If anything, the film serves as a case study of the distortions involved in collapsing aesthetics and biography into disability myth.

Notes

1. Immanuel Kant, in his *Anthropology from a Pragmatic Point of View*, maintains that a person born deaf "never arrives at real concepts" and at best can attain only "an analogon" of reason (51–52).

2. In his *Pilgrimage to Beethoven*, Wagner relates the fictional meeting of the protagonist "R" with Beethoven, describing the composer's appearance (clad in untidy house-clothes, disordered, long, and bushy grey hair, gloomy forbidding expression — and deafness): "I knew of Beethoven's deafness, and had prepared myself for it. Nevertheless it was like a stab through my heart when I heard his hoarse and broken words, 'I cannot hear.' [...] That moment gave me the key to Beethoven's exterior, the deep furrows on his cheeks, the somber dejection of his look, the set defiance of his lips — he heard not!" (38). Conversation at the meeting takes place by way of paper and pencil (38–39). Rose's script bears resemblance to Wagner's [fictional] description of Beethoven in *Pilgrimage*.

3. *Beethoven* is not a book that Adorno wrote and therefore must be approached with caution. All of the notes were intended for Adorno himself, and the sequence of their production is not that of their arrangement ("Editor's Preface" ix).

4. Colin Sample puts the point succinctly: "It is Hegel who forms for Adorno the deepest philosophical parallel with Beethoven" (382).

5. It would be fruitful to relate Adorno's interpretation of Beethoven's deafness to his writing on the phonograph and sound-recording technology, a study that, as far as I know, has not yet been done. For such an endeavor, Barbara Engh's essay on Adorno's "The Curves of the Needle" might provide a provocative point of departure, one that would bring sexual difference into the study of the historical ties of disability to "artificial" sound or "mechanical" music: Engh notes in her essay that Adorno in "The Curves" makes the "strange assertion" that "a woman's singing voice cannot be recorded well, because it demands the presence of her body. A man's voice is able to carry on in the absence of his body, because his self is identical to his voice; his body disappears" (120; see also Levin).

6. Even a critic as astute as K. M. Knittel is disappointing in her discussion of possible dates on which the public first became aware of Beethoven's hearing impairment, and on extant knowledge of his hearing loss progression, because she leaves all critical questioning aside ("Wagner"). Although no decisive date emerges as to when Beethoven's hearing loss became publicly known, Knittel considers a number of possibilities: the *Heiligenstadt Testament* (1802) was not known to the public until it was published in 1827; in 1816, the *Allgemeine musikalische Zeitung* informed readers of Beethoven's troubles; in 1828 the *Allgemeine Theaterzeitung und Unterhaltungsblatt* published Beethoven's 1801 letter to Franz Wegeler, in which he admitted that he had difficulty hearing; and, probably in 1826, Gerhard von Breuning recounted testing

Beethoven's hearing "by playing loudly on the piano when the composer's back was turned, which suggests that he did not believe Beethoven was truly deaf. He also reported a rumor circulating in Vienna that 'the great composer's hearing organs were only deaf to speech and noise, but not to music'" (58).

Why, in an essay that concerns itself centrally with deafness, does Knittel offer no comment on von Breuning's diagnoses, as if concurring with him that a "deaf" person cannot know, when his or her back is turned, that a piano is being played loudly? And why not respond to the suggestion that Beethoven was deaf to speech (and noise?) but not to music? More importantly, as Knittel goes on to document varying opinions on the progression of Beethoven's deafness, she either concurs with, or refrains from commenting on, the material she presents. Why would we assume that, once Beethoven began to use the Conversation Books in 1818, he could no longer hear speech (59)? Might he have been able to hear speech imperfectly, depending on the speaker? And if so, might this have contributed to the differing opinions Knittel outlines — disagreements on the part of eyewitnesses as to the severity of the impairment, as to the day-to-day changes in Beethoven's hearing, and as to his ability to hear, and converse with, persons with whom he was familiar (59)? If perceptions of Beethoven's deafness were incidental to reception of his late style, assessments of the kind and severity of his hearing loss might not be that important — but of course, this is not the case Knittel wants to make.

Works Cited

Adorno, Theodor W. *Beethoven: The Philosophy of Music*. Trans. Edmund Jephcott. Ed. Rolf Tiedemann. Stanford: Stanford University Press, 1993. Print.

Burnham, Scott. *Beethoven Hero*. Princeton: Princeton University Press, 1995. Print.

Cooper, Barry, "Review of *Diagnosing Genius: The Life and Death of Beethoven*." *Music & Letters* 90.1 (Feb. 2009): 156–58. Print.

___, ed. *The Beethoven Compendium*. London: Thames and Hudson, 1991. Print.

Dennis, David B. *Beethoven in German Politics: 1870–1989*. New Haven: Yale University Press, 1996. Print.

Eadie, Mervyn J. "Review of *Beethoven in Person: His Deafness, Illnesses and Death*." *Health and History* 4.1 (2002): 113–116. Print.

Ealy, George Thomas. "Of Ear Trumpets and a Resonance Plate: Early Hearing Aids and Beethoven's Hearing Perception." *19th Century Music* 17.3 (Spring 1994): 262–273. Print.

Engh, Barbara. "Adorno and the Sirens: Tele-phono-graphic Bodies." *Embodied Voices: Representing Female Vocality in Western Culture*. Eds. Leslie C. Dunn and Nancy A. Jones. Cambridge: Cambridge University Press, 1994. 120–135. Print.

Hegel, G. W. F. *Aesthetics: Lectures On Fine Art. Vol. II*. Trans. T. M. Knox. Oxford: Clarendon Press, 1975. Print.

Immortal Beloved. Dir. Bernard Rose. Perf. Gary Oldman, Jeroen Krabbé and Isabella Rossellini. Columbia Pictures, 1994. Film.

Knittel, Kristin M. "'Late,' Last, and Least: On Being Beethoven's Quartet in F Major, Op. 135." *Music and Letters* 87.1 (Jan. 2006): 16–51. Print.

_____. "Wagner, Deafness, and the Reception of Beethoven's Late Style." *Journal of the American Musicological Society* 51.1 (Spring 1998): 49–82. Print.

Kant, Immanuel. *Anthropology from a Pragmatic Point of View*. Trans. Robert B. Louden. Cambridge: Cambridge University Press, 2006. Print.

Levin, Thomas Y. "For the Record: Adorno on Music in the Age of Its Technological Reproducibility." *October* 55 (1990): 23–48. Print.

Lockwood, Lewis. "Film Biography as Travesty: 'Immortal Beloved' and Beethoven." *The Musical Quarterly* 81.2 (Summer 1997): 190–98. Print.

Mackowiak, Philip A. "Review of *Diagnosing Genius: The Life and Death of Beethoven*." *Journal of the History of Medicine and Allied Sciences* 63.3 (July 2008): 390–92. Print.

Mai, François Martin. *Diagnosing Genius: The Life and Death of Beethoven*. Montréal: McGill-Queen's University Press, 2007. Print.

Marvin, Clara. "Review of *Diagnosing Genius: The Life and Death of Beethoven*." *University of Toronto Quarterly* 78.1 (Winter 2009): 256–258. Print.

Maslin, Janet. "The Music Almost Tells the Tale." *The New York Times* (16 Dec. 1994): C4. Print.

Morgenstern, Leon. "The Bells Are Ringing: Tinnitus in their own words." *Perspectives in Biology and Medicine* 48.3 (Summer 2005): 396–407. Print.

Plantinga, Leon. *Romantic Music: A History of Musical Style in Nineteenth-Century Europe*. New York: W.W. Norton, 1984. Print.

Saffle, Michael, and Jeffrey R. Saffle. "Medical Histories of Prominent Composers: Recent Research and Discoveries." *Acta Musicologica* 65.2 (July–Dec. 1993): 77–101. Print.

Sample, Colin. "Adorno on the Musical Language of Beethoven." *The Musical Quarterly* 78.2 (Summer 1994): 378–93. Print.

Solomon, Maynard. "New Light on Beethoven's Letter to an Unknown Woman." *The Musical Quarterly* 58.4 (Oct. 1972): 572–587. Print.

_____. *Beethoven.* New York: Schirmer Books, 2001. Print.

Spitzer, Michael. *Music As Philosophy: Adorno and Beethoven's Late Style.* Bloomington: Indiana University Press, 2006. Print.

Stanley, J. Glenn. "Review of *Beethoven Hero.*" *Journal of the American Musicological Society* 50.2–3 (Summer–Autumn 1997): 464–483. Print.

Subotnik, Rose Rosengard. "Adorno's Diagnosis of Beethoven's Late Style: Early Symptoms of a Fatal Condition." *Journal of the American Musicological Society* 29.2 (Summer 1976): 242–275. Print.

Thayer, Alexander Wheelock. *Life of Beethoven.* Rev. and ed. Elliot Forbes. Princeton: Princeton University Press, 1967. Print.

Vazsonyi, Nicholas. "Beethoven Instrumentalized: Richard Wagner's Self-Marketing and Media Image." *Music and Letters* 89.2 (May 2008): 195–211. Print.

Wagner, Richard. *Beethoven.* Trans. William Ashton Ellis. Whitefish, MT: Kessinger, 2006. Print.

Witkin, Robert W. *Adorno On Music.* New York: Routledge, 1998. Print.

_____. *Pilgrimage to Beethoven and Other Essays.* Trans. William Ashton Ellis. Lincoln: University of Nebraska Press, 1994. Print.

"This isn't something I can fake"

The Discourse of Disability Surrounding *Glee!*

KATIE ELLIS

Social media allows communities to form quickly and communicate effectively. Communities share common interests, such as a favourite TV show.

— Antony Mayfield

[Watching Glee] makes me want to throw a big Slushee at my TV.

— Mina Asayesh-Brown

Fox Broadcasting's musical comedy-drama series *Glee!* (2009-present) features a competitive glee club at the fictional William McKinley High School in Lima, Ohio. Many of the characters in the club are disabled by the social world of high school: Kurt Hummel (Chris Colfer) is gay, Rachel Berry (Lea Michele) is an overachieving Jewish girl with two gay dads, gothic Tina Cohen-Chang (Jenna Ushkowitz) (supposedly) stutters and is also of Asian descent, and Mercedes Jones (Amber Riley) is overweight and black. Several more characters in the series are actually disabled, experiencing bodily impairment, including club member Artie Abrams (Kevin McHale), Becky Jackson (Laura Potter), a cheerleader, and the cheerleading coach Sue Sylvester's (Jane Lynch) elder sister Jean Sylvester (Robin Trocki). Guest stars have included a Deaf glee club from the fictional Haverbrook School for the Deaf ("Hairography," season 1, episode 11) and Sean Fretthold (Zack Weinstein), a high school footballer who sustained a spinal cord injury ("Laryngitis" season 1, episode 18). Such a popular show with both series regulars and guest characters with disability requires a critical interrogation, particularly since it has generated an online engagement from both mainstream media and bloggers identifying as disability activists. From its first episode, *Glee!* has drawn accusations of tokenism, particularly with regard to "Wheels" (season 1, episode 9), which incited a particularly vocal response for its examination of accessibility issues. My aim in this essay is to offer a critical analysis of the representation of disability in "Wheels" while exploring the discourses of disability that have emerged in online conversation around this episode. A consideration of narrative as well as style and *mise en scène* provides a comprehensive overview of the ways disability is culturally constructed within visual texts (Ellis 36) while an exploration of the critical response demonstrates the ways disability operates within culturally based paradigms (Quinlan and Bates 64). Blogging has created many possibilities for community creation amongst people with disability by providing an opportunity to further social movements of disability in ways that reflect their everyday experiences (Goggin and Noonan 165). While disability bloggers, for example on the popular culture blog *Feminists With Disabilities*, mobilized to respond negatively to the depiction of disability in "Wheels," the mainstream media interpreted the images of disability in this episode quite differently (Sheppard). Criticism of disability bloggers' claims that "Wheels" perpetuates disabling attitudes and stereotypes suggests that disability is still imagined by many viewers in culturally dominant ways that reflect the marginalization of disability on television and in other media. As a result, alternative views that critique these mainstream patterns of perception and narrative representation or that seek to improve the social position of people with disability may be strongly resisted.

Each episode of *Glee!* centers on a lesson or assignment given to members of the glee club by their teacher Will Schuester (Matthew Morrison). In "Wheels" the lesson is concerned with "accessibility." Will urges the group to go back to basics in their musical numbers because the judges at the sectional competition, at which they're about to compete, like "accessible songs"—ones they already know. Disability emerges as a narrative subplot from this central concept. Artie is unable to join the rest of the club in taking a bus to the sectionals because the club can't afford the $600 per week required to rent a "handicapable bus." Principal Figgins (Iqbal Theba) is characteristically unsympathetic, stating that Artie should be adept at overcoming obstacles. The rest of the glee club's reaction is that Artie's father will drive him, like he always does. Will insists the bus ride is an important team building experience in which Artie should be included. This leads to Artie's first solo number in the series, Billy Idol's "Dancing with Myself." In a visual style not unlike other solos by Rachel, Finn Hudson (Cory Monteith) or Quinn Fabray (Dianna Agron) featured in previous episodes, Artie is constructed as alienated and separated from everyone else throughout this solo. Arguably, in this instance a disabled character is represented in the same way as nondisabled characters. Nevertheless, the individualization of disability enacted through the characterization of Artie perpetuates many culturally disabling aspects of television representations of disability.

Disability on Television

Johnson Cheu suggests that critical analysis of the representational system of disability reveals the cultural discourses behind our understanding of disability (199). If we come to understand the social and cultural constructions of disability, especially in relation to stigma, then we are able to perceive that disability is more than a medicalized bodily impairment. Disability is the restriction of activity and denial of inclusion imposed on people who have impairments. The definition of disability as social oppression advanced by disability theorists such as Oliver (22) can be expanded to include images, characters and narratives that encourage negative attitudes towards disability. Early (Longmore) and recent (Richardson) disability scholarship has focused on the perpetuation of stereotypes, including for example the "evil disabled monster" figure (Richardson 176) and the overcoming all odds character who triumphs over physical limitations. The frequency of "evil avenger" and "supercripple" images of disability on television contributes to the underrepresentation and distorted representation of people with disability as these images are both inaccurate and unfair (Harnett 21). As disability media scholarship identifies persisting stereotypes of disability, it demonstrates that the media may function as a form of cultural oppression (Barnes 19).

Another trope that runs throughout much of the popular press and disability media scholarship is the discourse of normality. For example, Longmore suggests that advertising that depicts people with disability within paradigms of normal everyday life signifies a representational breakthrough on television. Positive images of people with disability who are "attractive, active, and *with it,* involved and competitive, experiencing 'normal' relationships [...] and smart about what they buy" negates the ubiquitous helpless and dependent stereotypes (Longmore 78). Guy Cumberbatch and Ralph Negrine argue that people with disability should be presented as part of ordinary life, not alien to it and that social change will occur when people with disability become among the leading characters on television because disability would come to be seen by the general public as an ordinary experience (141). Barnes, however, contends that depictions of people with disability as "normal" do not recognize the way social attitudes and organizational practices disable people who have bodily impairments. He argues that presenting people with disability as normal "perpetuates widespread ignorance about the realities of impairment" (18).

Social modelists suggest that the representation of disability on screen should challenge discrimination in overt ways. But would these ways involve "normalizing" disability within existing nondisabled environments or depicting the chasm between cultural constructions of "normal" and of "disability" alongside the realities of lived experience? When Artie is featured with any significance on *Glee!* he appropriates normality and his social alienation is attributed to being a teenaged outcast rather than a person with a disability. As blogger Gerrick Kennedy writes, "Him being in a wheelchair has zero to do with his personality, and as a viewer you don't notice it — and not that the kids didn't care because they loved him. They just never took the time to think how hard being disabled could be because Artie doesn't make it seem so bad after all." Kennedy's interpretation suggests that for some viewers Artie does embrace the ordinary. However, as Artie's characterization individualizes disability and does not address social discrimination it is unlikely that social change will occur through his mere presence as a positively viewed series main character.

Characters with disability have appeared among leading figures on television, but they represent less than 1 percent of series regulars (Gay). Although series regular characters with disability remain rare, disability itself frequently appears in various culturally determined ways. Cumberbatch and Negrine's study of six weeks of prime–time television highlighted stereotypes and revealed a stark contrast between the portrayal of disability and that of other social issues in many televisual genres (140). Audiences of people with disability have long noticed the frequent appearance of characters with disability on screen in stereotypical roles (Ross 669). Karen Ross' 1997 investigation of the perspectives of viewers with disability in "But Where's Me in It?: Disability, Broadcasting and the Media" was intended to balance the emphasis on content-analysis studies within disability studies. The participants in her study focused on common stereotypes of people with disability as criminals or outcasts, especially within soap operas. The participants saw these images as contributing to their social marginalization (Ross 669). As people with disability represent a disparate group with diverse perspectives, more recent analysis of disability on television has followed Ross' lead by turning to a consideration of audience response as articulated on Internet forums (see Johnson and Quinlan and Bates).

This essay takes *Glee!* as a case study because of the popularity *Glee!* has garnered amongst international audiences who meet online to discuss the issue of disability. The show has been honored with six Teen Choice awards, four Golden Globes and six Emmy Awards. It has been nominated for more than fifty other media awards and praised for its sensitive treatment of disability, including an interrogation of access issues in "Wheels." As *E!* columnist and television personality Kristin dos Santos writes, "'*Wheels*' is all about empowering people with disabilities and sends out an uplifting message to the disabled community. It should also be noted that the series now has a recurring character with Down syndrome, which I don't think has happened on network TV in a very long time." While the mainstream media found the portrayals in "Wheels" sensitive (Kennedy, dos Santos), disability bloggers almost unanimously criticized the episode as ableist in motivation, finding that it reinforces ableist myths surrounding the experience of disability that distort its representation. As blogger Wheelchair Dancer writes:

> So many of the newspaper articles call this episode of *Glee* a "game-changer." I don't see that immediately. It strikes me most clearly that *"Wheels"* is an example of lousy script writing, the usual inspirational over-acting, and pathetic choreography. It changes nothing; indeed, it only reinforces the able-bodied world's ideas about disability.

Throughout this chapter blogs written by Wheelchair Dancer, s.e.smith and Anna (from FWD—*Feminists with Disabilities*) have been selected for consideration as all three bloggers are prolific in the disability blogosphere. Their perspectives are often referred to in both academic and mainstream publications and hyperlinked on other blogs. Responses to "Wheels" by Kristin dos Santos on *E! Online* and Gerrick Kennedy in *The Los Angeles Times* are examined as representative of mainstream media and popular culture views. Taken together, these publications are considered in this discussion as indicative responses because they form what Benkler describes as a "cluster" within the blogosphere (252). A cluster emerges when a number of blogs on the same topic appear. Sites within a cluster become highly connected through hyperlinks and work together to filter views deemed relevant by the community. These clusters become highly specific in their views as groups of people with common interests to join together under "superstar" blogs. Superstar blogs such as Wheelchair Dancer, Feminists with Disability, *E! Online* and the *Los Angeles Times* articulate dominant views and create "shortcuts to wide attention" (Benkler 13). I also draw on academic interrogations of disability on screen to explore the ways television contributes to social disablement.

"Wheels": Narrative & Critical Response

Although Artie has been visible since the pilot episode he was not given a significant role, beyond the occasional one-liner, until "Wheels," which appears halfway through the first season. While Rachel's, Mercedes' and Kurt's auditions for the glee club at the beginning of the series gave insight into their personalities, Artie's audition wasn't given screen time. Disability bloggers have found the storyline tokenistic and argued that ultimately the episode actually did not focus on Artie; it focused primarily on the able-bodied characters. Conversely, Artie's absence from major storylines was not seen as much of an issue by journalist and *Los Angeles Times* blogger Gerrick Kennedy, who focused on the disappointment expressed within the disability blogosphere instead of the length of time it took to give Artie a storyline or the way in which his experiences are arguably stereotyped or used to achieve certain symbolic representations. Kennedy laments giving press coverage to disability activists' responses, believing it takes away from the sensitivity of the episode: "The episode, simply titled *"Wheels,"* finally addressed Artie's (brilliantly played by Kevin McHale) challenge of living life in a wheelchair. But of course we know in Hollywood that nothing you do is correct."

"Wheels" takes its name from one of the central plot conflicts of the episode: that the glee club will be enjoying the bonding experience of riding to sectionals on an inaccessible bus without Artie — their wheels and Artie's wheelchair are not compatible — and from the finale number that the group performs at sectionals in which Artie and Mercedes solo while the club sings their way through "Defying Gravity" from the musical *Wicked* while dancing a choreographed routine using wheelchairs.

When Artie admits to the group that he wants to ride on the bus with them to sectionals, Will announces that everyone in the Glee club must spent three hours each day in wheelchairs he has purchased from a tag sale being held by a local nursing home. He says this will offer them an insight into Artie's daily struggles. He also tells them that they must hold a bake sale to raise the funds needed to rent an accessible bus. The irony that the school cannot afford to rent a bus yet can afford to purchase wheelchairs for use by each member is left unexplained.

As the enthusiastic Glee club members embark on their wheelchair adventures a montage of everything being just out of reach follows — Rachel is unable to reach the lunch tray and Finn is hit in the face by sporting equipment attached to walking students' school bags. When Tina, on whom Artie is sweet, tells him that she didn't realize what his experience must be like with a disability, Artie draws a connection between his paralysis and her stuttering, only to have Tina confess that she'd been faking the stutter since seventh grade as a result of being too shy to want to interact with others. Artie clearly feels betrayed — taken in by someone he thought understood him because she also experiences an authentic impairment. He responds: "This isn't something I can fake." Eventually the glee club members are united at the end of episode in solidarity with Artie as they perform their "Defying Gravity" routine, which the DVD synopsis calls "their most unusual number" to date, using the wheelchair dancing skills he's ostensibly taught them.

The episode is arguably problematic in several different ways. First, Artie's "This isn't something I can fake" response, which is the most emotionally poignant moment of the episode, sits in stark contrast to the "disability drag" (Siebers) of the able-bodied actor Kevin McHale's performance as Artie (he is, in fact, faking it). As David Kociemba writes:

> When Kevin McHale's Artie says in this episode, "This isn't something I can fake," it has a doubled meaning. The experience of disability for the character isn't something he can fake because disability is located in social barriers, not individual physical impairments. But McHale is faking the mobility impairment. Woodlee [the choreographer] is faking dance choreography informed by disability culture, and badly. Clearly, the creators don't believe the lines they wrote, because they reinforce those social barriers for actors with mobility impairments and erase disability culture while pretending to celebrate it. "*Wheels*" reveals that its creators think that there's nothing very special for mainstream audiences to learn from the experience of those with disabilities in their Very Special Episode.

Secondly, the episode is problematic insofar as it attempts to raise awareness about disability by concentrating on what the restriction of activity entailed in using a wheelchair means to the able-bodied members of the group and the ways they exploit it, rather than on Artie's experiences. Inviting people without disability to spend a period of time in a wheelchair is a popular "disability awareness" training exercise that is tokenistic and ignores the realities of life using a wheelchair. Further, Wheelchair Dancer describes the show's choreography for the "Defying Gravity" number as reinforcing non-wheelchair users' misinterpretation of the competitive sport of wheelchair dancing:

> The one potentially interesting move that McHale supposedly "does" is a cut — he wheelies on one rear wheel. The rest is notable only for the way that it shows that able-bodied, non-wheelchair-using folk really do think of chairs as bicycles you move with your arms. There's absolutely no body-chair integration at all. They think of sitting in a chair as being only about

not being able to move their legs (and in Artie's case as being about having his hips and legs twisted to one side). That mistaken understanding leads to some very weird looking people in chairs. *On chairs* would be a better phrase for it. The fake paralysis of their legs somehow wends its way up their bodies so that they are really only able to push with their elbows (no wonder they have sore arms!).

For Wheelchair Dancer, the dancing "sucks."

Throughout "Wheels," the able bodied members of the glee club are constructed as socially disconnected. In relation to other students they are the quintessential high school out-group sitting in wheelchairs behind a bake sale table. Amongst themselves they are divided from the viewer's point of view by lies and bullying (Quinn is busy scamming Finn), inauthenticity and duplicity (Tina's stutter), disparities in popularity within the club (Rachel is less liked than Kurt), and unshared social stigma (Kurt silently throws his audition for his dream role when his father receives a threat targeting Kurt's homosexuality). Nevertheless, even at the end of the episode Artie's experience of disability continues to be individualized, making him the most socially separated peer as the other club members sit as a unified group in the auditorium to give Will the money they have made from their bake sale. While everyone else sits closely together on chairs, Artie remains isolated by inaccessible stairs that separate him from the rest of the group. Martin F. Norden describes this as a common use of environment to separate characters with disability in film: "[Directors] have used the basic tools of their trade—framing, editing, sound, lighting, set design elements (e.g., fences, windows, staircase banisters) to suggest physical or symbolic separation of disabled characters from the rest of society" (1).

Artie's separation from the other glee club members both physically and symbolically is reinforced when he decides to use the money for wheelchair access to the auditorium instead of the handicapable bus and have his father drive him to the sectionals. The lessons the group supposedly learned about accessibility and exclusion are quickly forgotten as they express relief that they won't have to carry Artie in and out of the auditorium, rather than disappointment that he will miss out on their team building bus ride. (In previous episodes Artie is carried up and down the stairs of the auditorium by Noah "Puck" Puckerman, played by Mark Salling, and Mike Chang, played by Harry Shum, Jr.) Despite this act for the "greater good" Artie is actually able to ride the bus due to an unexpected charitable donation from Sue Sylvester.

Sue's financing of accessible transportation for the glee club seems wildly out of character, especially since the episode features her opposition to Principal Figgins' accessibility initiatives. When Will realizes the only wheelchair entrance to the school is on the far side of campus, he takes his complaint to Principal Figgins who decides that Sue Sylvester, coach of the Cheerios cheerleading squad and Glee Club nemesis, must hold open auditions to appear more "accessible." Surprisingly, after humiliating everyone who auditions, Sue invites Becky, a girl with Down syndrome, onto the squad. Sue's strange change of heart is explained at the end of the episode when we learn that her older sister Jean has Down syndrome. This sister adds another dimension to the character of Sue as Jane Lynch articulates: "Sue Sylvester's sister, we find out has Down syndrome and is in a home, yes, so it's a more touching episode and we get to see a softer side of Sue" (Eastman). Presumably her donation for Artie's "handicapable" bus demonstrates that softer side, directly crediting reasonable environmental adaptation and basic civic inclusion to the admirable largesse of the nondisabled, thereby providing a feel-good ending for nondisabled viewers.

Prolific disability blogger s.e. smith saw the character of Becky as a continuation of this episode's exercise in tokenism:

Hiring an actress with Down syndrome for a single throwaway guest role is not including actors with disabilities. Centering a disability plot around able bodied characters is not including people with disabilities. Continuing to use crip drag (and having the actor unabashedly say "this isn't something I can fake") is not including people with disabilities.

Although Becky has in fact become a reoccurring character, smith's critique is still valid as Becky effectively functions as a character foil, providing viewers with more information about Sue Sylvester, an able-bodied character. Becky herself remains undeveloped; she is not afforded narratives focusing on her own experiences. When the media adopt these character portrayal techniques, disability is individualized as a narrative shortcut that relies on stereotypes and prejudicial attitudes (Ellis 53). s.e. smith's critique of "Wheels" tied the appropriation of disability characters in the episode to larger patterns of tokenistic dealing with minority groups:

> It hit a number of major tropes for pretty much a hat trick of disability fail. We got "disability is inspiring," "disability is a burden," "appropriation of disability for a Very Special Learning Experience," "faking disability," and "see my sister has a disability so I'm not a bigot." Here's the thing about tokenization, which is what this episode specialized in: It does nothing to advance the cause of people who live in marginalized bodies.... Painting accessibility as a hardship, a burden, and "special treatment" is also not including people with disabilities.

The tropes that smith highlights are frequently seen on television and have permeated cultural understandings of what the experience of disability is. Characters with disability are often one dimensional and used for emotional appeal, symbolism and dramatic effect (Harnett 21) and in turn are naturalized and adopted unproblematically by the media and viewers. A cultural interrogation of these issues within the disability blogosphere is crucial in offering a more nuanced cultural understanding of disability. To take one of smith's examples, disability as burden reinforces the assumption that people with disability are dependant and a drain on resources:

> The origins of social problems are located in the 'damaged' body, and society is absolved of responsibility. Meeting the differing needs of people who have impairments is viewed as a drain on resources by this stereotype. The character that is caring for the disabled character [often acts] as the site of burden. These characterisations are designed to bestow carers with 'saintly' qualities such as self-sacrifice [...] The disabled character is used to provide information about the more important able-bodied characters, ultimately perpetuating the belief that "society would be better off without disabled people" [Ellis 34].

Artie is constructed as somewhat of a burden to the rest of the glee club in "Wheels," both logistically (as he has to be carried up stairs into the auditorium for rehearsals) and emotionally (because they are expected by Will and by viewers to be touched by his condition). Kennedy implicitly recognizes this when he writes that his own "heart broke into little pieces when watching the kids be so passive to Artie and his issues." Yet the decision to structure the episode around the accessibility obstacles experienced by *able bodied* characters obscures the ways in which Artie's "issues" are created by a disabling world. The fact that Tina, the only other member of the glee club with a physical impairment, admits in this episode in a one-on-one conversation with Artie that she fakes her stutter to get out of stressful social situations and schoolwork further characterizes disability as a personal problem located (or not) in the individual. A challenging consideration of the social constructedness of disability is absent, despite the larger thematic focus on accessibility.

smith's arguments regarding crip drag in particular circulated the blogosphere, appearing on *This Aint Livin, Bitch Media* and *Feminists with Disabilities. The Guardian* also published a smith opinion piece. While some mainstream press articles covered smiths' and other disability bloggers' collective disappointment that an actor without disability had been cast in the role (Sheppard), others commenting on these sites failed to grasp the significance of crip drag. Below is an indicative comment:

> I'm not quite understanding the beef with "crip drag." It seems to me if you're going to have an issue with a non-disabled person playing the role of a disabled person, you cannot appreciate any level of acting because all acting is a lie. Maybe that's why it's called acting. Just sayin. So, you should also be up in arms about the actress who is portraying the pregnant teen because she's not pregnant in real life, and likewise, you should also feel your feathers ruffled by the cheerleading coach because she's not a coach in real life. See where I'm a-going with this? ["Anonymous" comment on smith "Glee"].

smith's and Wheelchair Dancer's analyses were also criticized by Kennedy whose response perpetuates the major tropes of disability smith is so critical of:

> I was very disheartened to see advocates for the disabled in an uproar about the episode. Here we have an episode bluntly addressing the complexities of disability and doing so with so much respect and dignity, and there are complaints about Artie not being wheelchair-bound in real life? [...] Must we always reach so far in Hollywood? [...] Acting is acting [Kennedy].

Kennedy suggests that the disappointment amongst the disability blogosphere has taken mainstream media attention away from the "boldness of the episode." It is true that several news articles concentrated on the activists' disappointment that a disabled actor was not cast in the role rather than on the content of the episode (see Grigsby Bates, Davis, Elber). Kennedy's indignation that people with disability would complain about the use of disability in a show that so clearly emotionally resonates with nondisabled viewers reveals the social pressure placed on people with disability to accept their disempowered social position by deferring to mainstream views. By comparison, Kennedy's article is a prominent example of the way mainstream media approaches disability with a condescending tone. Critiques of the disability bloggers' response to "Wheels" were combined with comments from the cast and crew of *Glee!* and spun to generate more publicity for the series. However, disability bloggers remained vocal in the debate and used the opportunity to interrogate images of disability on television:

> I didn't feel "empowered" by *Glee*, nor did most of the women with disabilities that I know. That said, my goal here isn't to tell you or anyone you know how to feel about the show. My objection [...] is not only the condescending tone and dismissal of everything that people who actually work in the industry are saying about representations of disability and how that *affects their work*, but also being told how I should feel about the show [Anna].

Conclusion

With the widespread popularity of Internet forums, Facebook fan pages, popular culture blogs, and twitter hashtags, watching television now involves a creative engagement with multiple screens. According to Margaret Quinlan and Benjamin Bates, one of the significant factors to emerge from the growth of audience blogging is that it captures both "empowering and disempowering potentialities" (64) regarding disability in the media. Through an analysis of blogger discourse regarding Heather Mills' appearance on *Dancing with the Stars,* Quinlan and Bates argue that disabling social values embedded in these exchanges are absorbed by the audience. Despite this, blogging also provides disability more media attention and allows people with disability a voice in debates from which they are usually excluded

(Haller 1). The availability of blogger responses to television representations of disability has implications for academic discussions of disability and television. Where previous theorization has largely been based upon the experience of a select group of disability scholars, we now have easy access to what a wide (albeit self-selected) spectrum of viewers with and without disabilities actually thinks about the way disability features on television.

Communities that emerge around similar interests such as television shows can be seen in the online conversations surrounding *Glee*. Similarly, people with disability have mobilized online to unite in their disappointment with *Glee*'s representation of disability. With its musical form and plot *Glee!* promised to be something very different from the usual narrative set in a high school. It has become a popular cultural phenomenon. This essay examined mainstream media and blogger responses to "Wheels" (season 1, episode 9) in order to explore the ways in which disability marginalization is both embraced and refuted by the audience and the resulting social media conversation amongst those with differing points of view. The episode received critical acclaim and numerous awards. A critical disability analysis of both the episode itself and the cultural criticism surrounding it allows us to consider discourses of disability that appear in the media.

Embraced as a "sensitive" portrayal of disability by mainstream media and bloggers, cultural commentators active in the disability blogosphere have slammed "Wheels" as exploitative, ableist and tokenistic. This in turn has led to passionate debate regarding the role of disability criticism. While some see this criticism as overshadowing the importance of the episode as a positive representation of disability (Kennedy), others emphasize the importance of offering a disability critical point of view (s.e. smith). As for Artie, following "Wheels" he returns to the background for most of season 1 until "Dream On," another highly controversial depiction of disability. "Dream On" sees Artie imagine that he has been cured and is able to achieve his dream of being a dancer. Although recognizing that some people with disability do dream of a miraculous cure, this episode is problematic because, like "Wheels," it fails to recognize either the highly competitive and elite field of wheelchair dancing or issues of social disablement inherent in the representation and cultural construction of disability, both within the story world of *Glee!* and in the very real social world of viewers.

Works Cited

Anna. "Glee: 'That's Why We Call It Dismissing Legitimate Concerns Instead of Acting.'" *Disabledfeminists.com*. FWD (Feminists with Disabilities) For a Way Forward. 16 Nov. 2009. Web. 8 Oct. 2011.
Asayesh-Brown, Mina. "Why I Hate *Glee*; Really, *Glee?* You Started Out So Hot. Now You're Just Wrong. It's Insulting." *St. Petersburg Times* 3 Feb. 2011: 8. Print.
Benkler, Yochai. *The Wealth of Networks: How Social Production Transforms Markets and Freedom*. New Haven: Yale University Press, 2006. Print
Barnes, Colin. "Disabling Imagery and the Media: An Exploration of the Principles for Media Representations of Disabled People." *Leeds.ac.uk*. The British Council of Organizations of Disabled People and Ryburn Publishing. 1992. Web. 8 Oct. 2011.
Cheu, Johnson. "De-Gene-Erates, Replicants and Other Aliens: (Re)Defining Disability in Futuristic Film." *Disability/Postmodernity*. Eds. Mairian Corker and Tom Shakespeare. New York: Continuum, 2002. 198–212. Print.
Cumberbatch, Guy, and Ralph Negrine. *Images of Disability on Television*. London: Routledge, 1992. Print.
Davis, Lennard. "Let Actors with Disabilities Play Characters with Disabilities." *Huffington Post*. 7 Dec. 2009. Web. 15 Jan. 2011.
dos Santos, Kristin. "Glee Boss Gets on Board with Puck and Rachel!" *E! Online*. 2009. Web. 8 Oct. 2011.
Eastman, Marc. "Glee's Jane Lynch Interview." *Are You Screening?* 11 Jan. 2010. Web. 8 Oct. 2011.
Elber, Lynn. "Glee" Wheelchair Episode Upsets Disabled." *Huffington Post*. 10 Nov. 2009. Web. 15 Jan. 2011.

Ellis, Katie. *Disabling Diversity: The Social Construction of Disability in 1990s Australian National Cinema.* Saarbrücken: VDM-Verlag, 2008. Print.

Gay & Lesbian Alliance Against Defamation. "Where We Are on TV Report: 2010– 2011." *Glaad.* 2011. Web. 8 Oct. 2011.

Grisby Bates, Karen. "Reclaiming Roles: Actors Play Beyond Disabilities." *National Public Radio.* 11 May 2010. Web. 15 Jan. 2011.

Goggin, Gerard, and Tim Noonan. "Blogging Disability: The Interface Between New Cultural Movements and Internet Technology." *Use of Blogs.* Eds. Axel Burns and Joanne Jacobs. New York: Lang, 2006. 161–72. Print.

Haller, Beth. *Representing Disability in an Ableist World: Essays on Mass Media.* Louisville, KY: Avocado Press, 2010. Print.

Harnett, Alison. "Escaping the 'Evil Avenger' and the 'Supercrip': Images of Disability in Popular Television." *Irish Communications Review* 8 (2000): 21–29. Print.

Johnson, Davi. "Managing Mr. Monk: Control and the Politics of Madness." *Critical Studies in Media Communication* 25.1 (2008): 28–47. Print.

Kennedy, Gerrick. "'Glee': Defying Gravity with Heart and Soul." *Los Angeles Times.* 12 Nov. 2009. Web. 8 Oct. 2011.

Kociemba, David "'Proud Mary': *Glee*'s Very Special Sham Disability Pride Anthem." *in media res: a mediacommons project.* Media Commons. 9 Apr. 2010. Web. 8 Oct.2011.

Longmore, Paul. "Screening Stereotypes: Images of Disabled People in Television and Motion Pictures." *Images of the Disabled, Disabling Images.* Eds. Alan Gartner and Tom Joe. New York: Praeger,1987. 65–78. Print.

Mayfield, Anthony. *What Is Social Media?* icrossing ebooks. 2008. Web. 15 Dec. 2011.

Norden, Martin F. *The Cinema of Isolation: A History of Physical Disability in the Movies* New Brunswick: Rutgers University Press, 1994. Print.

Oliver, Michael. *Understanding Disability: From Theory to Practice.* Hampshire: Palgrave, 1996. Print.

Quinlan, Margaret, and Benjamin Bates. "Dances and Discourses of (Dis)Ability: Heather Mills' Embodiment of Disability on Dancing with the Stars." *Text and Performance Quarterly* 28 1–2 (2008): 64–80. Print.

Richardson, Niall. *Transgressive Bodies: Representations in Film and Popular Culture.* Surrey: Ashgate, 2010. Print.

Ross, Karen. "But Where's Me in It? Disability, Broadcasting and the Media." *Media, Culture & Society* 19 (1997): 669–77 Print.

Sheppard, Alice. "Rockin' and Rollin' on Fox's Glee." *Disability Studies Quarterly* 31.1 (2011). Web. 15 Jan. 2011.

Siebers, Tobin. *Disability Theory.* Ann Arbor: University of Michigan Press, 2009.

_____. "Disability as Masquerade." *Disability Theory.* Ann Arbor: University of Michigan Press, 2008. 96–119. Print.

smith, s.e. "Glee: Wheels" *This Aint Livin.* 12 Nov. 2009. Web. 16 Jan. 2011.

_____. "No Glee for disabled people." *The Guardian.* 19 Aug. 2010. Web. 15 Jan. 2011.

_____. "The Transcontinental Disability Choir: *Glee*-Ful Appropriation." *Bitch Media.* 12 Nov. 2009. Web. 8 Oct. 2011.

Wheelchair Dancer. "*Glee.*" *Wheelchair Dancer.* 13 Nov. 2009. Web. 8 Oct. 2011.

Appendix I
Filmography

The Americas, Europe and Australia

TELEVISION

Battlestar Galactica (Sci-Fi 2004–2009)
Battlestar Galactica: Face of the Enemy (Syfy 2008)
Carnivàle (HBO 2003–2005)
Dancing with the Stars (ABC 2005-present)
Extraordinary People: The Twins Who Share a Body (BBC 2007)
Family Guy (20th Century–Fox 1999–2012)
Glee! (20th Century–Fox 2009–2012)

DOCUMENTARY

Best Boy (1979)
Best Man: "Best Boy" and All of Us Twenty Years Later (1997)
Blindsight (2006)
18q-: A Different Kind of Normal (2011)
Face to Face (2000)
The Girl with Eight Limbs (2007)
Joined for Life (2001)
Joined for Life: Abby and Brittany Turn Sixteen (2006)
Katie and Eilish (1992)
Murderball (2005)
Siamese Twins (1995)
Titicut Follies (1967)
Wigstock: The Movie (1995)

NARRATIVE FILM

Away from Her (2006)
Bad Boy Bubby (1993)
Bad Day at Black Rock (1955)
Born on the Fourth of July (1989)
The Bourne Series (2002, 2004, 2007, 2012)
Brothers of the Head (2005)
Coming Home (1978)
Control (2007)
Cutter's Way (1981)
The Eternal Sea (1955)
Fifty First Dates (2004)
Forrest Gump (1994)
Freaks (1932)
The Good Woman of Bangkok (Australia/Thailand 1991)
Hail the New Puritan (1987)
Heidi (1937)
Immortal Beloved (1994)
In the Land of the Deaf (*Au Pays des Sourds*, France 1992)
Interrupted Melody (1955)
Iris (2001)
The Majestic (2001)
Memento (2000)
The Miracle (2007)
My Left Foot (1989)
Night and Day (1946)
The Other Side of the Mountain (1975)
Rain Man (1988)
Read My Lips (*Sur Mes Lèvres*, France 2001)
The Saddest Music in the World (2003)
The Savages (2007)
Scent of a Woman (1992)
Son of the Bride (*El Hijo de la Novia*, Argentina 2001)
A Song for Martin (*En Sång för Martin*, Sweden 2001)
Soul Surfer (2011)
The Station Agent (2003)

The Stratton Story (1949)
Sunrise at Campobello (1960)
Temple Grandin (2010)
The Vow (2012)
The Wings of Eagles (1957)
With a Song in My Heart (1952)

Asia

Breaking the Silence (*Beautiful Mama*; *Pretty Mother*; *Piaoliang Mama*, China 2000)
Chocolate (Thailand 2008)
Colors of the Blind (*Hei Yanjing*, China 1997)
The Common People (*Guanyu Ai De Gushi*, China 1998)
The Good Woman of Bangkok (Australia Thailand 1991)
Happy Times (*Xingfu Shiguang*, China 2000)
A Moment to Remember (*Nae Meorisokui Jiwoogae*, South Korea 2004)
Poetry (*Shi*, South Korea, 2010)
Princess Mononoke (1999; *Mononoke Hime*, Japan 1997)
Shower (*Xizao*, China 1999)
Silent River (*Wu Sheng De He*, China 2000)
Sons (*Erzi*, China 1996)

India

Aa Gale Lag Jaa (1974)
Aadmi (1968)
Aai Phirse Bahaar (1960)
Aaj aur Kal (1963)
Aalayamani (1962)
Aap Ki Parchhaiyan (1964)
Abdullah (1980)
Adbhuta Dweepam (2005)
Ajooba (1991)
Allah Rakkha (1985)
Amar Akbar Anthony (1979)
Andipatti Arasampatti (2002)
Angel (2011)
Anjaam (1996)
Anuraag (1972; remade as *Aloy Phera*, 2007)
Apne Dushman (1975)
Apradhi (1947)
Arangetram (1973)
Arzoo (1965)
Athbhutha Dweepu (2005)
Athmakatha (2010)
Avtaar (1983)
Baat Ek Raat Ki (1962)

Badshah (1999)
Baga Pirivanai (1959; remade as *Khandan*, 1965)
Bahaaron Ke Sapne (1967)
Bairaag (1976)
Barsaat Ki Ek Raat (1983)
Basant (1942)
Basant (1960)
Bhairavi (1996)
Bharosa (1963)
Biradri (1966)
Black (2005)
Brashtachar (1989)
Cha Cha Cha (1964)
Chess (2006)
Chhodo Kal (2012)
Chup Chup Ke (2006)
Dada (1979)
Dariya Dil 1988)
Deedar (1951)
Devta (1956)
Dhanwaan (1981)
Dhoop Chhaon (1977)
Dil (1990)
Dil Tera Diwana (1962)
Do Badan (1966)
Don (1978)
Dosti (1964)
Dushman (1971)
Ek Chaddar Maili Si (1986)
En Mana Vaanil (2002)
Ennavale (2000)
Fanaa (2007)
Gauri (1968)
Gora Aur Kala (1972)
Guzaarish (2010)
Hawas (1974)
Hum Dono (1961)
Hum Hai Kamaal Ke (1993; remake of *See no Evil Hear no Evil*, 1989)
Humko Tumse Pyaar Hai (2006)
Insaaf (1987)
Insaan (1944)
Jailor (1958)
Jal Bin Machli Nritya Bin Bijli (1971)
Jalte Badan (1973)
Jaydaad (1989)
Jeevan Naiya (1936)
Jheel Ke Us Paar (1973)
Johar Mehmood in Hong Kong (1971)
Joshila (1973)
Kaalia (1982)
Kaasi (2003)

Kakakuyil (2001; remade as *London*, 2005; *Gol maal*, 2006)
Kalicharan (1978)
Kandaen (2010)
Kandukondain Kandukondain (2000)
Kannan en Kadhalan (1968)
Karma (1986)
Karumadikkuttan (2001)
Kasam (1988)
Kasauti (1974)
Kashmir ki Kali (1964)
Kasi (2001)
Katha Sangama (1975; remade as *Kai Kodukkum Kai*, 1984)
Khamoshi (1969)
Khamoshi: The Musical (1996)
Khandaan (1965)
Khandaan (1979)
Khilona (1970)
Khol de Meri Zubaan (1989)
Khuddar (1994)
Koshish (1972)
Koyla (1997)
Laadla (1994)
Lafangey Parindey (2010)
Lawaris (1981)
Major Chandrakanth (1966)
Mar Adentro (*The Sea Inside*, 2004)
Marte Dam Tak (1987)
Meerayude Dukhavum Muthuvinte Swapnavum (2003)
Mehboob ki Mehendi (1971)
Mera Dost Mera Dushman (1984)
Moondru Mudichu (1976)
Mother India (1957)
Mozhi (2007)
Mujhse Shaadi Karoge (2004)
Muqaddar Ka Sikandar (1975)
My Big Father (2010)
My Name Is Khan (2010)
Naan Kadavul (2009)
Naan Vaaza Vaippen (1979)
Naan Vazhavaippen (1979)
Naan yen Piranthen (1972)
Nadodigal (2009)
Nau Bahar (1952)
Neel Kamal (1984)
Nerum Neruppum (1971)
Netrikkan (1979)
Nuvvu Vasthavani (2000)
123 (2002)
Oomappenninu Uriyadappayyan (2002)
Paa (2009)

Paalum Palamum (1960)
Palum Pazhamum (1961)
Pandit aur Pathan (1977)
Parasakhti (1951)
Parineeta (1953)
Parthal Pasi Theerum (1962)
Parvarish (1977)
Pati Patni (1966)
Patita (1953)
Pattiyal (2006)
Payal (1957)
Perazhagan (2004)
Pithamagan (2003)
Poikkal Kuthirai (1983)
Prem Nagar (1940)
Prem Patra (1962)
Prem Pujari (1970)
Prince (1969)
Punjabi House (1998)
Punyam (2001)
Pyaar Diwana Hota Hai (2002)
Pyar Ka Mausam (1969)
Pyare Mohan (2006)
Qatl (1986)
Raaja Paarvai (1981)
Raji en Kanmani (1954)
Ram Tera Desh (1984)
Rascals (2011)
Ratha Kaneer (1954)
Roudram (2011)
Saajan (1991)
Saajan ka Ghar (1994)
Saathi (1968)
Saccha Jhootha (1970)
Saccha Jhutha (1978)
Sahara (1958)
Sangeet Samrat Tansen (1962)
Santhi (1965)
Sapnon Ka Mandir (1991)
Sati Sukanya (1959)
Satte Pe Satta (1982)
Shaan (1982)
Shadow (2009)
Sharaabi (1984)
Shiraz (1929)
Shirdi ke Sai Baba (1977)
Sholay (1975)
Shor (1972)
Shravan Kumar (1984)
Sollamale (1998)
Sone Ka Dil Lohe Ke Haath (1978)
Sparsh (1980)
Suhaag (1979)

Suhaag (1994)
Suhaag Raat (1968)
Sunayna (1979)
Taare Zameen Par (2007)
Thanmatra (2005)
Thokar (1974)
Thulladha Manamum Thullum (1999)
Tom, Dick, and Harry (2006)
Toofan (1989)
U Me aur Hum (2008)
Upkaar (1967)
Vaada (2005)

Vaali (1999)
Vakil Babu (1983)
Vasanthiyum Lakshmiyum Pinne Njaanum (1999)
Vazhayadi Vazhai (1972)
Veer Kunal (1925)
Vijaypath (1994)
Vinmeegal (2012)
Vishwanath (1978)
Waqt ka Shahenshah (1987)
Zakhmon ka Hisaab (1993)
Zameen Asmaan (1972)
Zordaar (1996)

Appendix II
Selected Readings in Disability Studies

For readers new to disability studies, the selected readings below are intended to provide an introduction to the field. The list is representative, not comprehensive. In the interest of limiting it to a manageable length, a number of key essays and significant volumes have been omitted, most notably histories and cultural studies of disability before 1960 and creative, autobiographical or reflective works by disabled writers and artists. The list is also primarily oriented to the United Sates, which reflects both its limits and the grounding of disability studies hitherto in that context as well as in the United Kingdom, Canada, Australia and New Zealand. Combining these texts with those listed in the Works Cited pages of the chapters in this anthology should provide a solid grounding from which to launch into disability studies and film. Happy reading and welcome to the field.

Contemporary History

Campbell, Jane, and Mike Oliver. *Disability Politics: Understanding Our Past, Changing Our Future.* New York: Routledge, 1996. Print.

Charlton, James I. *Nothing About Us Without Us: Disability Oppression and Empowerment.* Berkeley: University California Press, 2000. Print.

Fleischer, Doris, and Frieda Zames. *The Disability Rights Movement: From Charity to Confrontation,* 2d ed. Philadelphia: Temple University Press, 2011. Print.

Shapiro, Joseph P. *No Pity: People with Disabilities Forging a New Civil Rights Movement.* New York: Three Rivers Press, 1994. Print.

Concepts and Contexts

Barnes, Colin, and Geof Mercer. *Exploring Disability*, 2d ed. Cambridge: Polity Press, 2010. Print.

Bauman, H-Dirksen, ed. *Open Your Eyes: Deaf Studies Talking.* Minneapolis: University Minnesota Press, 2008. Print.

Baynton, Douglas C. "Disability and the Justification of Inequality in American History." *The New Disability History: American Perspectives.* Eds. Paul K. Longmore and Lauri Umansky. New York: New York University Press, 2001. 33–57. Print.

Brueggemann, Brenda Jo. *Lend Me Your Ear: Rhetorical Constructions of Deafness.* Washington, D.C.: Gallaudet University Press, 1999. Print.

Davis, Lennard J. "Bodies of Difference: Politics, Disability, and Representation." *Disability Studies: Enabling the Humanities.* Eds. Sharon Snyder, Brenda Jo Brueggemann and Rosemarie

Garland-Thomson. New York: Modern Language Association of America, 2002. 100–106. Print.

_____."Introduction: Disability, the Missing Term in the Race, Class, Gender Triad" and "Constructing Normalcy." *Enforcing Normalcy: Disability Deafness and the Body*. New York: Verso, 1995. 1–22, 23–49. Print.

Garland-Thomson, Rosemarie. "Integrating Disability: Transforming Feminist Theory." *Feminist Disability Studies*. Ed. Kim Q. Hall. Bloomington: Indiana University Press, 2011. 13–47. Print.

Goodley, Dan. *Disability Studies: An Interdisciplinary Introduction*. Thousand Oaks, CA: Sage, 2010. Print.

_____, Bill Hughes, and Lennard Davis, eds. *Disability and Social Theory: New Developments and Directions*. New York: Palgrave Macmillan, 2012. Print.

Ingstad, Benedicte, and Susan Reynolds Whyte, eds. *Disability and Culture*. Berkeley: University of California Press, 1995. Print.

Lane, Harlan. "Constructions of Deafness." *The Disability Studies Reader*. Ed. Lennard J. Davis. New York: Routledge, 1997. 153–171. Print.

Lane, Harlan, Robert Hoffmeister, and Ben Bahan, eds. *A Journey Into the Deaf-World*. San Diego: DawnSignPress, 1996. Print.

Linton, Simi. *Claiming Disability: Knowledge and Identity*. New York: New York University Press, 1998. Print.

McRuer, Robert. "Introduction: Compulsory Able-Bodiedness and Queer/Disabled Existence." *Crip Theory: Cultural Signs of Queerness and Disability*. New York: New York University Press, 2006. 1–32. Print.

McRuer, Robert, and Anna Mollow, eds. *Sex and Disability*. Durham, NC: Duke University Press, 2012. Print.

Mitchell, David T., and Sharon L. Snyder. "Introduction: Disability Studies and the Double Bind of Representation." *The Body and Physical Difference: Discourses of Disability*. Eds. David T. Mitchell and Sharon L. Snyder. Ann Arbor: University of Michigan Press, 1997. 1–31. Print.

Oliver, Michael. *Understanding Disability: From Theory to Practice*, 2d ed. New York: Palgrave Macmillan, 2009. Print.

Poore, Carol. *Disability in Twentieth-Century German Culture*. Ann Arbor: University of Michigan Press, 2007. Print.

Samuels, Ellen. "Critical Divides: Judith Butler's Body Theory and the Question of Disability." *Feminist Disability Studies*. Kim Q. Hall, Ed. Bloomington: Indiana University Press, 2011. 48–66. Print.

Shakespeare, Tom. *Disability Rights and Wrongs*. New York: Routledge, 2006. Print.

Siebers, Tobin. *Disability Theory*. Ann Arbor: University Michigan Press, 2009. Print.

Snyder, Sharon L., and David T. Mitchell. *Cultural Locations of Disability*. Chicago: Chicago University Press. Print.

Watson, Nick, Alan Roulstone, and Carol Thomas, eds. *Routledge Handbook of Disability Studies*. New York: Routledge, 2012. Print.

Wendell, Susan. "Toward a Feminist Theory of Disability." *The Disability Studies Reader*. Ed. Lennard J. Davis. New York: Routledge, 1997. 260–278. Print.

Critical Representation Studies

Bérubé, Michael. "Disability and Narrative." *PMLA* 120.2 (2005): 568–76. Print.

Davidson, Michael. *Concerto for the Left Hand: Disability and Defamiliar Body*. Ann Arbor: University of Michigan Press, 2008. Print.

Garland-Thomson, Rosemarie. *Extraordinary Bodies: Figuring Physical Disability in American Culture and Literature*. New York: Columbia University Press, 1996. Print.

_____. "Seeing the Disabled: Visual Rhetorics of Disability in Popular Photography." *The New Disability History: American Perspectives*. Eds. Paul K. Longmore and Lauri Umansky. New York: New York University Press, 2001. 335–374. Print.

Hevey, David. *The Creatures Time Forgot: Photography and Disability Imagery.* New York: Routledge, 1992. Print.

Mitchell, David T., and Sharon L. Snyder. "Representation and Its Discontents: The Uneasy Home of Disability in Literature and Film" and "Narrative Prosthesis and the Materiality of Metaphor." *Narrative Prosthesis: Disability and the Dependencies of Discourse.* Ann Arbor: University of Michigan Press, 2000. 15–46; 47–64. Print.

Quayson, Ato. "A Typology of Disability Representation." *Aesthetic Nervousness: Disability and the Crisis of Representation.* New York: Columbia University Press, 1997. 32–53.

Russell, Emily. *Reading Embodied Citizenship: Disability, Narrative and the Body Politic.* New Brunswick: Rutgers University Press, 2011. Print.

Siebers, Tobin. *Disability Aesthetics.* Ann Arbor: University of Michigan Press, 2010. Print.

Performance Studies

Kuppers, Petra. *Disability Culture and Community Performance: Find a Strange and Twisted Shape.* New York: Palgrave Macmillan, 2011. Print.

Sandahl, Carrie, and Philip Auslander, eds. *Bodies in Commotion: Disability and Performance.* Ann Arbor: University of Michigan Press, 2005. Print.

Film Studies

Cheu, Johnson. "De-gene-erates, Replicants and Other Aliens: (Re)defining Disability in Futuristic Film." *Disability/Postmodernity: Embodying Disability Theory.* Eds. Mairian Corker and Tom Shakespeare. London: Continuum, 2002. 198–212. Print.

_____, ed. *Diversity in Disney Films: Critical Essays on Race, Ethnicity, Gender, Sexuality and Disability.* Jefferson, NC: McFarland, 2012. Print.

Chivers, Sally. *The Silvering Screen: Old Age and Disability in Cinema.* Toronto: University Toronto Press, 2011. Print.

_____, and Nicole Markotić. *The Problem Body: Projecting Disability on Film.* Columbus: Ohio State University Press, 2010. Print.

Davidson, Michael. "Phantom Limbs: Film Noir's Volatile Bodies." *Concerto for the Left Hand: Disability and Defamiliar Body.* Ann Arbor: University of Michigan Press, 2008. 58–79. Print.

Enns, Anthony, and Christopher R. Smit. *Screening Disability: Essays on Cinema and Disability.* Lanham, MD: University Press of America, 2001. Print.

Fraser, Benjamin. *Disability Studies and Spanish Culture: Films, Novels, the Comic and the Public Exhibition.* Liverpool: Liverpool University Press, 2013. Print.

Goggin, Gerard and Christopher Newell. *Digital Disability: The Social Construction of Disability in New Media.* Lanham, MD: Rowman & Littlefield, 2003. Print.

Longmore, Paul K. "Conspicuous Contribution and American Cultural Dilemmas: Telethon Rituals of Cleansing and Renewal." *The Body and Physical Difference: Discourses of Disability.* Eds. David T. Mitchell and Sharon Snyder. Ann Arbor: University of Michigan Press, 1997. 134–158. Print.

_____. "Screening Stereotypes: Images of Disabled People in Television and Motion Pictures." *Why I Burned My Book and Other Essays on Disability.* Philadelphia: Temple University Press, 2003. 131–148. Print.

Molina, Caroline. "Muteness and Mutilation: The Aesthetics of Disability in Jane Campion's The Piano." *The Body and Physical Difference: Discourses of Disability.* Eds. David T. Mitchell and Sharon Snyder. Ann Arbor: University of Michigan Press, 1997. 267–282. Print.

Norden, Martin F. *Cinema of Isolation: A History of Physical Disability in the Movies.* New Brunswick: Rutgers University Press, 1994. Print.

Pointon, Ann, with Chris Davies, eds. *Framed: Interrogating Disability in the Media.* London: British Film Institute, 1997. Print.

Shakespeare, Tom. "Arts and Lies? Representations of Disability on Film." *Disability Discourse*. Eds. Mairain Corker and Sally French. Buckingham: Open University Press, 1999.

Snyder, Sharon L., and David T. Mitchell. "After the Panopticon: Contemporary Institutions as Documentary Subject." *Cultural Locations of Disability*. Chicago: Chicago University Press, 2006. 153–155. Print.

_____. "Body Genres and Disability Sensations: The Challenge of the New Disability Documentary Cinema." *Cultural Locations of Disability*. Chicago: Chicago University Press. 156–181. Print.

Smith, Angela. *Hideous Progeny: Disability Eugenics, and Classic Horror Cinema*. New York: Columbia University Press, 2012. Print.

About the Contributors

Johnson **Cheu** is an assistant professor in the Department of Writing, Rhetoric, and American Cultures at Michigan State University. He is the editor of *Diversity in Disney Films* (McFarland, 2012) and serves on the editorial board of *The Journal of Literary and Cultural Disability Studies*. He is editing a collection of scholarly essays on Tim Burton.

Sally **Chivers** is an associate professor in the departments of Canadian studies and English at Trent University in Ontario. The author of *From Old Woman to Older Women* (Ohio State University Press, 2003) and *The Silvering Screen* (University of Toronto Press, 2011), and the co-editor (with Nicole Markotić) of *The Problem Body* (Ohio State University Press, 2010), she researches the relationship between aging and disability in the Canadian public sphere and beyond.

David **Church** is a doctoral candidate at Indiana University in the Department of Communication and Culture, and the editor of *Playing with Memories: Essays on Guy Maddin* (University of Manitoba Press, 2009). His dissertation focuses on the intersection of nostalgia and home video technologies in the contemporary fandom of exploitation cinema. He has published in *Disability Studies Quarterly, Cinema Journal, The Journal of Film and Video, Senses of Cinema, The Encyclopedia of American Disability History* and edited collections on cinema culture.

Paul A. **Darke**, writer, cultural critic and originator of Normality Theory, has researched extensively with the issue of identity and culture. He earned his Ph.D. from the University of Warwick in England examining disability and its cultural specificities and impact in British cinema from the late 1960s to the early 1980s. He is the chief executive of one of the U.K.'s leading disability arts organizations and has produced innovative work with Simon McKeown shown in galleries worldwide.

Sarah **Dauncey** is a lecturer in Chinese studies at the University of Sheffield in England. Her current research, which has appeared in publications as diverse as *China Information* and *Disability and Society*, focuses on the representation of disability in Chinese film and literature, as well as life writing by and on behalf of disabled people in contemporary China.

Heath A. **Diehl** is on the faculty of the University Honors Program at Bowling Green State University where he has taught courses on the Harry Potter series, vampire fiction and film, the *Dexter* series, and "zombie literature." His work has appeared in *M/MLA: The Journal of the Midwest Modern Language Association, Studies in the Literary Imagination,* and *M/C: A Journal of Media and Culture.* He is also the author of *Stages of Sexuality: Performance, Gay Male Identity, and Public Space* (VDM, 2009).

Katie **Ellis** is a lecturer in media and communications at Murdoch University in Perth, Australia, where she received her doctorate. She is the author of *Disabling Diversity* (VDM, 2008) and co-author of *Disability and New Media* (Routledge, 2011). Her research focuses on disability, television, and digital and networked media, with attention to both representation and active possibilities for social inclusion. She has participated in several feature film and documentary productions in research and production roles.

Michelle **Jarman** is an assistant professor of disability studies at the Wyoming Institute for Disabilities at the University of Wyoming. She received her Ph.D. in English with concentrations in disability studies and women's studies from the University of Illinois–Chicago. Her essays have appeared in *The Review of Disability Studies, Disability and Society, MELUS* (Multi-Ethnic Literature of the U.S.) and in disability studies and literary anthologies.

Eunjung **Kim** is an assistant professor in the Department of Gender and Women's Studies at the University of Wisconsin with a joint appointment in rehabilitation psychology and special education. Her work has appeared in *Disability and Society and Sexuality Research and Social Policy*, and several anthologies, including *The Problem Body: Projecting Disability on Screen* (Ohio State University Press, 2010). She holds a Ph.D. in disability studies from the University of Illinois–Chicago.

Nicole **Markotić** is an associate professor of English at the University of Windsor in Ontario. She is the author of several books including two volumes of poetry and the co-edited (with Sally Chivers) *The Problem Body* (Ohio State University Press, 2010). She has edited special issues on disability for *Canadian Journal of Film Studies / revue canadienne d'études cinématographiques* and *Tessera*. Her novella *Yellow Pages* focuses on Alexander Graham Bell and Deaf culture.

Dawne C. **McCance** is a university distinguished professor in the Department of Religion, and editor of *Mosaic: A Journal for the Interdisciplinary Study of Literature*, at the University of Manitoba. She has published several books, including *Medusa's Ear* (State University of New York, 2004), a study of the trope of female deafness in the philosophy of the Western research university, and numerous papers on ethics, continental philosophy, critical animal studies, disability, and the work of Jacques Derrida.

Simon **McKeown** is an artist and reader in animation at Teesside University in the U.K. His degree was in Fine Arts. His interests center on the discourse of the cultural representation of disability. His work Motion Disabled (www.motiondisabled.com) was exhibited globally and shown at the Smithsonian International Gallery. An accomplished animator with more than twenty years of experience in animation and special effects, he has made films on Deafness, disability, dance and the institutionalization of disability.

Russell **Meeuf** is an assistant professor in the School of Journalism and Mass Media at the University of Idaho. His work on masculinity, disability, and global cinema has appeared in *Cinema Journal, The Journal of Popular Film and Television, Third Text*, and *Jump Cut*. He is the author of *Wayne's World: John Wayne and Transnational Masculinity in the Fifties* (University of Texas Press, 2013) and is the co-editor (with Raphael Raphael) of *Transnational Stardome* (Palgrave Macmillan, 2013).

Marja Evelyn **Mogk** is an associate professor of English at California Lutheran University, where she teaches courses in writing, film and drama. She holds a Ph.D. in English with an interdisciplinary dissertation in disability studies from the University of California-Berkeley. She is the co-author (with Lylas G. Mogk) of *Macular Degeneration: The Complete Guide to Saving and Maximizing Your Sight* (Ballantine, 2003).

Martin F. **Norden** teaches and writes about film as a professor of communication at the University of Massachusetts–Amherst. He is the author of *The Cinema of Isolation* (Rutgers University Press, 1994) and many other publications. He has lectured across North America and Europe on the movie representation of people with disabilities and is writing a book on the early screenwriter-director Lois Weber.

Joyojeet **Pal** is an assistant professor at the University of Michigan's School of Information. His broad area of interest is in technology and economic development. His publications on disability-related issues include vision impairment and workplace accommodation and technology adoption issues related to screen readers. He is also interested in film, and has written the documentary film *For the Love of a Man* on fan clubs in Tamil Nadu, and published extensively on the portrayal of technology as aspirational in South Indian cinema.

Alyson **Patsavas** is pursuing a doctorate in disability studies at the University of Illinois–Chicago.

Her research focuses on the cultural discourses of pain and representations of disability in film. She is one of several collaborators on a feature-length documentary film project with the working title *Code of the Freaks*, which examines representations of disability in film across history from the perspective of people with disabilities.

Ellen **Samuels** is an assistant professor of English and gender and women's studies at the University of Wisconsin-Madison. Her critical writing has been published in numerous journals and anthologies, including *Signs: Journal of Women in Culture and Society*, *The Oxford Handbook of Nineteenth-Century American Literature*, *Feminist Disability Studies*, *GLQ: Journal of Lesbian and Gay Studies,* and *Leviathan: A Journal of Melville Studies*. Her first book, *Self Evident: Disability and Bodily Identity*, is forthcoming; and she is writing a book on "Double Meanings: Representing Conjoined Twins."

Terri **Thrower** is actively involved in the disability arts and culture movement in Chicago, serving as a board member for Tellin' Tales Theater and a consortium member for Bodies of Work. She has also served as director of disability and learning resources at the School of the Art Institute of Chicago, has taught seminars to medical and art therapy students about disability arts and culture, and has co-taught "Foundations of Disability," a graduate course at the University of Illinois–Chicago, where she is completing her doctorate in disability studies.

Veronica **Wain** holds a doctorate from the Griffith Film School in Queensland, Australia. Her first short documentary, *The Creek*, was purchased by national broadcaster SBS and screened on Global Village in 2003. She has made a number of award-winning films including *Car Pool*, which won the prestigious St. Kilda Best Comedy Award in 2007, and *Shorn*, selected to screen at the Hollywood Film Festival. Her debut feature documentary *18q-: A Different Kind of Normal* screened at the SURGE International Film Festival in Austin, Texas, and at Handicapable in New Caledonia.

Heather **Warren-Crow** is an assistant professor of interdiscplinary arts at Texas Tech University. She has published articles on animation, dance film, and performance-based photography and is completing her first book, *Girlhood and the Plastic Image*. She is also collaborating on transdisciplinary research about synthesized speech and communication disability. Both a theorist and a practicing performance artist, she has exhibited her artwork across the United States and abroad. She has a Ph.D. in performance studies from the University of California–Berkeley.

Timothy E. **Wilson** is completing his doctorate in French at the City University of New York (CUNY) Graduate Center, where his dissertation is a cultural history of children's television in France. His primary interests include twentieth-century French literature, cinema, television, and popular culture, Indian Ocean literature, disability studies, and foreign language pedagogy. He has taught at Hunter College and the College of Staten Island. In 2011–12, he served as a Writing Fellow at LaGuardia Community College.

Index

Numbers in **bold italics** indicate pages with photographs.